THE COMPLETE IDIOT'S GUIDE® TO

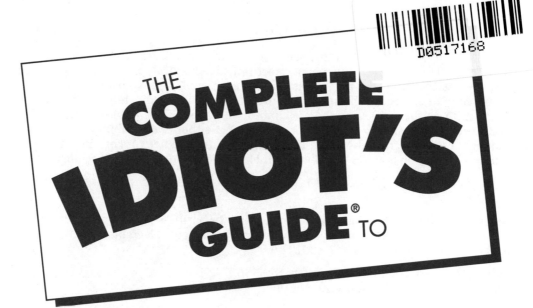

Alternative Medicine

by Dr. Alan H. Pressman and Sheila Buff

alpha
books

A Division of Macmillan General Reference
A Simon & Schuster Macmillan Company
1633 Broadway, New York, NY 10019

Macmillan Publishing books may be purchased for business or sales promotional use. For information please write: Special Markets Department, Macmillan Publishing USA, 1633 Broadway, New York, NY 10019.

International Standard Book Number: 0-02-862742-3
Library of Congress Catalog Card Number: 98-87598

01 00 99   8 7 6 5 4 3 2 1

Interpretation of the printing code: the rightmost number of the first series of numbers is the year of the book's printing; the rightmost number of the second series of numbers is the number of the book's printing. For example, a printing code of 99-1 shows that the first printing occurred in 1999.

Printed in the United States of America

The Complete Idiot's Guide to Alternative Medicine Reference Card

The World of Alternative Medicine

Acupressure—In traditional Chinese medicine (TCM), gentle but firm hand or finger pressure on particular healing points.

Acupuncture—In TCM, the insertion of very fine needles into selected parts of the skin to relieve pain and other symptoms of illness or injury.

Aromatherapy—The use of pleasant-smelling essential oils to treat physical and emotional problems.

Biofeedback—Learning to use internal signals from your body as a way to improve your health.

Chiropractic—Healing art that gives special attention to the role of the skeleton and muscles in health. Chiropractic care works with your body's natural strengths to restore and maintain your health—without drugs or surgery.

Guided imagery—Technique of imagining sights, sounds, emotions, and other sensations in order to affect your body, help you relax, and promote healing.

Herbalism—The use of traditional healing herbs from Europe and the Americas.

Homeopathy—The use of very, very tiny doses of a healing remedy. In larger doses, the remedy would cause symptoms similar to those the patient has; in homeopathic doses, the remedy relieves the symptoms.

Hypnotherapy—Use of hypnosis—a state of deep relaxation, altered perceptions, focused concentration, and greater openness to sensations and feelings—to treat specific health problems.

Macrobiotics—A dietary and philosophical approach to life that emphasizes balance and simplicity. The macrobiotic diet emphasizes whole grains and vegetables.

Naturopathy—A medical system that treats health problems by using the body's natural ability to heal. Modern naturopathy includes a wide range of therapies, such as herbs, homeopathy, acupuncture, and nutrition.

Osteopathy—A branch of medicine that believes your body structure—your bones and muscles—and the rest of your body functions operate together. Osteopathy is based on the belief that imbalances in your body structure cause disease and that restoring the balance will restore health.

Reflexology—A form of touch therapy that uses pressure on specific points of the feet (and also hands) to affect other parts of the body.

Reiki—A form of natural healing that uses patterns of touch to channel energy through the hands of the healer to the patient.

Rolfing—A form of deep-tissue massage that realigns and balances your body.

Transcendental Meditation™—A simplified form of meditation using a mantra that you repeat silently.

Yoga—An ancient Indian technique combining physical exercise, breathing techniques, and meditation.

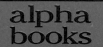

alpha
books

tear here

Take This to Your Health-Food Store

Herbs

➤ Buy only herbs that are fresh and aromatic.

➤ Be sure you know what you're getting. Buy accurately labeled products from reputable manufacturers.

➤ Standardized herbs have been lightly processed to make sure they always contain the same amount of the herbs' most active ingredient(s).

➤ Herbs can be made into drinks—teas, decoctions, and infusions. Strong-tasting herbs are best swallowed in capsules.

Homeopathic Remedies

➤ Buy homeopathic remedies only from reputable manufacturers.

➤ Homeopathic remedies are available in chewable pills or as liquids. Choose whichever you prefer.

➤ The usual remedy strengths for home use are 6c and 12c.

➤ Homeopathic remedies can be used along with herbal treatments and even medical drugs.

➤ Homeopathic remedies should be taken only as needed and for the shortest possible time. Stop taking them as soon as you feel better.

➤ Homeopathic remedies are very safe—it's impossible to overdose.

Vitamins and Minerals

➤ Buy vitamin and mineral supplements only from reputable manufacturers.

➤ If you want to take a multivitamin with minerals, choose one that contains all the B vitamins and trace minerals such as selenium. Older adults should avoid multisupplements that contain iron.

➤ Women should get at least 1,000 mg of calcium every day. If you don't get that much from your diet, consider taking a supplement made with calcium citrate.

➤ Older adults don't absorb B vitamins from their food very well. Consider taking a complete B supplement.

Alpha Development Team

Publisher
Kathy Nebenhaus

Editorial Director
Gary M. Krebs

Managing Editor
Bob Shuman

Marketing Brand Manager
Felice Primeau

Senior Editor
Nancy Mikhail

Editor
Jessica Faust

Development Editors
Phil Kitchel
Amy Zavatto

Assistant Editor
Maureen Horn

Production Team

Development Editor
Joan Paterson

Production Editor
Christy Wagner

Copy Editor
Fran Blauw

Cover Designer
Mike Freeland

Photo Editor
Richard H. Fox

Illustrator
Jody P. Schaeffer

Designer
Glenn Larsen

Indexers
Chris Barrick, Sandra Henselmeier, Nadia Ibrahim

Layout/Proofreading
David Faust, Angel Perez, Heather Pope

Contents at a Glance

Contents

7 Holistic Dentistry: Sinking Your Teeth into Health 85

8 Chelation: Grabbing for Good Health 93

ix

Foreword

The quality of your life depends on alternative medicine. Ignoring its benefits deprives you of optimizing your health to help you live better longer.

Supplements or procedures outside the mainstream of allopathic medicine, called "alternative medicine" or "alternative therapy," are becoming known as "complementary therapies" as more and more healthcare practitioners realize their value. Medical journals solicit articles on alternative medicine; medical schools request speakers to lecture on the subject; and the media reports on the success of alternative therapies.

It's not a matter of being against allopathic medicine and in favor of alternative medicine—it's not one or the other. Using the guidelines in this book, you can take advantage of the best that each has to offer. One weakness of allopathic medicine is that its approach is more toward masking symptoms than curing the underlying cause. As a result, allopathic medicine relies heavily on powerful drugs. It was reported in a medical journal in 1998 that prescribed drug interactions were responsible for about 100,000 deaths per year. This makes drug side effects one of the leading causes of death! No wonder that people are demanding more natural treatments with fewer side effects.

Alternative medicine offers therapies for several problems that aren't adequately responsive to allopathic medicine. It's a matter of utilizing the best that each has to offer, and this is where *The Complete Idiot's Guide to Alternative Medicine* shines. Dr. Pressman's thorough understanding of the strengths and weaknesses of each technique enables him to clearly guide the reader through complicated disciplines.

You are responsible for your health. Use your various healthcare professionals as consultants to optimize your health. When investing money for retirement, most people prefer a balanced portfolio of financial instruments to optimize their financial picture for retirement. Should your health be treated any less wisely?

Optimizing your health means more than just being free of disease—it means having a better quality of life. Optimal health involves more than the statistics of morbidity and mortality—it means a healthier body, a more agile mind, and a fulfilled spirit. Invest a little time in reading this book now, and you will be rewarded with learning how to plan for achieving optimal health.

Richard A. Passwater, Ph.D.

Richard A. Passwater is the Director of the Solgar Nutritional Research Center in Berlin, Maryland. Dr. Passwater discovered the synergism of antioxidant nutrients in 1965, was the first to report that antioxidant nutrients reduced the incidence of cancer in laboratory animals in 1972, and the first to show that vitamin E reduced the incidence of heart disease in a 1976 epidemiological study. Dr. Passwater has authored more than 35 books and more than 400 articles on nutrition.

Introduction

Have you ever had a nice cup of hot mint tea before bed or to soothe an upset stomach? Have you ever visited a chiropractor or had a massage? Have you ever taken a vitamin pill? If you have, you've used alternative medicine.

Whatever your reason, you've got plenty of company. A landmark study of alternative medicine appeared in 1993 in the *New England Journal of Medicine*. The study showed an astonishing one in three of all adult Americans had used an alternative therapy in the past year. The cost for all this added up to a whopping $13.7 billion, most of which the patients paid out of their own pockets. By 1998, a study in the *Journal of the American Medical Association (JAMA)* showed that amount had jumped to over $21 billion. Why? Because they're seeking better health and more compassionate healthcare. They're tired of drugs that don't help or only mask symptoms, and they want to avoid unnecessary surgery.

Does alternative medicine help? Yes—in many cases, it works as well as or even better than standard medicine, without expensive drugs and their side effects. We can't promise, though, that alternative medicine helps every health problem, and there are certainly many cases where standard medical treatment is your best bet. But even then, combining alternative treatments with standard medical treatments may well help you get better faster.

Talk to Your Doctor!

We urge you to discuss any alternative medicine treatment with your doctor before you try it. There could be good reasons for not using the alternative approach. And if your doctor has prescribed medicine (even an over-the-counter one), it could react badly with any drugs, herbs, supplements, or other substances you take as part of the alternative treatment. *Never* stop taking a drug your doctor has prescribed. *Never* change the dosage on your own—*always* talk to your doctor first.

Your Health Is in Your Hands

Many people turn to alternative medicine because they're fed up with today's hurried, impersonal doctors and hospitals. They're tired of being treated as nothing but a bunch of symptoms to be dealt with and hustled out of the office as quickly as possible.

Alternative medicine takes a different approach. Because healing comes from within, you're responsible for your own health. Your alternative medicine practitioner will spend a lot of time with you helping you find ways to heal yourself.

How to Use This Book

We've divided this book into eight parts. In Part 1, "Choosing Health," we explain the basic concepts of alternative medicine and self-healing. In Part 2, "What's Up, Doc? Alternative Medical Practices," we discuss the various alternative medical therapies and approaches, like osteopathy, naturopathy, and Ayurvedic medicine—treatments provided by trained physicians. In Part 3, "Acupuncture and Energy," we get charged up about treatments meant to restore the proper energy flow in your body. Part 4, "Homeopathy and Herbs," looks at some of the most popular alternative treatments, including traditional herbal medicine, flower remedies, and traditional Chinese herbs. Part 5, "You Are What You Eat," discusses nutritional supplements, vitamin megadoses, juice therapy, macrobiotics, and other ways to improve your health through your diet. In Part 6, "Getting in Touch," we look at the hands-on approach to alternative medicine. Here we discuss chiropractic, massage, various forms of bodywork (such as the Alexander Technique and Rolfing), and more. Part 7, "Making Sense of It All," explores the worlds of aromatherapy, light therapy, and sound therapy. In Part 8, "It's All in Your Mind," we look at the mind/body connection by examining yoga, hypnosis, meditation, and a range of other approaches, including biofeedback.

We urge you to read the first two chapters of this book to get an idea of the basic ideas behind alternative thinking. After that, feel free to skip around. Check out the therapies that intrigue you, or look up the therapies that might help your personal health. Look up the medical terms in the glossary. If you want to know more about any particular alternative treatment, we've given you names and addresses of professional organizations and associations wherever possible. We've also included a section of World Wide Web sites worth visiting.

We've used lots of charts and tables, some pictures and diagrams, and even some recipes to help make this book as complete and thorough as possible. We've also used four kinds of sidebars to give you extra information.

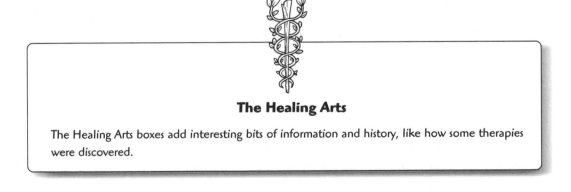

The Healing Arts

The Healing Arts boxes add interesting bits of information and history, like how some therapies were discovered.

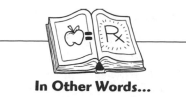

In Other Words...

In Other Words... boxes define treatments, medical terms, and other concepts.

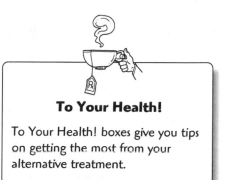

To Your Health!

To Your Health! boxes give you tips on getting the most from your alternative treatment.

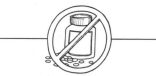

Hazardous to Your Health!

Hazardous to Your Health! boxes are warnings. Take these boxes seriously, please. They help you avoid problems, like dangerous drug interactions, and tell you when to consult your doctor.

Acknowledgments

We'd like to thank the many, many friends and colleagues who have shared their knowledge with us as we researched this book. We'd especially like to thank all the staff members of the many professional organizations and associations we contacted, who generously supplied us with the latest research in their fields. Thanks again to Hope Gillerman for her help on the Alexander Technique, Dr. Vasant Lad of The Ayurvedic Institute for permission to reprint his dosha questionnaire, and Nelson Bach USA for permission to reprint the Bach Flower Essences questionnaire. Thanks to Michael Edan and Laura Norman of Laura Norman Associates for their help with the foot reflexology charts.

Thanks also to Martin Kohl for research assistance, sage advice, and some good laughs. At Macmillan, we'd like to thank Gary Krebs for getting us started again, Nancy Mikhail for keeping us at it again, and Joan Paterson for once again working her editorial magic. Special thanks to Maureen Horn and Christy Wagner for their help with the production end and to Fran Blauw for her copyediting.

Special Thanks to the Technical Reviewer

The Complete Idiot's Guide to Alternative Medicine was reviewed by an expert who double-checked the accuracy of what you'll learn here to help us ensure that this book gives you everything you need to know alternative medicine. Special thanks are extended to Stuart Fischer, M.D., for his careful review of the manuscript and useful comments. We were fortunate to have the advice of such a well-informed and caring physician.

Dr. Stuart Fischer, born in Brooklyn, New York, completed an Internal Medicine residency at Maimonides Hospital. He worked for four years as an Emergency Room Attending Physician at Cabrini Medical Center. Dr. Fischer is currently in private practice in New York City and has hosted WEVD's *Vital Signs* for five sessions.

Part 1
Choosing Health

Are you sick of being sick? Does the medicine you take make you sicker? Are you ready to take charge of your health? If your answers are yes, read on—alternative medicine may be the cure for what ails you.

Which alternative treatment is best for you? We can't say, but in this section we can tell you the basic ideas behind alternative therapies, what the researchers and the government have to say about them, and how to talk to your doctor.

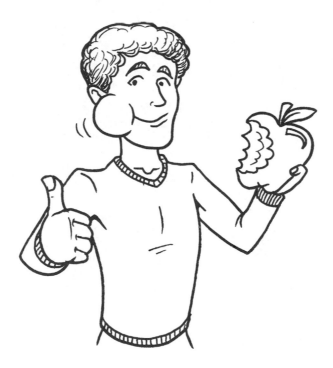

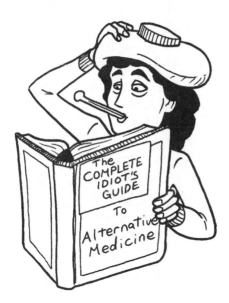

Alternative Medicine: In Sickness and in Health

In This Chapter

➤ Standard medicine versus alternative treatments

➤ Why people are turning to alternative medicine

➤ The wellness model

➤ Healing yourself

➤ Alternative medicine enters the mainstream

In the course of a typical year, Americans visit alternative healthcare providers about 629 million times. They visit primary care physicians only 386 million times. What's going on here? Not much—just a revolution in how we take care of our health.

In Sickness and in Health

You can look at your health in one of two ways. There's the standard medical model, which says that health is simply the absence of disease. Then there's the *alternative medicine* model, which says that health is much more than that. It's wellness—feeling your best in body, mind, and spirit. It's also prevention—keeping yourself healthy through diet, exercise, relaxation, and more. And when you do get sick, practitioners of alternative medicine believe that you have the power to heal yourself.

Let's look more closely at the basic ideas behind alternative medicine:

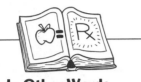

In Other Words...

Alternative medicine is a broad term that covers a range of healing therapies. It's usually defined as those treatments and healthcare approaches not generally used by doctors and hospitals and not generally reimbursed by medical insurance companies.

➤ **Healing comes from within.** Your own body has the power to heal itself, often without drugs or surgery. Treatment is designed to stimulate your natural self-healing powers.

➤ **A holistic approach.** Alternative medicine looks for the root cause of the problem and treats the whole person, not just the symptoms.

➤ **Your mind matters.** There's no artificial distinction between your body and your mind in alternative medicine.

➤ **Nutrition matters.** Eating right is central to alternative medicine, both as a treatment and as a way to promote health.

➤ **Prevent disease.** Alternative medicine focuses on prevention as much as treatment.

As you'll discover in this book, some alternative therapies, such as osteopathy and chiropractic, are pretty compatible with *standard medical treatment*—so much so that they've become widely accepted as part of mainstream medicine. Others, such as acupuncture and Ayurvedic medicine, are way outside the Western approach to medicine and are more controversial.

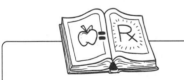

In Other Words...

Standard medicine, also called **allopathic medicine, mainstream medicine,** or **orthodox medicine,** is the medicine medical doctors learn in medical school and practice in hospitals. It's oriented toward treating illness, usually through drugs or surgery.

Going the Alternative Route

Why go the alternative medicine route? Maybe you're looking for relief from a chronic illness or chronic pain, treatment for a specific problem, or a wellness approach to your health. Maybe you're seeking an alternative to treatment that uses powerful drugs or surgery. Or maybe you want a more personal approach from your healthcare provider—someone who'll take the time to understand you and your health.

Whatever your reason, you have plenty of company. A landmark study of alternative medicine appeared in 1993 in the prestigious *New England Journal of Medicine*. The study showed that an astonishing *one in three* of all adult Americans had used an alternative therapy in the past year. The cost for all this added up to a whopping $13.7 billion, most of which the patients paid out of their own pockets. By 1998, a study in the equally prestigious *Journal of the American Medical Association* showed that amount had jumped to over $21 billion.

What was all that money going for? As you can see from Table 1.1, back pain topped the list, followed by a lot of other chronic problems that standard medicine doesn't always do much to help.

Table 1.1   Top 10 Reasons for Seeking Alternative Treatment

Condition	Percent of Alternative Treatments
Back problems	36
Anxiety	28
Headaches	27
Sprains or strains	22
Depression	20
Insomnia	20
Arthritis	18
Digestive problems	13
High blood pressure	11
Allergies	9

Source: "Unconventional Medicine in the United States," David M. Eisenberg, M.D., et al., New England Journal of Medicine, *Jan. 28, 1993.*

Looking at some of the health problems on the list, it's easy to see why the patients turned to alternative medicine. Take insomnia, for example—a problem that affects some 65 million Americans. The usual medical approach is to prescribe sleeping pills. The pills may help in the short run, but they're expensive, can be addictive, can interact badly with other drugs you might need, and often leave you feeling groggy in the morning. Worse, a prescription for pills doesn't deal with the basic question of what's keeping you up at night.

Alternative medicine takes a different approach—one that helps the patient cope with the problem from within. For insomnia, that might mean teaching the patient a simple relaxation technique that works just about 100 percent of the time (see Chapter 29, "Relaxation and Meditation: Rising Above It All," for the details).

In 1998, another survey—this one conducted for Landmark Healthcare, Inc., a managed alternative care company—showed that the percentage of adult Americans using alternative medicine had jumped to 42 percent. Check Table 1.2 to see which therapies they preferred.

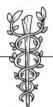

The Healing Arts

According to a 1998 study in *Journal of Clinical Oncology*, the leading cancer journal, nearly half of all cancer patients turn to some kind of alternative medicine in an effort to cure their disease. Although using alternative medicine doesn't improve their survival rate, the study suggests that it may help improve their quality of life. Is this bad news or good? The doctors say bad: Alternative medicine raises false hopes. The alternative practitioners say good: Alternative medicine improves the quality of life for dying patients. Who's right? Both—alternative medicine doesn't work miracles, but improving the quality of life for someone's final days certainly seems worthwhile to us.

Table 1.2   Top 10 Alternative Care Choices

Therapy	Percent Using in Past Year
Herbs	17
Chiropractic	16
Massage	14
Vitamins	13
Homeopathy	5
Yoga	5
Acupressure	5
Acupuncture	2
Biofeedback	2
Hypnotherapy	1

Source: "The Landmark Report on Public Perceptions of Alternative Care," 1998.

Of the people surveyed, 44 percent said they'd use an alternative method if standard medical treatment wasn't helping.

Alternative Medicine: The Smart Choice

Another 1998 study in *JAMA* looked at who uses alternative medicine—and why. Here too the results were surprising. The number of adult Americans who had used an alternative therapy in the past year jumped to 40 percent. Why? Interestingly, not because they were dissatisfied with conventional medicine. Instead, they saw alternative treatment as more compatible with their own values regarding the meaning of health and illness. People who wanted to be responsible for and involved in their own health chose alternative medicine.

Another interesting thing came out of the *JAMA* survey: Only 4.4 percent of the respondents used alternative medicine exclusively. Everyone else combined conventional medicine with alternative approaches. The people most likely to use alternative medicine are well educated and have less-than-optimal health. In other words, they're smart enough to know that conventional medicine isn't helping them and smart enough to find alternatives that do.

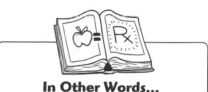

In Other Words...

Complementary medicine (sometimes called **integrative medicine**) is the use of alternative treatments in addition to—not instead of—standard medical treatment. Complementary medicine usually means the alternative practices, such as acupuncture and chiropractic, that are most widely accepted by medical doctors and health insurers.

Studies like these make the medical community pay attention. In 1997, the American Medical Association decided to encourage medical schools to offer courses in alternative medicine. The schools responded with enthusiasm. As of 1998, nearly two-thirds of the 125 American medical schools offer courses in alternative or *complementary medicine.*

The Operation Was a Success...

Standard medicine does some things very, very well. Trauma, for instance. If you're ever hurt in an accident, the well-trained staff at the well-equipped emergency room will know exactly what to do— they might well save your life. In plenty of other areas (cancer treatment, for instance), today's high-tech medicine can work wonders.

In Other Words...

An **adverse drug reaction (ADR)** is any unpleasant, unintended, and undesired effect of a drug used as a medical treatment. A serious ADR puts you in the hospital or keeps you there longer and could be permanently disabling or even kill you.

There's a big catch to all this, though—today's medicine could also kill you by mistake. In April 1998, *JAMA* published a very disturbing study of *adverse drug reactions* (ADRs) among hospitalized patients. The authors estimated that in any recent year, 2,216,000 hospital patients had ADRs—and 106,000 died from them. That makes adverse drug reactions one of the top killers in the country—just behind heart disease, cancer, stroke, lung disease, and accidents.

If an ADR doesn't get you in the hospital, there's a fair chance a serious infection will. Every year, some two million patients catch serious infections while they're in the hospital—and nearly 100,000 die from them. And easily one-quarter of all deaths from heart attack, stroke, and pneumonia trace straight back to medical error.

Alternative Therapies: The Wellness Model

Hazardous to Your Health!

If you are currently taking any drug—prescription or over-the-counter—that your doctor has recommended, don't stop! Alternative treatments may help you need less of the drug or even stop taking it eventually, but never change the dose or stop taking a drug on your own! Always talk to your doctor before starting an alternative treatment, and always talk to your doctor about changing your medication.

Here's where alternative medicine can make the difference. Almost all alternative treatments are drug-free—no side effects, no bad reactions, and no expense. You still might need to take pills, but they'll be vitamins, herbs, and other supplements meant to boost your own healing powers, not just to suppress your symptoms. And rather than just prescribe a pill, alternative health practitioners look at your whole lifestyle. Their prescriptions are much more likely to be for dietary improvements, more exercise, and finding ways to reduce the stress in your life.

Alternative medicine might also keep you out of the hospital. As Dr. Dean Ornish has proven, diet, exercise, stress reduction, and meditation can actually reverse heart disease, without bypass surgery or powerful drugs. Chiropractic treatment might keep you out of the hospital for back surgery. Patients of osteopathic physicians typically have shorter hospital stays than patients of medical doctors.

PG-Rated

Alternative medicine can be helpful for kids with health problems. Naturopathic physicians, for example, claim that treating middle-ear infections with diet is more effective than treating them with antibiotics—and they have the stats to back them up. A 1997 study in the journal *Pediatrics* showed that half of American parents turn to alternative therapies to help their children fight illness. The therapies most often include spiritual healing and prayer, massage therapy, acupuncture, medicinal herbs, and megavitamins. Do they help? The study couldn't say, but it did point out that using the alternative therapies did no harm and made the parents feel less helpless in the face of their child's illness.

The Office of Alternative Medicine

Alternative medicine formally entered the mainstream in 1992, when Congress created the *Office of Alternative Medicine* (OAM) as part of the *National Institutes of Health* (NIH). (The NIH is, in turn, part of the Public Health Service, which is part of the Health and

Human Services Department.) The OAM's primary job is to evaluate alternative treatments and determine how well they work.

So far, expert panels organized by the OAM have looked carefully at alternative treatments such as acupuncture and chiropractic for lower-back pain and given them the thumbs up. The OAM is also sponsoring ongoing university studies on alternative approaches to AIDS, women's health issues, stroke, asthma, cancer, aging, chronic pain, and more. The results down the road should be very interesting. We're sure the studies will scientifically prove the value of many alternative treatments.

To request information from the OAM, contact:

Office of Alternative Medicine
National Institutes of Health
OAM Clearinghouse
P.O. Box 8218
Silver Spring, MD 20907
Phone: (888) 644-6226

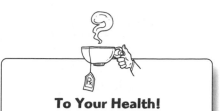

To Your Health!

The Office of Alternative Medicine is a research agency only. Unlike some other arms of the NIH, the OAM is not a treatment center and can't answer specific medical questions. It can provide you with plenty of useful information about the alternative treatments under study, and it can tell you how to learn more, but it can't refer you to individual practitioners or recommend a particular therapy.

What's in a Name?

One of the most important things the OAM has done is sort out some of the confusion about different types of alternative treatments. As you can see from Table 1.3, there are a lot of treatments, and they fall into several broad categories.

Table 1.3   Types of Alternative Health Practices

Alternative Systems of Medical Practice

Acupuncture	Native American practices
Anthroposophically extended medicine	Natural products
Ayurveda	Naturopathic medicine
Community-based healthcare practices	Past-life therapy
Environmental medicine	Shamanism
Homeopathic medicine	Tibetan medicine
Latin American rural practices	Traditional Oriental medicine

continues

Table 1.3   Types of Alternative Health Practices   (continued)

Bioelectric Applications

Blue-light treatment and artificial lighting	Electrostimulation and neuro-magnetic stimulation devices
Electroacupuncture	Magnetoresonance spectroscopy
Electromagnetic fields	

Diet, Nutrition, Lifestyle Changes

Changes in lifestyle	Macrobiotics
Diet	Megavitamins
Gerson therapy	Nutritional supplements

Herbal Medicine

Echinacea (purple coneflower)	Wild chrysanthemum flower
Ginger	Witch hazel
Ginkgo biloba extract	Yellowdock
Ginseng	

Manual Healing

Acupressure	Osteopathy
Alexander Technique	Reflexology
Biofield therapeutics	Rolfing
Chiropractic medicine	Therapeutic Touch
Feldenkrais Method	Trager Approach
Massage therapy	Zone therapy

Mind/Body Control

Art therapy	Meditation
Biofeedback	Music therapy
Counseling	Prayer therapy
Dance therapy	Psychotherapy
Guided imagery	Relaxation techniques
Humor therapy	Support groups
Hypnotherapy	Yoga

Table 1.3   Types of Alternative Health Practices

Pharmacological and Biological Treatments

Antioxidizing agents

Cell treatment

Chelation therapy

Metabolic therapy

Oxygen therapies

Source: Office of Alternative Medicine

There's some disagreement about all this, and the OAM points out that the classification and listing of therapies is neither complete nor authoritative. It's a good starting point, though, and we'll be discussing most of the therapies later on in this book.

The Least You Need to Know

➤ Every year, at least one in three adult Americans visits an alternative practitioner. The most common problem is back pain, followed by anxiety and headaches.

➤ Alternative medicine takes a wellness-based, holistic approach to your health, looking at you as a whole person and not just a group of symptoms.

➤ The goal of most alternative treatments is to treat the underlying problem by activating your own self-healing abilities.

➤ Alternative therapies avoid drugs and surgery and focus on nutrition, stress reduction, herbs, and other gentle treatments.

➤ The Office of Alternative Medicine at the National Institutes of Health was formed in 1992 to study alternative treatments and has already given positive assessments to chiropractic treatment for lower-back pain and acupuncture. Other studies are underway.

Chapter 2

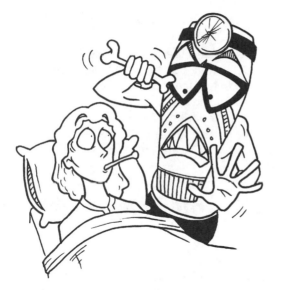

Myths and Realities

In This Chapter

➤ Can alternative medicine help you?

➤ When you need a medical doctor

➤ Who's in charge here?

➤ Finding—and paying for—alternative treatments

➤ Avoiding quackery

A lot of medical doctors dismiss alternative therapies, saying "It's just the placebo effect." What they're really saying is, "You got better from the alternative treatment and I don't really know why, so I'm saying it's all in your head rather than admit that the treatment might actually help."

Sounds like sour grapes to us. As a chiropractor and nutritionist, Dr. Pressman has helped thousands of patients over the years—patients whose doctors couldn't do anything more for them. We think his results, and the results of many alternative practitioners, are very far from being "just the placebo" treatments.

Why Alternative Medicine Works

Far from being a *placebo effect*, alternative medicine works for the same reasons standard medicine works—it finds the cause of the problem and treats it. The difference is how. Alternative medicine practitioners and medical doctors alike know that many health problems are caused by stress and that almost all health problems can be

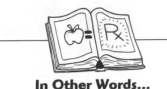

In Other Words...

The **placebo effect** happens when you get better from a harmless treatment or dummy drug that has no real action. The word comes from the Latin word meaning "I will please."

helped by diet, exercise, and lifestyle changes. The difference is that alternative practitioners really *listen* to their patients and help them find practical, drug-free ways to deal with stress and really make those lifestyle changes. They help their patients feel in control of their health and be active participants in the treatment. And feeling positive about your treatment does a lot to aid healing.

Is Alternative Medicine Right for Me?

Only you can decide that—and only after talking with your doctor. But as we'll discuss throughout this book, even people with very serious illnesses can benefit from some alternative treatments along with standard medical care. For example, hypnosis has been shown to help people facing surgery come through the operation better and recover faster.

In general, alternative therapies are very helpful for people with chronic diseases such as asthma, diabetes, heart disease, and high blood pressure. They're also very helpful for stress-related problems such as migraines, tension headaches, irritable bowel syndrome, insomnia, depression, and anxiety. Alternative therapies can also help people with chronic pain manage it better and improve the quality of their lives.

Talking to Your Doctor About Alternative Medicine

A big reason medical doctors object to alternative medicine is that most practitioners aren't qualified to diagnose your problem. Sure, osteopaths, chiropractors, and naturopaths have the medical training to tell if that cough that won't go away is from bronchitis or from lung cancer, but you certainly wouldn't want to leave that decision to your massage therapist or a homeopath.

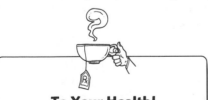

To Your Health!

If you're not sure what's wrong with you, we strongly urge you to see your doctor. They're very good at diagnosis—and they have all the tests and equipment of modern high-tech medicine to help them.

Treatment is where you and your doctor may disagree. He or she may want to follow the standard medical route—and you may want to try alternative therapies along with or instead of that treatment. Today more and more doctors are willing to discuss and even recommend alternative therapies—but usually only if they're in addition to standard treatment. The docs have a good point. Take high blood pressure, for instance. Even moderate high blood pressure sharply raises your risk of a heart attack or stroke. Your doctor will recommend diet and lifestyle changes, but he or she will probably also prescribe one of the very effective drugs that lower blood pressure. If you then want to try an alternative therapy such as chelation or biofeedback to lower it even more, discuss it with your doctor first. These treatments might help to the point where you need less medication or can stop taking it altogether, but they don't work for everyone, and the effects don't always last.

Many patients don't bother to tell their doctors about visits to alternative health practitioners. They also don't mention any vitamins, herbs, or other supplements they might be taking. We urge you to be open with your doctor about any other treatments you're using.

If you're worried that your doctor will disapprove, you might be in for a surprise. Doctors today are a lot more open-minded about alternative approaches.

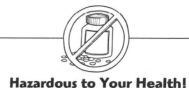

Hazardous to Your Health!

Never stop taking your medicine on your own. Never change your dosage on your own. Always discuss any changes in your medication with your doctor.

The Regulatory Picture

There's a regulatory picture, all right, but it looks a lot more like abstract art than a simple landscape. The reason is that every state has its own set of rules about healthcare. And as we'll discuss throughout this book, those rules can vary quite a bit. Before we get into the details, let's clarify how states look at credentials:

➤ **Certification.** Professional certification uses a formal process to show that a practitioner has met a recognized standard of training, experience, and knowledge in his or her field. Certification is a voluntary process in which a nongovernmental professional organization grants recognition to an individual who has met certain qualifications.

➤ **Licensure.** A nonvoluntary process by which a government agency regulates a profession. If the practitioner meets the standards set by the agency, he or she is granted a license—permission to practice in that state. Licensure is always based on laws passed by the legislature of that state. So, if a particular type of healthcare—acupuncture, say—is licensed in your state, it's illegal to practice it without a license.

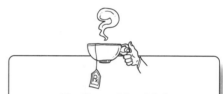

To Your Health!

Always ask an alternative health provider about his or her education. If you think the practitioner went to a, shall we say, uncompetitive school or might have a mail-order degree (you can buy these for your pets), look up the program in *Accredited Institutions of Postsecondary Education*, a reference book that's found in most libraries. If the school or program isn't there, find another practitioner.

➤ **State certification and registration.** These processes are less restrictive than licensing, but how each is defined can vary a lot from state to state. Don't confuse state certification with professional certification.

➤ **Accreditation.** A voluntary nongovernmental process that evaluates institutions, agencies, and education programs. To be accredited, a training program—a massage school, say—must meet standards set by an independent professional association or agency.

Throughout this book, we give you the general guidelines for certification and licensing for many aspects of alternative medicine. We also give you the names and addresses of certifying organizations so you can contact them directly.

State Regulatory Agencies

Finding out if your state regulates a particular alternative treatment can be a little complicated. A good place to start is the State Government section of your phone book. You can often figure out which branch of your state government is in charge of licensing what. In general, medical doctors and osteopaths are licensed by a state medical board, and you can contact your county medical society for more information. Other types of healthcare licenses aren't so easy. In our home state of New York, for example, nutritionists and many others are licensed by the department of education. We recommend a visit to your local public library. The librarian can help you use your state's government manual—often called a *red book* or *blue book*—to figure it out.

For information about a hospital, clinic, or treatment center, contact the state or local health authorities where the center is located.

Finding Qualified Practitioners

You've heard about an alternative therapy that could help your health problem. You've researched it, discussed it with your doctor, and decided to go ahead. Now what?

Finding a qualified practitioner in alternative medicine is actually pretty easy. In fact, your doctor may be able to refer you—a recent study showed that well over half of all primary care doctors either recommend alternative therapies to their patients or use them themselves. If your doctor can't help, try these steps:

➤ Ask friends and relatives for the names of local alternative practitioners they've used.

➤ Check around locally: the phone book, nearby alternative health centers, the bulletin board at your local health-food store, ads in the community paper.

➤ Contact professional organizations for referrals to practitioners in your area. We list these in each chapter where relevant; you can also call the national umbrella organizations listed in Appendix C, "National Organizations."

➤ Contact your local hospital and ask about support groups for various ailments. Chances are someone in the group can recommend a good alternative practitioner.

➤ Go online and search the World Wide Web. There's tons of great information out there. Try visiting the sites we list in Appendix E, "Alternative Health Online"—they're a good way to locate practitioners near you.

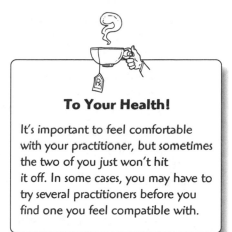

To Your Health!

It's important to feel comfortable with your practitioner, but sometimes the two of you just won't hit it off. In some cases, you may have to try several practitioners before you find one you feel compatible with.

Once you've located a practitioner, check him or her out. Don't be embarrassed to ask about the practitioner's education, training, experience, and any relevant licensing and certification requirements. Also ask for references of satisfied clients—and be sure to check them. Outstanding providers are proud of their skills and good reputation and will be happy to provide the information.

Alternative medicine doesn't mean sloppy medicine. Alternative practitioners should be professional in appearance and manner, keep good records, have clean, well-equipped offices with trained support staffs, and be businesslike about fees and handling your insurance paperwork.

One of the best things about alternative medicine is that the providers are generally far less harried than today's doctors and can spend time getting to know you and discussing your health. That sort of caring attention is all but lost in today's managed-care medicine. On average, an alternative practitioner spends about 30 minutes with a patient—or about four times the amount the average doctor spends.

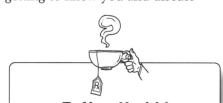

The Cost of Care: Will Insurance Cover It?

Maybe yes, maybe no. If you choose an alternative treatment that's widely accepted by the medical world, you'll probably be covered, at least in part. Osteopathic physicians, for example, are considered completely mainstream; their bills are treated exactly like the bills from a medical doctor. Chiropractic treatment for lower-back pain is generally covered without question. Also, you're usually covered for the more mainstream alternative treatments, like acupuncture, if your doctor recommends it.

To Your Health!

Most alternative health providers have a pretty good understanding of the health-insurance maze and can advise you on whether their services are usually covered. Even so, check with your insurer first. If you're turned down, ask about the procedure for appealing the decision. Be persistent and provide as much evidence as you can for the value of the treatment.

You may be covered in part for some alternative treatments if they're meant to help a specific health problem. A good example would be hypnosis as a way to stop smoking.

Where the picture gets murky is for less standard treatments, like chelation or reflexology. Your insurer may refuse to pay, saying that the treatments aren't usual and haven't been proved to work. In some states, though, "freedom of choice" laws have been passed that force insurers to cover some alternative treatments.

Whatever the alternative treatment, you can make a much better case for insurance coverage if it's given by a trained and licensed professional who meets all the requirements for practicing in your state and is certified by a recognized professional organization. We've given more detailed information in many chapters later on in this book—check under the heading "Rules, Rules, Rules."

More and more health insurers are starting to realize that the wellness approach of alternative medicine saves money in the long run. We feel that as more and more alternative treatments are shown to work, coverage will improve. In the meantime, coverage varies widely—always check before you start any alternative treatment.

Quacks, Kooks, and Fringe Treatments

Sick people are easy targets for *quacks* and kooks pushing weird treatments that don't work. Use your common sense and these guidelines to avoid being taken in:

➤ **Check credentials.** As we discussed earlier, ask about the provider's education, professional training, and if he or she is certified and licensed to provide the service in your state. If you have any doubts, stay away.

➤ **Look for the weasel words.** If the pitch includes words like "miraculous," "special," "scientific breakthrough," "instant relief," "secret," "quick and easy," "rediscovered," or "ancient," beware! The only thing miraculous about these treatments is how fast your money will vanish.

➤ **Ask how it's sold.** If a "miracle cure" is an "exclusive product" that's "not sold in stores," stay away.

➤ **Look for conspiracy claims.** Statements like "the government doesn't want you to know this" or "the secret doctors (or drug companies) won't tell you" should raise large red flags for you.

➤ **Be suspicious of testimonials.** Anecdotes are nice, but hard facts are a lot better. If the main selling point for the product or service is testimonials from satisfied customers, skip it.

If you feel that any healthcare practitioner has acted improperly toward you, bring the matter to the appropriate regulatory agency in your state. For physicians, that will probably be your county or state medical board. For other healthcare providers, it will be the agency that licenses or regulates them. You can also report the provider to any relevant professional organizations.

Health fraud is big business. The FDA estimates that 38 million Americans used a fraudulent health product within the last year—at a cost of some $27 billion! Here's a list of top health frauds:

➤ **Fraudulent arthritis products.** Are you willing to try snake venom?

➤ **Spurious cancer clinics.** Laetrile, one of the drugs used at these clinics, has been proven time and again not to work.

➤ **Bogus AIDS cures.** Don't trust an "underground" or "guerrilla" clinic.

➤ **Instant weight-loss schemes.** Need we say more?

➤ **Fraudulent sexual aids.** Trust us—weird stuff like Chinese crocodile penis pills doesn't work.

➤ **Baldness cures and other appearance modifiers.** Some people will believe anything.

➤ **False nutritional schemes.** There's no substitute for a good, balanced diet.

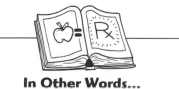

In Other Words...

A **quack** is anyone who pushes false or useless health treatments or remedies. The word comes from the older word *quacksalver*, meaning someone who hawks useless ointments in public places like fairs and markets. The old expression "snake-oil salesman" once meant someone who sold worthless remedies, but today it means someone who sells any phony product.

Most of the people and companies you'll encounter in the world of alternative medicine are well-trained, sincere, and honest. You shouldn't put up with someone who makes bogus claims or sells you worthless products. To report a company for falsely labeling its products or to report a problem related to a dietary supplement, call your local Food and Drug Administration office (check the Government pages of your phone book under U.S. Department of Health and Human Services for the number). To report a false advertising claim, contact:

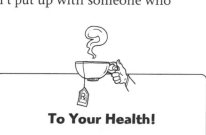

To Your Health!

A recent study by the U.S. Office of Technology Assessment suggests that only about 20 percent of modern medical remedies in common use have been scientifically shown to be effective.

Consumer Response Center
Federal Trade Commission
Washington, DC 20580
Phone: (202) 326-2222

You can also report false advertising claims to your state Attorney General and Better Business Bureau.

If you're unhappy with a quack product you bought through the mail, complain to your local postmaster.

If you want to take legal action against a quack, you may be able to get help from the National Council Against Health Fraud. For more information, contact:

Stephen Barrett, M.D.
National Council Against Health Fraud
P.O. Box 33008
Kansas City, MO 64114
Phone: (610) 437-1795

Having said all this about quacks and frauds, we hope we haven't scared you. If you follow the guidelines we've outlined here, use your common sense, and talk with your doctor before you try an alternative therapy, the chances are good that you'll be helped.

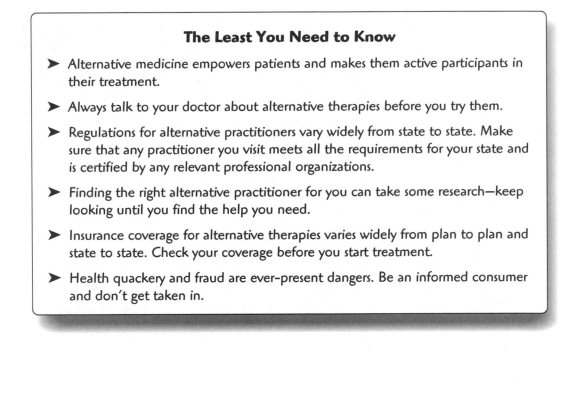

The Least You Need to Know

➤ Alternative medicine empowers patients and makes them active participants in their treatment.

➤ Always talk to your doctor about alternative therapies before you try them.

➤ Regulations for alternative practitioners vary widely from state to state. Make sure that any practitioner you visit meets all the requirements for your state and is certified by any relevant professional organizations.

➤ Finding the right alternative practitioner for you can take some research—keep looking until you find the help you need.

➤ Insurance coverage for alternative therapies varies widely from plan to plan and state to state. Check your coverage before you start treatment.

➤ Health quackery and fraud are ever-present dangers. Be an informed consumer and don't get taken in.

Part 2

What's Up, Doc? Alternative Medical Practices

Plenty of well-trained physicians and other medical types offer alternative therapies. Osteopathy, for instance, takes a hands-on approach to your health, but osteopathic physicians are, for all intents and purposes, medical doctors—even your insurance company will agree. Naturopathic physicians combine modern medical training with holistic treatments, including nutrition and herbs, while Ayurvedic physicians combine the ancient healing tradition of India with Western medicine. Then there's traditional Chinese medicine. Here, too, thousands of years of experience combine with modern ideas and holistic treatments.

Treatments such as chelation therapy, oxygen therapy, and holistic dentistry are controversial—read what we have to say and talk it over with your doctor before you try any of these.

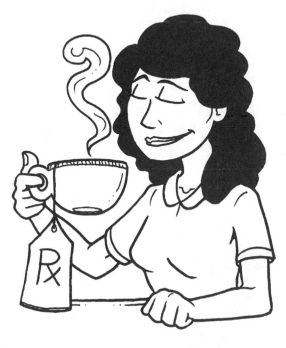

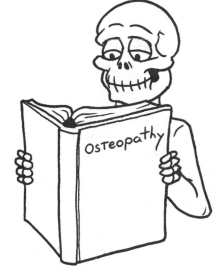

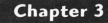

Chapter 3

Osteopathy: Boning Up

In This Chapter

➤ Basic concepts of osteopathy

➤ Differences and similarities between osteopathy and standard medicine

➤ How osteopathy helps lower-back aches and other painful problems

➤ Why osteopathy is becoming more popular

➤ Finding a qualified osteopath

Modern medicine has lots of great tools—things like CAT scans, miracle drugs, and advanced microsurgery. Osteopathic medicine uses them all but adds a couple more: the doctor's own two hands.

That's because osteopathic medicine believes that most illnesses can be traced back to an imbalance in the bones and muscles that form the basic framework of your body. To straighten you out again, osteopathic doctors use gentle touch and manipulation on your muscles and joints.

They don't stop there, though. Osteopathic doctors look at you as a whole person, not just a set of symptoms. They realize that your diet, your lifestyle, and your emotional health are all important to your overall health. That's why a lot of people call osteopathy the original holistic medicine—and that's why osteopathy is one of the fastest-growing areas in healthcare.

Frontier Medicine in the Modern World

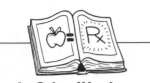

In Other Words...

Osteopathy, also known as **osteopathic medicine**, is a branch of medicine that believes that your body structure—your bones and muscles—and the rest of your body functions operate together. The word comes from the Greek word *osteo-*, meaning *bone*, and *pathy*, meaning "disease." Those who practice osteopathy believe that imbalances in your body structure cause disease and that restoring the balance will restore health.

Osteopathic medicine, or *osteopathy*, began back in the 1870s with a frontier doctor named Andrew Taylor Still. Back then, doctors were more likely to harm or even kill their patients than to help them. Dr. Still decided that the best way to help his patients was to help them help themselves. He believed that the body's *musculoskeletal system*—your bones, muscles, joints, ligaments, and connective tissues—is crucial to good health. It's the framework that supports your entire body; in fact, it makes up about 60 percent of your weight. And if your musculoskeletal system gets out of whack, other parts of your body—even organs like your heart or lungs—are affected. Dr. Still began to develop methods to find the problems in his patients' musculo-skeletal systems. Once he found the abnormality or imbalance, he would use touch and gentle manipulation of the muscles and joints to get them realigned. He found that his manipulations helped to stimulate the body's own self-healing powers. His patients improved, often without the use of drugs or surgery.

Dr. Still founded the first college of osteopathy in 1892. Naturally, he ran into a lot of opposition from the medical establishment, but his methods were so successful and popular that osteopathy became the first true form of alternative medicine. That's mostly because students

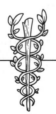

The Healing Arts

When Andrew Taylor Still, M.D. (1828–1917), was a doctor on the Missouri frontier in the 1870s, standard medical practice was downright dangerous to your health. Doctors routinely prescribed potent drugs that contained mercury, arsenic, calomel, and other poisonous substances. They scoffed at the idea that microscopic germs could cause disease and saw nothing wrong with using the same unwashed scalpel over and over again. After losing his wife and three of his children to serious disease, Dr. Still decided there had to be a better way. He went back to a basic principle of medicine—helping patients heal themselves from within.

at osteopathic colleges got pretty much the same scientific training as medical doctors—but they also learned the techniques of osteopathic touch.

For a long time, osteopathy ran on a parallel track to conventional medicine. Graduates of osteopathic colleges got the degree *D.O.*, for *doctor of osteopathy*, instead of *M.D.*, or *medical doctor*. They had their own practices and sent their patients to osteopathic hospitals. They did a lot of touching and manipulating, and they didn't prescribe drugs or surgery very often.

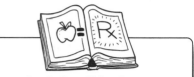

Over the years, the two tracks got much closer. In the late 1930s, osteopathic training got a lot tougher. By 1972, regulatory changes made D.O.s and M.D.s essentially equal. These are the only types of complete physicians in the United States. Both types of doctors do four years of basic medical education and then go on for several years of additional training as interns and residents. Both D.O.s and M.D.s have to pass comparable types of state licensing exams. Today osteopathic physicians practice in every area of medicine, from gynecology to surgery to psychiatry. Even so, about half of all osteopathic doctors put their holistic training to use as primary care physicians rather than choose narrow specialties.

In Other Words...

The abbreviation **D.O.** stands for **doctor of osteopathy**. For all practical purposes, it's the equivalent of the more traditional **M.D.**, or **medical doctor**, degree. A D.O., also called an **osteopath**, can do everything an M.D. can, including prescribe drugs, perform surgery, and admit you to the hospital.

Osteopathy on the Rise

In the past few years, osteopathy has become a lot more popular—to the point of more than 100 million visits to D.O.s every year. Why? Many patients prefer the personal, hands-on (literally) approach of osteopaths. They also like the holistic approach of osteopathy, with its emphasis on wellness and a healthy lifestyle. Osteopaths believe that the body heals itself, not that drugs or surgery do the healing—a belief that more and more patients agree with.

At a time when traditional medical schools are cutting back on graduates, osteopathic medical schools are growing. In 1968, there were just five osteopathic colleges; in 1998, there were 19, with several more in the planning stages. In 1975, there were only around 15,000 osteopathic physicians; in 1989, there were still only 25,000. In 1999, there are about 40,000, and there'll probably be more than 45,000 by 2005.

Because osteopathy takes the holistic approach and stresses both good body motion and good nutrition, it has become very, very popular with athletes—both the professional and the weekend-warrior kind. A lot of team physicians these days are osteopaths.

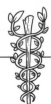

The Healing Arts

As of 1998, there were about 48,000 osteopaths in the United States. Although they make up only about 5 percent of all the 700,000 or so doctors, D.O.s make up almost 10 percent of all primary care doctors. Because many D.O.s feel a doctor should have a personal relationship with his or her patients, they prefer to practice in small towns and medically underserved communities. In rural areas with populations of less than 10,000, D.O.s provide about 15 percent of the primary care.

Hands-On Medicine

According to osteopathic thinking, physical or emotional stress, an injury, or poor posture affects your musculoskeletal system. Some part of your body then tenses up and gets painful. The pain makes you tense up even more, which pulls your body even more out of line, which makes it even more painful. You get the picture: A nasty pain-tension cycle sets in. If it goes on long enough, it starts to affect not just your muscles and joints but also your organs. By the same token, a problem with an organ—kidney trouble, say—could first show up as back pain. An osteopath can usually tell where the pain comes from and why—which could get you the right diagnosis and treatment faster.

To break the pain-tension cycle, a D.O. uses *osteopathic manipulative therapy* (OMT). The idea is to correct the problem by gently getting the affected area back into line.

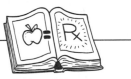

In Other Words...

Osteopathic manipulative therapy (OMT) is the overall term for a variety of hands-on physical techniques used to diagnose and treat musculoskeletal problems.

Osteopathic manipulative therapy has three basic goals:

➤ Relieving tension in your musculoskeletal system so that the muscles, ligaments, and joints return to their proper alignment.

➤ Improving your blood circulation and stimulating your nervous system. The pain-tension cycle tightens your musculoskeletal system so much that it reduces blood flow in the affected area and presses painfully on nerves.

➤ Improving body mechanics. Poor posture and other imbalances in your body can cause health problems.

If you need OMT, your osteopath will use one or more of several manipulation techniques:

➤ **Mobilization.** Gently moving a painful joint to give it greater mobility.

➤ **Soft-tissue techniques.** Methods that use rhythmic stretching, deep pressure, pushing or pulling, and tensing and releasing to relax muscles.

➤ **Functional and positional release.** The osteopath moves your body into particular positions that let the tense muscles relax.

➤ **Thrust technique.** Sometimes, when you really can't move some part of your body, the osteopath uses a quick push, sometimes called a *high-velocity thrust*, to get it moving again. The thrust is painless, but you may hear a perfectly normal clicking sound as the joint moves into a better position.

➤ **Lymphatic technique.** This technique is said to help your immune system by improving the circulation of the lymph fluids. It's sometimes used in cases of illness and infection—along with, not instead of, any necessary antibiotics.

OMT works painlessly and well—sometimes amazingly well—on people with knee problems, lower-back pain, neck problems, headaches, and chronic pain. Many patients say it helps with other problems, such as migraines and menstrual pain.

It's less clear how helpful OMT is for a lot of problems. An osteopath would treat a case of pneumonia, for example, with regular medical methods, including any needed drugs, along with special attention to your nutrition and possibly the lymphatic technique.

Overall, osteopaths use OMT on only about a quarter of their patients—or even fewer. Some osteopaths use OMT so rarely that you can hardly tell them from a regular M.D.

In addition to OMT, osteopaths also teach their patients relaxation techniques, better breathing methods, and ways to improve their posture and working positions. They often provide nutritional counseling and recommend supplements.

It's All in Your Head: Cranial Osteopathy

Cranial osteopathy is a controversial offshoot of regular osteopathy. Practitioners of cranial osteopathy believe that the bones of your skull, rather than being fused solidly together, actually are flexible and can move to some extent. (Remember that the next time someone calls you a blockhead!) The movement of the skull bones has an effect on the flow of the fluid that bathes your brain and spinal column. In addition, the fluid is said to have its own pulse, separate from your heartbeat or breathing. Cranial osteopaths claim that they can feel the cranial pulse and detect subtle changes and blockages in the motion of your skull bones.

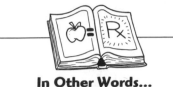

In Other Words...

Cranial osteopathy, also sometimes called craniosacral therapy or cranial therapy, focuses on the bones of your skull. Cranial osteopaths claim that they can gently manipulate your skull to diagnose illness, relieve pain, and even cure problems such as chronic fatigue and hyperactivity.

By using very gentle OMT and massage, osteopaths say they can relieve the blockages and help problems such as headaches, the effects of stroke, spinal cord injuries, depression, and many other ailments. Cranial osteopathy is also said to help children who have learning disabilities such as attention deficit disorder (ADD).

The evidence for cranial osteopathy is a little sketchy, although the existence of the cranial pulse has recently been proven. What still hasn't been proven is whether the cranial pulse has anything to do with your health.

Most mainstream osteopaths don't use the technique. A lot of osteopaths, dentists, and physical therapists have been taught how to do it, though, and they claim that it can really benefit some patients. Dentists in particular say cranial osteopathy can be very helpful, especially for people with jaw pain (you'll learn more about this in Chapter 7, "Holistic Dentistry: Sinking Your Teeth into Health").

A Visit to the Osteopath

Going to an osteopathic physician is very much like going to any doctor. You might go because it's time for a checkup, or because you're not feeling well, or because you've injured yourself somehow. Whatever the reason, your osteopath will do all the usual medical things, like draw blood for diagnostic tests, that any doctor would. Unlike most medical doctors, however, an osteopath will also look at your body framework—the way you stand, walk, sit, and hold your head. He or she will do a structural examination of your body to find any tenderness or loss of motion in your soft tissues and joints. If necessary, your treatment will include OMT and other treatments to correct any imbalances.

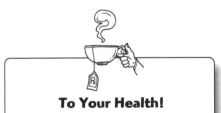

To Your Health!

Many muscle and joint problems are helped quickly by OMT—back pain from a muscle spasm could be gone in just one visit. It's more likely that you'll need three to six visits of about 20 to 30 minutes each to resolve the problem, though.

Your medical insurance will pay for your treatment exactly as if you had gone to see an M.D. In fact, the insurance company may prefer that you see an osteopath. That's because in some cases osteopaths deliver more bang for the buck than medical doctors. Their patients tend to get over problems like back injuries faster, which cuts down on disability costs. If your osteopath sends you to the hospital, you're likely to have a slightly shorter stay—and given today's hospital costs, even a day less saves a lot of money. Insurance companies aren't too keen on craniosacral osteopathy, however, and your insurer may not want to pay for it. Check before you get started.

Finding an Osteopath

Osteopaths today are well trained in basic medicine and osteopathic techniques. Most have done internships and residencies at teaching hospitals and can handle any sort of medical problem. To find an osteopath near you, contact:

American Osteopathic Association
142 East Ontario Street
Chicago, IL 60611
Phone: (800) 621-1773
Fax: (312) 202-8204
E-mail: osteomed@wwa.com

For varying reasons, not all osteopaths use a lot of OMT. If you'd like to find one who makes it an important part of his or her practice, contact:

American Academy of Osteopathy
3500 DePauw Boulevard, Suite 1080
Indianapolis, IN 46268-1136
Phone: (317) 879-1881
Fax: (317) 879-0563

Both organizations can give you useful information about osteopathy and help you decide if a particular osteopath is the right one for you.

Are You Being Manipulated?

Today the parallel universes of the D.O.s and the M.D.s are converging closer and closer. Some M.D.s remain dubious. They point out that the admission standards for osteopathic colleges are slightly lower than those for medical colleges. Frankly, that criticism sounds a little feeble to us. Another education criticism, one that carries more weight, is that osteopathic colleges have much smaller faculties, so students get less direct attention and supervision.

Many medical doctors feel that OMT is useful only for the relief of back pain and that it shouldn't be used to diagnose or treat anything else. They point out, rightly, that there just aren't enough good studies to justify a lot of the OMT claims. Most osteopaths agree and use OMT only where they feel it will really help. They're also trying hard to design and carry out better studies.

The biggest medical objection to osteopathy today is aimed at craniosacral therapy. There's very little proof that it works or that the separate craniosacral pulse has any relation to your health. The medical doctors—and, to be honest, a lot of osteopaths as well—say it's nothing but quackery.

The Least You Need to Know

➤ Osteopathic medicine takes a holistic approach to health that emphasizes wellness and prevention.

➤ Osteopaths believe that your musculoskeletal system—the bones and muscles that are the framework of your body—is crucial to good health. Imbalances in the framework are painful and can lead to problems in other parts of the body.

➤ Today osteopaths (D.O.s) and medical doctors (M.D.s) have very similar training and qualifications. Osteopaths can do anything medical doctors can, including prescribing drugs and performing surgery.

➤ In addition to standard medical therapies, osteopaths often use osteopathic manipulative treatment (OMT).

➤ Osteopathic manipulation is often very helpful for treating lower-back pain, joint problems, sports injuries, headaches, and other problems.

Chapter 4

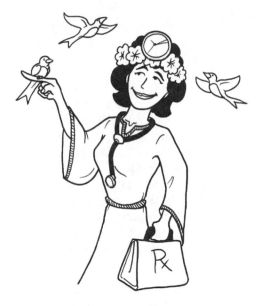

Naturopathy: The Healing Power of Nature

In This Chapter

➤ Why an old idea is new again

➤ Basic principles of naturopathy

➤ The road to wellness

➤ Alternative methods used in naturopathy

➤ Finding a naturopathic physician

More than two thousand years ago, Hippocrates, the father of modern medicine, taught that people naturally heal themselves—all a doctor does is gently help the process along. Good diet, rest, and exercise, said Hippocrates, help patients heal from within. Makes sense, right? Well, somewhere along the line, Hippocrates' message got lost and didn't surface again until the 1890s. Now, a century later, we're hip to Hippocrates all over again. Naturopathy—natural treatments that stimulate the patient's own healing—is one of today's most popular approaches to alternative medicine.

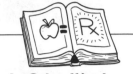

In Other Words...

Naturopathy or **naturopathic medicine** treats health problems by using the body's natural ability to heal. The terms come from the word *natural*, as in the methods used, and *-path*, the Greek word for "disease." Modern naturopathy includes a wide range of therapies, such as herbs, homeopathy, acupuncture, and nutrition.

What's Old Is New

Nature cures—treatments like hydrotherapy, gentle exercise, vegetarian diets, and fresh air—became popular in Europe in the 1850s. Fashionable people went to spa towns to "take the waters." By the 1890s, the nature-cure idea had reached the United States, brought by a pioneer from Germany named Benedict Lust. One of the first physicians to grasp the idea was Dr. John Scheel of New York. In 1895, he invented the word *naturopathy* to describe the new approach. Naturopathy caught on fast, and by 1920, there were thousands of *naturopathic physicians* and about 20 naturopathic colleges in the United States.

But when sulfa, the first "miracle drug," was discovered in the 1930s and when penicillin came along in the 1940s, naturopathic treatment began to lose ground. By the 1950s, new drugs, better surgical techniques, and high-tech machinery made conventional medicine seem invincible. Naturopathy faded so fast that all the naturopathic medical schools closed.

By the 1970s, though, things like antibiotic-resistant bacteria were making conventional medicine look a lot less miraculous. Patients weren't too happy with the high cost of high-tech medicine, and they didn't like being seen as just a bunch of symptoms instead of people. Naturopathic medicine slowly started to come back as a reasonable alternative. Today the move toward naturopathy is snowballing as more and more evidence shows that in a lot of cases it works just as well as conventional medicine. There are a couple of big differences, though: Naturopathic medicine costs less and patients are generally more satisfied.

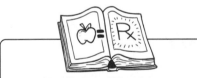

In Other Words...

Naturopathic physicians are general practitioners trained as specialists in natural medicine. After four years of undergraduate college and four more years at an accredited naturopathic college, a student earns the degree **Doctor of Naturopathic Medicine** and can put the letters **N.D.** after his or her name. Naturopathic doctors are also called **naturopaths**.

Whole-Body Health

The guiding principles of naturopathic medicine start with one really basic idea—the same one that Hippocrates had way back: the healing power of nature. It's the slogan and rallying cry of naturopathic medicine. Your body and mind have their own powerful healing mechanisms that help you heal yourself from within. Your naturopathic physician's job is to help you heal yourself using methods and medicines that are in harmony with your natural processes.

Going beyond the fundamental concept of the healing power of nature, naturopathic medicine also follows these guiding principles:

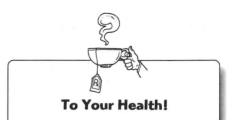

➤ **First do no harm.** If everyone followed this idea in everything, not just medicine, we'd all be a lot better off. To a naturopathic physician, this means choosing treatments that are as noninvasive as possible and have the least chance of side effects.

➤ **Find the cause.** Naturopaths believe that every illness has an underlying cause—and it's usually something to do with your diet or lifestyle. By dealing with the basic cause, not the effect or the symptoms (although they treat those too), naturopaths treat the illness and keep it from coming back.

To Your Health!

In 1994, the Office of Alternative Medicine at the National Institutes of Health began funding research into alternative treatments for HIV/AIDS. It was the first formal recognition of naturopathic medicine by the federal government.

➤ **Treat the whole person.** Your health—and your illnesses—come from a complex mixture of your physical makeup, your environment, your diet, your lifestyle, and more. Naturopathic doctors look at everything about you, not just your symptoms, when they treat you.

➤ **Prevention is the best cure.** If you treat a minor problem or change a bad health habit, you could prevent more serious or chronic problems down the line. Prevention through education is a major principle of naturopathic medicine.

What do you get when you combine these principles? A holistic approach to medicine to help you get over health problems and achieve new levels of well-being.

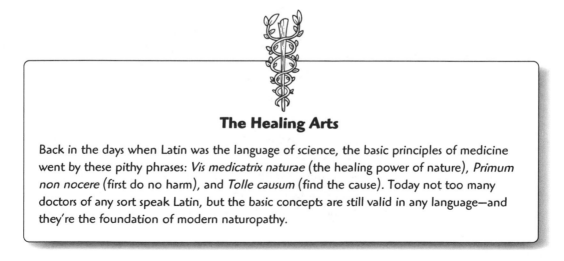

The Healing Arts

Back in the days when Latin was the language of science, the basic principles of medicine went by these pithy phrases: *Vis medicatrix naturae* (the healing power of nature), *Primum non nocere* (first do no harm), and *Tolle causum* (find the cause). Today not too many doctors of any sort speak Latin, but the basic concepts are still valid in any language—and they're the foundation of modern naturopathy.

Natural Cures

Naturopathic medicine is helpful for all sorts of health problems, but many patients find it most valuable for chronic diseases and conditions. The naturopathic approach to things like ulcerative colitis, arthritis, high blood pressure, migraines, chronic fatigue syndrome, allergies, and asthma can do a lot to relieve the symptoms and put you on the road to better health. And when it comes to nonemergency surgery for problems such as enlarged prostate or middle-ear infections, naturopathic medicine often has safer, less-expensive alternatives.

Naturopathy can also be a complementary treatment to conventional medicine. People getting radiation treatments for cancer, for example, might see a naturopathic physician for advice on nutrition, herbs, and other remedies to help them deal with the treatment better.

There are a lot of naturopathic therapies to choose from, but five are especially important:

➤ **Clinical nutrition.** Naturopaths firmly believe that many medical conditions can be treated with foods and nutritional supplements like vitamins. Nutritional treatment often works just as well as standard medical treatment, without the complications and side effects. And improving your diet overall can help prevent many health problems down the line.

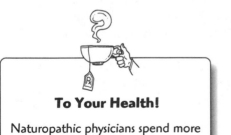

To Your Health!

Naturopathic physicians spend more than 140 hours in the classroom learning about nutrition. The average medical doctor spends less than 20.

➤ **Physical medicine.** Also known as *naturopathic manipulative therapy*, this is a general term for various hands-on treatments, including hydrotherapy, ultrasound, exercise, massage, and so on. We'll talk more about some of the treatments, like hydrotherapy and massage, in other chapters of this book.

➤ **Homeopathic medicine.** Homeopathic remedies are used to strengthen the immune system and treat some symptoms. They're such an important part of naturopathic medicine that we've given them their own chapter—see Chapter 13, "Homeopathy: Let Like Cure Like," for more.

➤ **Herbal medicine.** Also called *botanic medicine*, herbal medicine is another area that's so important we had to give it its own chapter—see Chapter 15, "Traditional Herbal Medicine," for more.

➤ **Counseling and stress management.** A lot of health problems are caused by stress and other negative emotions. Naturopaths are trained to understand how your emotions and mental attitudes affect your health. They're also trained in

ways to help, including biofeedback, hypnotherapy, stress management, and counseling.
(We'll talk more about biofeedback and
hypnotherapy in Chapter 30, "Use Your
Head.")

Depending on your condition, your naturopath
might recommend other treatments, such as
acupuncture or Ayurvedic herbs. Because they
have a good understanding of all the various types
of alternative medicine, they can choose the
treatments most likely to help you.

Learning to Be an N.D.

Today's naturopathic physicians are very well-
trained—if they've graduated from an accredited
naturopathic college. Unfortunately, there are a lot of people out there with bogus
mail-order naturopathic degrees from correspondence schools. These people aren't
really trained at all.

How can you tell who's qualified and who isn't? It's easy: There are only two accredited naturopathic medical colleges in the United States, and only two others that are
on the verge of being accredited. So far, the Council on Naturopathic Medical Education, the accrediting organization, has recognized only two colleges: Bastyr University
in Bothell, Washington, and the National College of Naturopathic Medicine in Portland, Oregon. The Southwest College of Naturopathic Medicine and Health Sciences in
Tempe, Arizona, and The Canadian College of Naturopathic Medicine in Toronto,
Ontario, are awaiting accreditation.

To find out more about becoming a naturopathic
physician, contact:

> **Bastyr University**
> 14500 Juanita Drive, NE
> Bothell, WA 98011
> Phone: (425) 823-1300
> Fax: (425) 823-6222
> E-mail: conted@bastyr.edu
>
> **National College of Naturopathic Medicine**
> 49 SW Porter
> Portland, OR 97201
> Phone: (503) 499-4343
> Fax: (503) 499-0027
> E-mail: communication@ncnm.edu

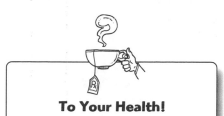

To Your Health!

Naturopathic medicine is safe—so
safe that malpractice suits against
naturopathic physicians are very
rare. In fact, less than 1 percent of
naturopathic physicians have been
sued for malpractice. By contrast,
about one medical doctor in five is
sued each year in the United States.

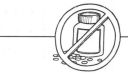

Hazardous to Your Health!

In a lot of states, anyone can claim
to be a naturopathic doctor. Don't
be fooled by a "doctorate" degree
from a mail-order diploma mill. If
you're in doubt about someone's
credentials, check with your state
regulators.

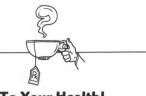

Southwest College of Naturopathic Medicine and Health Sciences
2140 East Broadway, Suite 703
Tempe, AZ 85251
Phone: (602) 858-9100
Fax: (602) 858-9116

The Canadian College of Naturopathic Medicine
2300 Yonge Street, 18th Floor
Toronto, Ontario M4P 1E4
Phone: (416) 486-8584
Fax: (415) 484-6821
E-mail: info@ccnm.edu

To Your Health!

In 1996, the Natural Medicine Clinic in Kent, Washington, became the first tax-supported community health clinic in the country devoted to natural medical treatments. Bastyr University was selected over several Seattle-area hospitals to operate the clinic.

To get into a naturopathic medical college, students have to complete the usual pre-med studies in basic sciences as an undergraduate. After that, the four-year curriculum at the naturopathic school is tough—just as tough as any conventional medical school. That's because basically it *is* the curriculum of a medical school, along with courses in naturopathic subjects like herbal medicine, homeopathy, Oriental medicine, nutrition, and lots more. Naturopathic students spend a lot of time in the classroom and also in clinics getting practical experience. After graduation, new N.D.s get more experience by doing internships in clinics. After all that training, an N.D. is well qualified to do just about anything a medically trained family doctor can do.

Some N.D.s go on for extra training in naturopathic obstetrics. In the states that allow it, they then are qualified to deliver babies by natural childbirth at home or in birth centers.

From A to Z with Your N.D.

Actually, that's from *A* for *acupuncture* to *Y* for *yoga*—we can't think of an alternative therapy that begins with *Z*. Regardless, your naturopathic doctor is your gatekeeper to the world of alternative medicine. He or she knows all about alternative therapies—and standard therapies—that work. If you have a medical problem, your N.D. can point you in the right treatment direction. And even if you're healthy now, your N.D. can do a lot to help you stay that way.

A typical first visit to a naturopathic physician lasts about an hour. That's because naturopaths look carefully at your whole lifestyle to understand your problems and find good treatments. As part of your first visit, you'll have the usual physical exam—the doctor will listen to your heart and lungs, test your reflexes, and probably take blood and urine samples just as any medical doctor would. The difference is that he or she will really *talk* with you about your eating habits, how much exercise you get, your job, your family life, even your spirituality. The goal is to understand and treat the whole person, not just a collection of symptoms.

If you have a particular health problem, your N.D. will take a holistic approach to it. Your treatment will probably include dietary and exercise recommendations, along with herbs and maybe acupuncture, homeopathic remedies, hydrotherapy, or whatever else might help. In states where they're licensed, N.D.s can generally also do minor surgery and X rays and prescribe drugs. Of course, if you really need surgery or a treatment your N.D. can't give you, you'll be referred to a medical doctor.

As your body starts to recover, you may actually find your symptoms getting worse for a day or two. This is what naturopaths call a *healing crisis*, and it's perfectly normal. Your body is just getting itself back into balance. Grin and bear it—in almost all cases, you'll start feeling a lot better once the crisis is over.

The goal of naturopathy is to keep you healthy, not just treat you when you're sick. Your naturopathic physician will spend a lot of time talking to you about healthier ways to handle your nutrition, exercise, stress, and other parts of your lifestyle.

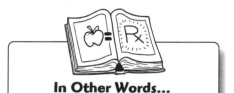

In Other Words...

After a few days of naturopathic treatment, you might feel worse, not better. You're going through a perfectly normal **healing crisis**. A healing crisis usually lasts for only a day or two—after that, you'll probably start to feel much better.

Finding an N.D.

To find a naturopathic physician in your area, contact the *American Association of Naturopathic Physicians* (AANP). Founded in 1986, the AANP is the professional organization that represents licensed N.D.s in the United States. Not every N.D. belongs to the AANP, but most do, so it's a good starting point.

> **American Association of Naturopathic Physicians (AANP)**
> 601 Valley Street, Suite 105
> Seattle, WA 98109
> Phone: (206) 298-0216
> Fax: (206) 298-0129
> E-mail: webmaster@naturopathic.org

Don't hesitate to ask anyone with an N.D. degree about where he or she went to school. If it's not one of the accredited naturopathic schools we discussed earlier, you can't be sure of getting care from someone who is well trained.

Rules, Rules, Rules

Right now, naturopathic physicians are licensed to practice in 11 states: Alaska, Arizona, Connecticut, Hawaii, Maine, Montana, New Hampshire, Oregon, Utah,

Vermont, and Washington. N.D.s are also legally allowed to practice in Idaho and the District of Columbia. In the states with licensing, N.D.s have to pass a tough exam to be allowed to practice. Exactly what they can do varies a bit from state to state. In some states, for instance, N.D.s can prescribe any drugs; in others, they can only prescribe some drugs or can't prescribe at all.

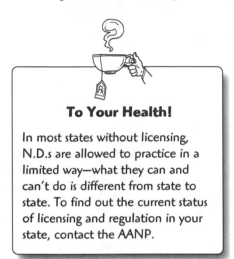

To Your Health!

In most states without licensing, N.D.s are allowed to practice in a limited way—what they can and can't do is different from state to state. To find out the current status of licensing and regulation in your state, contact the AANP.

You don't have to live in a licensing state to see an N.D. Trained N.D.s practice in most states—they just do it under other medical licenses, like licensed acupuncturist or registered dietitian.

Even if you live in a state where naturopaths are licensed, your health insurance might not cover your visits to an N.D. Read the "Definition of Physician" part of your policy. If N.D.s aren't specifically excluded, or if the definition isn't limited to specific providers other than N.D.s, you're probably covered. If your policy covers naturopathic services, just file your claim as you usually do. If your policy doesn't cover naturopaths, or if your insurance company or HMO gives you a hard time, contact the AANP and ask for their helpful brochure, "How to Get Reimbursement for Naturopathic Services."

The good news is that more than 90 insurance companies cover naturopathic medicine in the United States and Canada.

Mail-Order Medicine?

Conventional doctors are very wary of naturopaths. They say naturopaths are too likely to diagnose you with something vague or according to the medical fad of the month. The M.D.s also point out that a lot of naturopathic methods, like homeopathic and herbal remedies, are unproved or untested. On the other hand, a lot of what naturopaths have been saying for years about diet, exercise, and stress management are now part of standard medicine. We think that other naturopathic ideas will find their way into mainstream medicine soon.

What really burns M.D.s are the mail-order N.D.s. They're not the only ones—licensed N.D.s who are graduates of accredited naturopathic colleges don't like the mail-order types either. To help eliminate the problem of unqualified practitioners, the AANP is working closely with state governments to set high standards for licensing.

The Least You Need to Know

➤ The basic principle behind naturopathy is the healing power of nature. Your natural healing mechanisms restore your health.

➤ Naturopathic treatments are gentle, natural, and noninvasive. They're meant to stimulate your own natural healing.

➤ Standard naturopathic treatments include herbs, nutrition, homeopathy, acupuncture, and relaxation techniques. Drugs are rarely used.

➤ Naturopathy is very helpful for people with chronic conditions like arthritis, high blood pressure, asthma, chronic fatigue syndrome, and digestive problems.

➤ Today's naturopathic physicians are very well trained. The courses they take at an accredited naturopathic medical school are a lot like those at a standard medical school.

➤ Many naturopathic ideas, like the importance of diet, exercise, and stress management, are now part of mainstream medicine.

Chapter 5

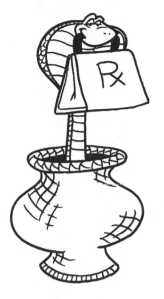

Ayurvedic Medicine: Health from India

In This Chapter

➤ Why the ancient art of Ayurveda is popular today

➤ How your dosha affects your health—and vice versa

➤ Eating right the Ayurvedic way

➤ Ayurvedic herbs for good health

➤ Health problems Ayurveda may help

You know how you keep that old shirt in your closet because you're sure someday it'll be back in style again? That's a lot like today's new interest in Ayurveda, the traditional medicine of India. It began more than five thousand years ago and went strong for millennia. Starting in the 1800s, Ayurveda in India was suppressed by foreign rulers and faded in popularity. Today it's roaring back—not just in India, but everywhere.

Why? Because Ayurveda is a complete system of alternative medicine that is often very helpful for chronic health problems. It takes an all-natural approach that treats the whole person, not just a collection of symptoms or body parts. By stressing diet and prevention, Ayurveda helps you get well and stay that way.

The Ayurvedic Tradition

Ayurveda is the ancient Indian art of holistic healing. The emphasis in Ayurveda is on health and longevity through prevention. In the Ayurvedic tradition, health problems are helped by finding the underlying cause of the ailment and removing it. And according to Ayurvedic thinking, the underlying cause of almost all health problems is an imbalance in your system.

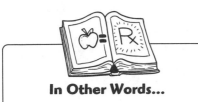

In Other Words...

Ayurveda is a Sanskrit word meaning "longevity knowledge." In practical terms, Ayurveda is a traditional medical system from India based on disease prevention through balance and harmony. Sanskrit is the ancient language of India and Hinduism; now it is used only for sacred and scholarly writings.

To solve your health problem, then, you need to restore that balance—generally by changing your diet and your daily activities to bring them back into line.

One reason Ayurvedic medicine is getting more popular is that it combines modern medical treatment with ancient holistic ideas. If you have diabetes, for instance, an Ayurvedic doctor would use standard tests to diagnose it and standard medication to treat it—but he or she would also put much more emphasis on diet and lifestyle changes to help you manage the disease by restoring the proper balance. And restoring your balance could help you need fewer drugs.

In general, Ayurveda can be really helpful for people with chronic illnesses. That's because Ayruveda takes a holistic approach that combines medical treatment with diet and lifestyle changes to help you handle your disease as well as possible.

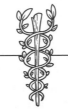

The Healing Arts

Ayurveda, the traditional medical system of India, can be traced back more than five thousand years. The earliest written references come from **vedas**, or Sanskrit holy writings, that date to about 1500 B.C. Ayurveda isn't a religion, though—people of all faiths benefit from its many centuries of collected wisdom. Ayurveda first came to the West back in the psychedelic '60s, when the **yogi** (wise teacher) Maharishi Mahesh brought transcendental meditation and other wisdom from India to America. In recent years, Ayurveda got a giant boost from the very popular inspirational writings of Dr. Deepak Chopra, a physician who combines Western medicine with Ayurvedic thinking.

The basic concepts of Ayurvedic medicine may seem a little complex and weird-sounding at first. Once you understand the ideas, though, they make a lot of sense.

The Doshas

The crucial first step in restoring balance is understanding your personal constitution. Once you know your body type according to Ayurvedic principles, you'll understand what you need to do to restore your balance and health.

The three *doshas* are the heart of Ayurvedic healing, so we'll start by explaining what they are and why they matter so much.

The word *dosha* is often translated as "vital energy" or "governing principle." Westerners often find it easier to think of dosha as meaning "metabolic body type." Your dosha is much more than just your body type, though—it's the physical, mental, and emotional characteristics that make up your individual Ayurvedic constitution.

In Ayurvedic thinking, there are three basic body types, or doshas. Everybody has some characteristics of each dosha, but in varying proportions. Most people are a mixture of doshas, with one main dosha and one secondary dosha. It's rare for someone to be exclusively one dosha or to have all three.

Let's look at the three basic doshas:

> **Vata** is cold, dry, light, and mobile. *Vata* people tend to be slim, with prominent features and dry skin. They're imaginative, energetic, active, and changeable, with a tendency toward moodiness. They also tend to have ups and downs of energy over the day. Stress affects their nervous system. Vata people tend toward insomnia and anxiety. They also tend toward arthritis and lung problems, such as pneumonia.

> **Pitta** is warm, oily, and intense. The basic *pitta* person is medium—medium height, medium build, medium weight. Pitta people lead regular lives, sleeping a solid eight hours every night and eating three square meals a

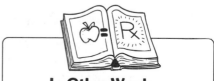

Hazardous to Your Health!

Ayurvedic treatment isn't always a good substitute for standard medical treatment, especially in a medical emergency or where surgery is needed. If you have a serious health problem, talk to your doctor before you try Ayurvedic herbs or other treatments. Never stop taking your medicine without talking to your doctor first!

In Other Words...

The three basic doshas are **vata**, **pitta**, and **kapha**. Each dosha has a separate function in your system. The vata dosha controls your movement, the pitta dosha controls your metabolism, and the kapha dosha controls your structure. Being alive requires all three doshas.

43

day. They tend to be fair-skinned, with blond or reddish hair. Pittas are often competitive types with sharp tempers. They're alert and intelligent. When they get sick, they tend to get stomach ailments, sore throats, and skin rashes.

➤ **Kapha** is cool, damp, and slow. *Kapha* people have heavy, solid bodies and a tendency to put on weight. Kaphas are often warm and thirsty. They're relaxed and slow to anger, but they also tend to procrastinate. Kaphas sleep heavily. They're more likely to get the flu, sinus problems, high cholesterol, and high blood pressure.

Everybody's got a different balance of doshas. Knowing your dosha type helps you understand your basic constitution.

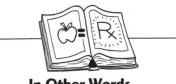

In Other Words...

Your **prakruti** is your natural dosha or combination of doshas—your inborn, natural constitution. Put more philosophically, your prakruti is your essential nature. Your **vikruti** is your daily constitution.

Constitutional Issues

Once you've figured out your mix of doshas, you've discovered your *prakruti*—your natural constitution, the one you were born with. Everyone is a unique mix of vata, pitta, and kapha—that's why everybody is different and has a different prakruti. That's also why you might catch a lot of colds but hardly ever get a stomach bug, while someone else has a delicate digestion but never so much as a sniffle.

Your prakruti basically stays the same throughout your life. But ordinary daily living constantly affects your prakruti, changing the balance. Your daily constitution is called your *vikruti*.

What's Your Dosha?

So which dosha are you? Take the quiz in Table 5.1 and add up your scores. You'll probably find that you're mostly one dosha, with some strong characteristics of a second dosha as well. You might decide you're a pitta-vata type, for example, or that you're mostly vata with some pitta as well. Remember, no one dosha or dosha combination is better than another.

Here's how to answer the quiz questions. Answer the questions as honestly as you can and be open to the results. First answer the questions according to how you ordinarily feel over the long run—this is your prakruti. Then do the questions again according to how you've been feeling for the past month or so—this is your vikruti. For some extra insight, you might also want to ask a friend to fill out the chart for you.

Table 5.1 What's Your Dosha?

Observations	V	P	K	Vata	Pitta	Kapha
Body size	❑	❑	❑	slim	medium	large
Body weight	❑	❑	❑	low	medium	overweight
Skin	❑	❑	❑	thin, dry, cold, rough, dark	smooth, oily, warm, rosy	thick, oily, cool, white, pale
Hair	❑	❑	❑	dry, brown, black, knotted, brittle, scarce	straight, oily, blond, gray, red, bald	thick, curly, oily, wavy, luxuriant
Teeth	❑	❑	❑	stick out, roomy, thin gums	medium, soft, tender gums	healthy, white, strong gums
Nose	❑	❑	❑	uneven shape, deviated septum	long, pointed, red at tip	short, rounded, button nose
Eyes	❑	❑	❑	small, sunken, dry, active, black, brown, nervous	sharp, bright, gray, green, yellow/red, sensitive to light	big, beautiful, blue, calm, loving
Nails	❑	❑	❑	dry, rough, brittle, break easily	sharp, flexible, pink, lustrous	thick, oily, smooth, polished
Lips	❑	❑	❑	dry, cracked, black/brown tinge	red, inflamed, yellowish	smooth, oily, pale, whitish
Chin	❑	❑	❑	thin, angular	tapering	rounded, double
Cheeks	❑	❑	❑	wrinkled, sunken	smooth, flat	rounded, plump
Neck	❑	❑	❑	thin, tall	medium	big, folded
Chest	❑	❑	❑	flat, sunken	moderate	expanded, round
Belly	❑	❑	❑	thin, flat, sunken	moderate	big, pot-bellied
Bellybutton	❑	❑	❑	small, irregular, herniated	oval, superficial	big, deep, rounded, stretched
Hips	❑	❑	❑	slender, thin	moderate	heavy, big
Joints	❑	❑	❑	cold, cracking	moderate	large, lubricated

continues

Table 5.1   What's Your Dosha?   (continued)

Observations	V	P	K	Vata	Pitta	Kapha
Appetite	❏	❏	❏	irregular, scanty	strong, unbearable	slow but steady
Digestion	❏	❏	❏	irregular, forms gas	quick, causes burning	prolonged, forms mucous
Taste	❏	❏	❏	sweet, sour, salty	sweet, bitter, astringent	bitter, pungent, astringent
Thirst	❏	❏	❏	changeable	surplus	sparse
Elimination	❏	❏	❏	constipation	loose	thick, oily, sluggish
Physical activity	❏	❏	❏	hyperactive	moderate	slow
Mental activity	❏	❏	❏	hyperactive	moderate	dull, slow
Emotions	❏	❏	❏	anxiety, fear, uncertainty	anger, hate, jealousy	calm, greedy, attachment
Faith	❏	❏	❏	variable	extremist	consistent
Intellect	❏	❏	❏	quick but faulty response	accurate response	slow, exact
Recollection	❏	❏	❏	recent good, remote poor	distinct	slow and sustained
Dreams	❏	❏	❏	quick, active, many, fearful	fiery, war, violence	lakes, snow, romantic
Sleep	❏	❏	❏	scanty, broken up, sleeplessness	little but sound	deep, prolonged
Speech	❏	❏	❏	rapid, unclear	sharp, penetrating	slow, monotonous
Financial	❏	❏	❏	poor, spends on trifles	spends money on luxuries	rich, good money preserver

Source: Reprinted with permission from Ayurvedic Cooking for Self-Healing, *by Usha and Dr. Vasant Lad (Albuquerque, NM: The Ayurvedic Press, 1994).*

Add up your quiz scores. How many Ps do you have? How many Ks? How many Vs? If one dosha is much higher than the others, you are a single-dosha type. If your scores for two doshas are roughly equal, you are a two-dosha type. The dosha with the higher score is more dominant. The dosha with the highest score is also the one that probably needs balancing.

If your prakruti and vikruti answers are different, your doshas could be out of balance. For example, if your vikruti shows more pitta than your prakruti, you might need to follow a pitta-calming diet (we'll get into that a little further on).

Other Aspects of Dosha

Dosha is much more than your physical body. Each dosha has a *seat* in the body—an organ that copes with small changes in the dosha. Depending on the dosha, different foods can have an aggravating (increasing) or pacifying (decreasing) effect. Each dosha is also affected by the season and even the time of day. Your dosha even changes as you get older. Check out Table 5.2 for a breakdown of what affects which dosha.

Table 5.2   You and Your Dosha

Vata Characteristics	
Seat	Colon
Season	Autumn, early winter
Time of day	Early morning best; late afternoon good
Aggravating tastes	Pungent, bitter foods; avoid raw foods
Pacifying tastes	Sweet, sour, salty foods; choose cooked foods and root vegetables
Pitta Characteristics	
Seat	Stomach
Season	Summer
Time of day	Noon best; middle of the night good
Aggravating tastes	Sour, salty, pungent foods; avoid red meat
Pacifying tastes	Sweet, bitter, astringent foods; choose salads, fish, chicken, mushrooms
Kapha Characteristics	
Seat	Lungs
Season	Mid-winter
Time of day	Late evening best; mid-morning good
Aggravating tastes	Sweet, sour, salty; avoid dairy products
Pacifying tastes	Bitter, pungent, hot and spicy; choose beans, lentils, leafy vegetables, apples

For optimal health, you need to understand your prakruti and live a lifestyle that's in harmony with it. If you don't, your doshas get aggravated or excited, your prakruti gets out of balance, and health problems start up.

What makes your doshas get imbalanced? A big difference between your prakruti and your vikruti. Small, natural imbalances happen all the time—when the seasons change, for example, and even over the course of a day. If you're in good health, you can handle the imbalances easily. If you've been eating the wrong foods or living the wrong lifestyle for your dosha, you won't handle the imbalances well at all. In fact, your diet and lifestyle could be causing serious imbalances. Other major causes of imbalances include trauma (like being in a car crash), stress, illness, and surgery.

Getting your doshas back into balance—*pacifying them*, as an Ayurvedic practitioner would say—helps you get well again. As we'll discuss in the rest of this chapter, how you do that will depend on your prakruti. What works well for one dosha type may not work for another. Use Table 5.3 just as a general guideline.

Table 5.3   Balancing the Doshas

Vata	Pitta	Kapha
Keep warm.	Avoid excessive heat.	Get plenty of exercise.
Keep calm.	Avoid excessive oil.	Avoid heavy foods.
Avoid raw foods.	Avoid excessive steam.	Keep active.
Avoid cold foods.	Limit salt intake.	Avoid dairy.
Eat warm foods.	Eat cooling, nonspicy foods.	Avoid iced foods.
Keep a regular routine.	Exercise during the cooler part of the day.	Avoid fatty, oily foods.
		Eat light, dry foods.

Source: Dr. Vasant Lad, Ayruvedic Institute.

The Healing Elements

What exactly happens when your doshas get out of balance? The answer is a little complicated and involves even more Sanskrit, so stick with us as we explain it.

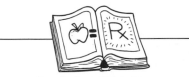

In Other Words...

Prana in Sanskrit means "life energy" or "life force." Prana enters your body through your food and through your breathing.

Agni is not just your digestive ability but also the way you absorb other things, like air or experiences.

Ama means waste or impurity.

If your doshas get out of balance, the *prana*, or life energy, in your body doesn't flow smoothly. And when your prana isn't flowing, your *agni*, or digestive ability, is disrupted. Blocked agni means that *ama*, or body waste, builds up in your system. An excess of ama leads to illness by blocking your channels of digestion and energy. Think of yourself as a flowing stream (prana) blocked by a pile of debris (ama). Instead of flowing, the water (agni) backs up into a stagnant pool. Remove the debris, and the stagnant water is carried away as the flow of clear water is restored.

How do you get rid of all that ama and get your doshas back into balance? Since in Ayurvedic thinking most imbalances are caused by your diet and lifestyle, changing them will do a lot to restore the balance. The two most important approaches are changing your diet and using herbal remedies.

Just a Taste

In Ayurvedic thinking, there's no one diet that works for everyone. Instead, you need to select the foods that are best for your particular prakruti. If you're in good health, you want to eat foods that will help keep you that way. If your doshas are out of balance, you need to choose foods that will stabilize them.

Which foods? This gets a little complicated. In Ayurveda, foods have six tastes—and each dosha does best with a particular combination.

Let's start with the six tastes:

➤ **Sweet.** Sugar and honey, and also water, milk, butter, grains, pasta, and most fruits.

➤ **Sour.** Citrus fruits, sour-tasting fruits, and fermented foods like yogurt and cheese.

➤ **Salty.** Salt and watery vegetables such as zucchini, tomatoes, and cucumbers.

➤ **Pungent.** Spicy foods in general are in the pungent category, especially if they use garlic, ginger, pepper, or cumin.

➤ **Bitter.** Dark, leafy greens such as spinach and dark lettuces.

➤ **Astringent.** Various herbal teas, beans, lentils, potatoes, and apples.

Each dosha has its natural tastes. In other words, if you're strongly pitta, you'll naturally prefer to eat sour foods. Each dosha also has its naturally beneficial tastes. For pitta people, bitter is very helpful. Table 5.4 sorts it all out.

Table 5.4   The Taste of Your Dosha

Dosha	Natural Tastes	Beneficial Tastes
Vata	bitter	salty
	astringent	sour
	pungent	sweet
Pitta	sour	bitter
	salty	astringent
	pungent	sweet
Kapha	sweet	pungent
	salty	bitter
	sour	astringent

Depending on your prakruti, the different food tastes will have different effects on you, as shown in Table 5.5.

Table 5.5   The Effects of Taste

Taste	Increases	Decreases
Sweet	kapha	vata, pitta
Sour	kapha, pitta	vata
Salty	kapha, pitta	vata
Pungent	pitta, vata	· kapha
Bitter	vata	pitta, kapha
Astringent	vata	pitta, kapha

Got all that? Now let's look at two other important aspects of your food: heating and cooling.

➤ Heating foods are pungent, sour, or salty. Pungent foods have the most heating power.

➤ Cooling foods are bitter, sweet, or astringent. Bitter foods have the most cooling power.

A basic principle of Ayurveda is that like increases like, while unlike (the opposite) decreases like. In other words, if you are a strong vata dosha and eat a lot of vata foods, you increase your vata. But increasing your vata too much could really aggravate it and knock your doshas completely out of balance. Instead, a vata person may need to eat a lot of pitta or kapha foods to pacify the doshas and get them balanced again. The goal is always to achieve calm, happy, and balanced doshas.

The Ayurvedic dietary system makes a lot of sense, but it's too complicated to go into in depth here—you'll need to work with your Ayurvedic practitioner. In general, you can use Table 5.6 to find basic dietary guidelines for your dosha.

Table 5.6   Your Ayurvedic Diet

Dosha	Eat	Avoid
Vata	warm foods	cold foods
	warm drinks	cold drinks
	oily foods	dry foods
	sweet foods	pungent foods
	sour foods	bitter foods
	salty foods	astringent foods
Pitta	cool foods	pungent foods
	cool drinks	sour foods
	sweet foods	
	bitter foods	
	astringent foods	

Dosha	Eat	Avoid
Kapha	warm foods	cold foods
	warm drinks	cold drinks
	pungent foods	oily foods
	bitter foods	sweet foods
	astringent foods	sour foods
		salty foods

In Ayurveda, the tastes and effects of foods are determined according to a complex system that takes into account each food's shape, size, color, taste, smell, and texture. Again, it's way too complex to go into in detail here. Instead, check Table 5.7 for foods that are good or bad for your dosha. If you're a vata type and you hate Brussels sprouts, you're in luck! At last you have a great reason not to eat them.

Foods that aren't specifically good or bad can be eaten, but only in moderation. Animal foods are listed in the table, but you don't have to eat them. In fact, as millions of people in India prove every day, you can be perfectly healthy and never eat any animal foods at all.

Table 5.7 Eating for Your Dosha

Vata Types

Vegetables to Eat	Vegetables to Avoid
asparagus	beans
carrots	bell peppers
green beans	Brussels sprouts
sweet potatoes	cabbage
tofu (bean curd)	cauliflower
winter squash	celery
zucchini	eggplant
	lentils
	mushrooms
	peas
	potatoes
	tomatoes
	turnips

continues

Table 5.7   Eating for Your Dosha   (continued)

Vata Types

Fruits to Eat	Fruits to Avoid
apricots	prunes
bananas	watermelon
berries	
cherries	
citrus	
mango	
melons	
pineapple	
plums	

Grains to Eat	Grains to Avoid
rice	buckwheat
wheat berries	corn
	millet
	oats
	rye

Animal Foods to Eat	Animal Foods to Avoid
buttermilk	cheese
cottage cheese	goat's milk
eggs	ice cream
fish	pork
milk	sour cream
shellfish	
yogurt	

Pitta Types

Vegetables to Eat	Vegetables to Avoid
asparagus	beets
beans	eggplant
bell peppers	hot peppers
broccoli	onions
Brussels sprouts	radishes
cabbage	Swiss chard

Vegetables to Eat	Vegetables to Avoid
cauliflower	tomatoes
cucumber	turnips
green beans	
kale	
lentils	
lettuce	
mushrooms	
okra	
peas	
potatoes	
winter squash	

Fruits to Eat	Fruits to Avoid
apples	bananas
apricots	grapefruit
berries	papaya
grapes	peaches
mangos	persimmon
melons	
oranges	
pears	
pineapple	
plums	
raisins	
watermelon	

Grains to Eat	Grains to Avoid
barley	buckwheat
oats	corn
rice	millet
wheat	rye

Animal Foods to Eat	Animal Foods to Avoid
butter (sweet)	cheese
chicken	eggs
cottage cheese	goat's milk
fish	ice cream

continues

53

Table 5.7 Eating for Your Dosha (continued)

Animal Foods to Eat	Animal Foods to Avoid
milk	red meat
	shellfish
	yogurt

Kapha Types

Vegetables to Eat	Vegetables to Avoid
asparagus	avocados
beans (except kidney and soy)	cucumbers
beets	pumpkin
bell (sweet) pepper	sweet potatoes
broccoli	tomatoes
Brussels sprouts	winter squash
cabbage	
carrots	
cauliflower	
celery	
eggplant	
green beans	
kale	
leeks	
lentils (red only)	
lettuce	
mushrooms	
okra	
onions	
peas	
spinach	
split peas	
turnips	

Fruits to Eat	Fruits to Avoid
apples	bananas
apricots	cranberries
berries	grapefruit
cherries	melons

Fruits to Eat	Fruits to Avoid
peaches	pineapple
pears	plums
pomegranates	watermelon
raisins	

Grains to Eat	Grains to Avoid
barley	oats
buckwheat	rice
corn	wheat
millet	
rye	

Animal Foods to Eat	Animal Foods to Avoid
chicken	eat dairy foods as little as possible
goat's milk	butter
turkey	buttermilk
	cheese
	fish
	ice cream
	milk
	red meat
	seafood
	sour cream
	yogurt

The cooking of India is healthful, varied, and delicious—and you can do it easily using ingredients found in the supermarket. There are lots of good Indian cookbooks at any bookstore. One we like is *Classic Indian Vegetarian and Grain Cooking*, by Julie Sahni (Morrow, 1985). An excellent guide to Ayurvedic eating is *A Life of Balance*, by Maya Tiwari (Healing Arts Press, 1995). In addition to detailed charts of the right foods for your dosha, it has great recipes. Another excellent guide is *Ayruvedic Cooking for Self-Healing*, by Usha and Dr. Vasant Lad (Ayurvedic Press, 1994).

Spicing Up Your Life

In Ayurvedic thinking, herbs and spices are used to flavor foods and make teas taste delicious, but that's not their main purpose. Instead, they're meant to balance your doshas, give you energy, and strengthen your immune system. Good taste is the bonus you get along with good health.

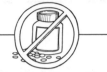

Hazardous to Your Health!

Kapha people should avoid dairy foods—but milk and other dairy foods are an important source of calcium, which you need to keep your bones strong throughout your life. If you skip the dairy foods, talk to your doctor about taking a calcium supplement.

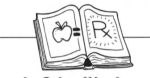

In Other Words...

Triphala means "three fruits" in Sanskrit. It's a popular Ayurvedic herbal remedy made from the dried, powdered fruits of three different Indian herbs.

As with foods, Ayurvedic herbs and spices can be sweet, sour, astringent, and so on. Different herbs have different effects on your dosha:

➤ **To calm vata.** Basil, cardamom, cinnamon, coriander, cumin, fennel, ginger, oregano, sage, tarragon, thyme.

➤ **To cool pitta.** Cardamom, chamomile, cilantro, cinnamon, coriander, cumin, fennel, ginger, mint, nutmeg, turmeric.

➤ **To stimulate kapha.** Black pepper, cardamom, cayenne, cilantro, cinnamon, cloves, coriander, cumin, garlic, ginger, mustard.

Several different Ayurvedic herbal mixes are used as general tonics to help keep you healthy. The most common and popular is one called *triphala*. This is actually a mixture of three different Indian fruits that have been dried and powdered. Triphala is good for balancing the doshas and treating minor ailments, like a slight cold or a mild stomach flu. Most people mix half a teaspoon or so into some warm water and have it at night before going to bed and again in the morning when they get up. The usual daily dose works out to about 1,000 mg. If you prefer, you can get it in capsules. In large doses, triphala acts as a mild laxative.

Each of the three fruits in triphala is important in Ayurveda:

➤ **Amalaka** (*Emblica officinalis*) rejuvenates and is a good source of vitamin C. It's good for the blood, bones, liver, and heart.

➤ **Bibitaki** (*Terminalia belerica*) removes toxins. It's good for the lungs, throat, voice, eyes, and hair. It's also good for the digestive and urinary tracts.

➤ **Haritaki** (*Terminalia chebula*) is said to increase mental awareness.

Some other standard Ayurvedic herbs or herbal mixtures are helpful for other conditions or as general tonics:

➤ **Abana** is a mixture of herbs and minerals that is often prescribed for heart problems, especially angina. Discuss abana with your doctor before you try it.

➤ **Ashwaganda** (*Withania somnifera*) is used as an overall male tonic that enhances stamina. It's often combined with licorice and turmeric. The usual dose is 1,000 mg a day.

➤ **Gasex**, a combination of several herbs, is helpful for nausea, gas, heartburn, and motion sickness. Chewing a few tablets relieves the discomfort. A tea made from the bark and leaves of the *neem tree* can also be helpful.

➤ **Gotu kola** or **brahmi** (*Hydrocoytle asiatica*) improves brain function, memory, concentration, and mental alertness.

➤ **Gugulipid** or **Indian bdellium**, made from the resin of the *Commiphora mukal* tree, helps lower high cholesterol. Some studies suggest that it works as well as standard drugs, without the side effects. Discuss gugulipid with your doctor before you try it.

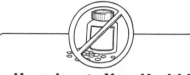

Hazardous to Your Health!

If you want to try an Ayurvedic herb or herbal mixture to help a serious health problem such as heart disease or high cholesterol, discuss it with your doctor first, especially if you are already taking prescription drugs. Do not stop taking your medicine on your own!

➤ **Shatavari** (*Asparagus racemosus*) is used as an overall female tonic. It's often helpful for premenstrual syndrome (PMS) and menstrual cramps. It's often combined with licorice and turmeric. The usual dose is 1,000 mg a day.

➤ **Turmeric** (*Curcuma longa*), also sometimes called **curcumin**, is a bright-yellow powder that's helpful for a wide range of ailments, especially if there's swelling and redness (inflammation). It's often used to treat arthritis and may help lower your cholesterol. It's helpful for digestive ailments such as gas, colic, and liver and gall bladder problems. The usual dose is 1,000 mg a day, usually in capsule form.

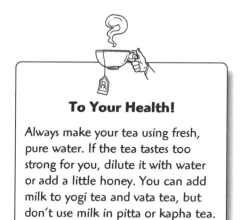

To Your Health!

Always make your tea using fresh, pure water. If the tea tastes too strong for you, dilute it with water or add a little honey. You can add milk to yogi tea and vata tea, but don't use milk in pitta or kapha tea.

➤ **Boswellia**, made from the *Boswellia serrata* tree, is used as an anti-inflammatory to help arthritis and muscle pain. It's sold in tablets or as a cream that's rubbed into the painful part.

You'll probably find other Ayuvedic herbal blends on the shelves at your health-food store. They're usually promoted as helping a particular body organ or health problem; a mixture might be said to help the liver or be good for people under stress. Unfortunately, you can't always tell exactly what's in these mixtures—avoid them.

Hazardous to Your Health!

Be extremely cautious with all herbal remedies. If you take any medications or are being treated for a specific medical problem, talk to your doctor before you try any herbs. Always start with small doses, and stop taking the remedy if you have any sort of bad reaction, such as nausea, vomiting, diarrhea, a rash, hives, or a headache.

Can't find an Ayurvedic herbal remedy or tea mixture at your local drugstore? Not even at your health-food store? You may need to get it from a mail-order source. Catalogs of Ayurvedic products are available from:

Infinite Possibilities
60 Union Avenue
Sudbury, MA 01776
(800) 858-1808

Ayurvedic Institute
11311 Menaul NE, Suite A
Albuquerque, NM 87112
(505) 291-9698

Ayurvedic medicine often uses herbal teas. Many practitioners recommend drinking these mixtures on a regular basis to promote good health. You can buy premixed tea bags, or you can make your own blends, as explained in the following recipes. All doshas benefit from yogi tea, a sort of all-purpose herbal blend. Vata types might benefit from a vata-soothing tea, while pitta types might need a calming, cooling blend. Kapha types often benefit from spicy, invigorating blends.

Ayurvedic Herbal Teas

Yogi Tea

4 cups water	1 cinnamon stick
2 tsp. freshly grated ginger	8 cloves
6 cardamom pods	

Combine ingredients in saucepan and bring to boil. Lower heat and simmer 20 minutes. Strain before drinking.

Vata-Calming Tea

4 cups water	10 cardamom pods
2 tsp. freshly grated ginger	2 cinnamon sticks

Combine ingredients in saucepan and bring to boil. Lower heat and simmer 10 minutes. Turn off heat and steep 10 minutes. Strain before drinking.

Pitta-Stabilizing Tea

4 cups water	2 tsp. dried peppermint or spearmint leaves
2 tsp. freshly grated ginger	2 cinnamon sticks
10 cardamom pods	$1/4$ tsp. fennel seeds

Combine ingredients in saucepan and bring to boil. Lower heat and simmer five minutes. Turn off heat and steep five minutes. Strain before drinking.

Kapha-Stimulating Tea

4 cups water	$1/2$ tsp. black peppercorns
10 cardamom pods	1 Tbsp. freshly grated ginger
10 whole cloves	

Bring water to boil in saucepan. Remove from heat and add remaining ingredients. Steep for 10 minutes. Strain before drinking.

Other Ayurvedic Remedies

Ayurvedic treatment goes beyond diet and herbs. Breathing exercises and yoga exercises are standard parts of Ayurvedic treatment (see Chapter 28, "Yoga: Exercise Your Body—and Your Mind"). In Ayurvedic theory, all your senses affect your dosha and should be used in healing. *Five-senses healing*, as this approach is called, uses herbs, spices, and foods along with aromatherapy, color therapy, massage, and music as important elements of treatment. In addition, your Ayurvedic doctor may suggest cleansing treatments such as enemas.

Conditions Ayurvedic Medicine May Help

Ayurveda helps lots of health problems. It's often very helpful for ailments that are chronic or stress-related, such as these:

➤ Digestive problems, especially bowel problems.

➤ Arthritis—Ayurveda often helps improve mobility and reduce pain and swelling.

➤ Skin problems such as psoriasis, eczema, and rashes.

➤ Anxiety and insomnia.

➤ Wound healing—Ayurveda may help you recover faster from surgery.

➤ Liver problems, especially hepatitis.

➤ Chronic fatigue syndrome—Ayurveda is often very helpful for this frustrating disease.

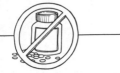

Some diabetics say that Ayurvedic treatment helps them reduce the amount of insulin they need. Ayurvedic treatment may also help patients better tolerate chemotherapy or radiation treatment for cancer. Women who have PMS often find that Ayurveda helps relieve their symptoms.

Finding a Qualified Practitioner

If you lived in India or Sri Lanka, you'd have no trouble finding a well-trained Ayurvedic doctor—there are more than a hundred Ayurvedic medical schools in India, more than 300,000 Ayurvedic doctors, and many Ayurvedic hospitals. Students study for at least five years and earn either a BAMS (Bachelor of Ayurvedic Medicine and Surgery) or DAMS (Doctor of Ayurvedic Medicine and Surgery). Unfortunately, these degrees aren't recognized in the United States. In fact, Ayurveda isn't even recognized as a therapy here, and there are no licensing boards or certification procedures. It's also unlikely that your insurance will cover Ayurvedic treatment unless it's given by a licensed physician—and even then, you may not be covered.

Many medical doctors who trained in India and then moved to the United States are knowledgeable about Ayurveda. They combine standard medical treatment with Ayurvedic treatment, taking the best of both approaches. A lot of American-trained doctors have started to take an interest in Ayurveda and have taken courses in the basics.

How can you find one of these experts? Check out the referral services from these leading training centers:

> **Ayurvedic Institute**
> 11311 Menaul NE, Suite A
> Albuquerque, NM 87112
> (505) 291-9698
>
> **Chopra Center for Well-Being**
> 7630 Fay Avenue
> La Jolla, CA 92037
> (888) 4-CHOPRA
>
> **Educational Service of Maharishi Ayurved International**
> P.O. Box 49667
> Colorado Springs, CO 80949
> (800) 843-8332

Going to the Ayurvedic Doctor

Your first visit to an Ayurvedic doctor will probably be totally unlike any doctor's visit you've ever had. The biggest difference is how much time the doctor spends with you. He or she has to understand your dosha and prakruti thoroughly, and that could take up to an hour of asking you detailed questions about your health and lifestyle and giving you a physical exam. Later visits usually take about 20 to 30 minutes.

As part of the physical exam, an Ayurvedic doctor will do all the standard things—like ask for a urine sample, take blood, and listen to your heart with a stethoscope—that a regular medical doctor would do. Things start to get a little different when the Ayurvedic doctor takes your pulse. In Ayurvedic theory, you have three different kinds of pulses, based on the doshas, that can be felt on each side of your wrist—a total of 12 pulses in all. An Ayurvedic doctor uses the different pulses to help diagnose problems.

Things start to get really different when the Ayurvedic doctor asks you to stick out your tongue. By looking at your tongue, he or she can tell if your doshas are out of whack and, if so, which organs are to blame. If your tongue is whitish, for instance, it could mean that your kapha is disturbed. If the whitish area is toward the central back part of your tongue, the problem could lie in your intestines.

Your Ayruvedic doctor will also look carefully at your skin, lips, nails, and eyes and will probably also feel your abdomen and listen to your intestines with a stethoscope.

The goal is always to understand your dosha, find the imbalance, and get you back into balance. For a minor problem, that could take just a couple of visits a week or so apart. For more serious problems, you might need to return once a week for several months.

A Dosha Reality?

If they stopped to think about it, most Western doctors would agree with the Ayurvedic idea that a lot of disease is caused by bad diet and a lousy lifestyle. Western doctors have a lot of trouble with the dosha concept, though, and think the whole business is way too vague to be meaningful. They also point out that some Ayurvedic remedies contain potentially harmful herbs or small amounts of dangerous substances such as mercury. Some Ayurvedic practitioners do make pretty wild claims for longevity, saying that people in India have used Ayurveda to reach the age of 200! Then there's the motives of Ayurveda popularizers like Maharishi Mahesh and Deepak Chopra. Opponents note that there's plenty of money to be made selling Ayurvedic training classes and remedies. (It's true that Deepak Chopra's books have been mega best-sellers, but as writers, we think that's great!) Even so, today a lot of doctors are cautiously starting to include Ayurvedic ideas in their treatments. Some Ayurvedic treatments are now being scientifically investigated to see if they really work. Stay tuned—Western doctors could be in for some big surprises.

The Least You Need to Know

➤ Ayurvedic medicine is a holistic approach to health from India. It's based on five thousand years of experience and tradition.

➤ Your dosha—your physical, mental, and emotional makeup—plays a major role in your health.

➤ Imbalances in your dosha are the root cause of poor health.

➤ Diet, herbs, and other treatments help balance your dosha and return you to good health.

➤ Ayurvedic treatment can be very helpful for people with chronic health problems, such as arthritis, digestive problems, chronic fatigue syndrome, skin problems, anxiety, and insomnia.

Chapter 6

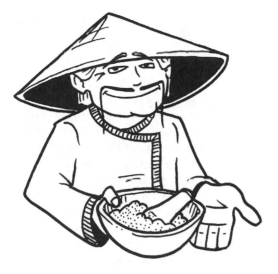

Traditional Chinese Medicine

In This Chapter

➤ Energy flows and your health

➤ The basics of traditional Chinese medicine

➤ Understanding health problems the traditional Chinese way

➤ Conditions traditional Chinese medicine may help

➤ The Chinese way to eat right for health

➤ Traditional Chinese medicine and today's healthcare

The roots of traditional Chinese medicine trace all the way back to the legendary Yellow Emperor, a powerful ruler who lived nearly five thousand years ago. More than two thousand years ago, his ideas were written down in *The Yellow Emperor's Classic of Internal Medicine*—a book that is still central to Chinese medicine. We've learned a lot since then, of course, but the Yellow Emperor's basic ideas still apply. Prevention, harmony, and balance have always been the foundation of Chinese medicine.

Today traditional Chinese medicine is still widely used in China—there are more than two thousand hospitals that use mostly traditional methods. And even in "modern" Chinese hospitals, traditional methods are used right alongside the latest medical technology. Doctors trained in traditional medicine and doctors trained in Western medicine often cooperate to give their patients the best of both approaches.

Can one billion Chinese people be wrong? Not in this case. The traditional medicine of China has a lot to offer the world.

The Medicine of the Mysterious East

The thinking behind *traditional Chinese medicine* (TCM) is different—way, way, different—from the sort of thinking you're used to. In Western medicine, you're seen as a machine made up of different body parts that can break down and need repair. In TCM, you're seen as an integrated web of systems that can get out of balance and need to be restored. In Western medicine, doctors use drugs and surgery to repair problems; in TCM, herbs, diet, and acupuncture are used to rebalance your system. (In fact, acupuncture—painlessly inserting very thin needles into special points along your body—and herbs are so important to TCM that we give them their own chapters later on in this book.) Just as important, in TCM every case is different, even when the symptoms seem the same, because everyone's internal balance is different.

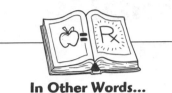

In Other Words...

Traditional Chinese medicine (TCM) is the system of medicine that has been used in China and other parts of Asia, including Japan and Korea, for thousands of years. It's also sometimes called **Oriental medicine**.

The two approaches are so fundamentally different that we're going to have to do a lot of explaining in this chapter. Many of the concepts may seem illogical, unscientific, or more like philosophy or mysticism than medicine. Stick with us. The basics are important, but don't worry if you don't get them right away. Even if you don't really grasp why in TCM your ears are connected to your kidneys, your *Oriental medicine practitioner* (OMP) does and knows what to recommend.

Yin, Yang, and You

The idea of balance is the basic idea behind all traditional Chinese medicine—and Chinese thinking in general. The Chinese use the concept of *Yin* and *Yang* as a fundamental way of looking at all things, including your body and your health.

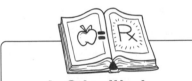

In Other Words...

An **Oriental medicine practicioner (OMP)** is a healthcare professional trained in traditional Chinese medicine. In the United States, most OMPs are licensed acupuncturists.

Everything in the world contains aspects of both Yin and Yang—the two are necessary and inseparable. To get a better grasp on the concept, imagine a beautiful hill in the countryside. On the sunny south-facing side, it's covered with heat-loving plants that do well in dry weather; on the shady north-facing side, it's covered with cool-loving plants that do well in rainy weather. The hill is like Yin and Yang. The sides are different but equal—neither one is better or worse. To have the shady side, you have to have the sunny side, and vice versa. The two sides exist in harmony with each other.

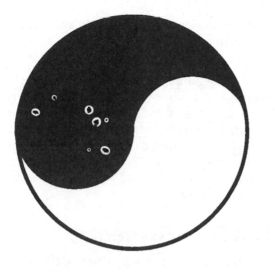

The ancient symbol for Yin and Yang represents both the sunny and shady sides of the same hill.

We Western types tend to think of Yin and Yang as opposing or competing forces. That's not quite right. Although Yin and Yang do represent opposites—male and female, dark and light, and so on—they don't compete. They coexist and counterbalance each other. Just as you can't have left without right, or up without down, you can't have Yin without Yang. The following table explains the basic relationships of Yin and Yang.

Yin and Yang Relationships

Yin Aspects	Yang Aspects
Inside	Outside
Descending	Ascending
Contracting	Expanding
Heavy	Light
Dark	Bright
Solid	Hollow
Cold	Hot
Water	Fire
Passive	Active
Female	Male
Winter	Summer
Moon	Sun

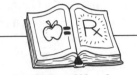

Here's another way to look at Yin and Yang. Yin is cold; Yang is hot. As a cup of hot tea cools, it changes from Yang to Yin—but it's still tea.

Yin and *Yang* apply to everything, but they have special roles in TCM. When your Yin and Yang get out of balance, you get sick. Exactly what kind of sickness you get depends on the kind of imbalance. Too much Yin leads to cold symptoms, like chills; too much Yang leads to heat symptoms, like fever. In addition, some organs, such as your liver, are Yin, while others, such as your stomach, are Yang.

The Five Elements

Yin and Yang are dynamic—they're always changing and moving. Traditional Chinese medicine sees five different changing aspects within the great web of Yin and Yang. The Five Elements, as they're called, are Earth, Fire, Metal, Water, and Wood. Each element corresponds to things in both the natural world, like the seasons and colors, and within your body, like your organs. Check out the table for details.

The Five Elements

Element	Season	Climate	Color	Taste	Yin Organ	Yang Organ	Opening	Tissue
Earth	Late summer	Dampness	Yellow	Sweet	Spleen	Stomach	Mouth	Muscles
Fire	Summer	Heat	Red	Bitter	Heart	Small intestine	Tongue	Blood vessels
Metal	Autumn	Dryness	White	Pungent	Lungs	Large intestine	Nose	Skin
Water	Winter	Cold	Blue/ black	Salty	Kidney	Bladder	Ears	Bones
Wood	Spring	Wind	Blue/ green	Sour	Liver	Gall bladder	Eyes	Tendons

The Five Elements support and interact with each other as part of a complex system. For example, Water helps Wood grow; Fire burns Wood; Water puts out Fire. In traditional Chinese medicine, these ideas are applied to your organs. Disharmonies among your Five Elements cause an imbalance in your Yin and Yang that could make you sick. For example, Fire controls Metal, because heat melts metal. In your body, your heart and small intestine (Fire organs) affect your lungs and large intestine (Metal organs). So, if your Fire organs are weak, your Metal organs may get out of hand, and you might develop lung problems.

In TCM, the relationships among the Five Elements are often seen as fanciful metaphors. A good example is *Wood insults Earth*, meaning your liver (a Wood organ) dominates your spleen (an Earth organ). When that happens, you get headaches, gas, poor appetite, weakness, and maybe sore eyes and dizziness.

The Five Elements idea can be applied to your body type and personality. Some people are Wood types, others are Water types, and so on. Because each type has a particular area that's likely to cause problems, the Five Elements are sometimes used for diagnosis. Metal types, for example, tend to have large intestine and lung problems. We could go on for many more pages about the Five Element body types. We won't, though, especially because not all OMPs use the theory in practice.

Qi: The Chinese Theory of Energy

With us so far? Now it's time for the next big idea in traditional Chinese medicine: the concept of *Qi*. For a concept that's so important, this one is awfully hard to translate. (It's easy to pronounce, though—just say *chee*.) Qi can be translated as "vital substance" or "life force," but the most usual translation is "life energy" or sometimes just "energy."

Qi is the energy that flows through all things, even nonliving ones like rocks. In the larger sense, Qi is the organizing force of the universe. Qi is invisible and can't be measured. It flows through your body along pathways called *meridians*. Like Qi, the meridians are invisible. We'll get into meridians in detail in a little bit. For now, let's just say you have 12 regular meridians, each relating to one of the 12 major organs in traditional Chinese medicine, and you have eight extraordinary meridians that tie in closely to the regular ones.

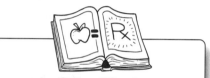

In Other Words...

Qi (sometimes written *chi* or *ch'i* and pronounced *chee*) is the invisible but fundamental energy that flows through everything and everyone in the universe. It's usually translated as "energy," but Qi is more than that. It's the life force of all living things, but it's also the energy found in all nonliving things.

When your Qi flows nicely through your meridians, you have good health. That's because Qi has five major functions in your body:

➤ **Movement** (sometimes called *impulsing*). Qi makes your body move in every sense of the word. It controls your physical activity, your internal processes (digestion, heartbeat, and so on), and your mental activity.

➤ **Warmth.** Qi keeps your body temperature normal.

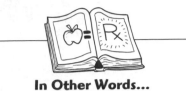

In Other Words...

Your Qi flows through invisible pathways or channels in your body called **meridians**. Blockages in the meridians interrupt the smooth flow of Qi and cause illness.

➤ **Protection** (sometimes called *defending*). Your Qi protects you from disease, stress, and injury. In this sense, Qi is roughly the same as your immune system.

➤ **Transformation.** Qi changes air, water, and food into vital substances that keep you alive. This is roughly comparable to respiration and digestion.

➤ **Retention and containment.** Qi holds your organs and other body parts in place and keeps them working right.

If the meridians are blocked for some reason, your Qi doesn't flow smoothly and you have health problems. So, the fundamental goal of traditional Chinese medicine is to keep your Qi flowing smoothly and to remove any blockages that might develop.

Qi Disharmonies

What happens if your Qi gets blocked? In TCM, there are four basic types of Qi disharmony:

➤ **Deficient Qi.** If you don't have enough Qi, it can't do its job. You might feel cold all the time, for instance, because you don't have enough Qi to keep you warm.

➤ **Sinking Qi.** Sinking Qi usually affects retention and containment.

➤ **Stagnant Qi.** When the normal flow of Qi in the meridians is slowed or blocked, it is said to be stagnant. Swelling is a good example of stagnant Qi.

➤ **Rebellious Qi.** When Qi flows in the wrong direction, it's being rebellious. Your stomach Qi, for instance, should flow downward toward your intestines. When it flows upward instead, you feel nauseous or even vomit.

The major treatment goal of traditional Chinese medicine is to restore harmony to your Qi. When that happens, health and well-being are restored as well.

The Three Treasures

In traditional Chinese medicine, three basic substances circulate in your body and carry energy. The first and most important is Qi. The next is *jing*, another one of those untranslatable concepts. Jing is usually translated as "vital essence," but what it really means is your

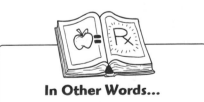

In Other Words...

Your **jing** is your "vital essence," or your ability to change, grow, and adapt on a long-term basis. Your **shen** is your "spirit" or "mind."

ability to change and adapt. To a degree, you're born with the jing you inherit from your parents, but what you eat and drink also affects your jing. Your jing affects your ability to learn, grow, reproduce, and develop.

The third treasure is *shen*. This is best translated as "spirit" or "mind" and means your spiritual aspect. It also reflects your personality and keeps your mind alert.

Two More Treasures

Two more substances circulate in your body and are essential to your health. The first is *Blood*, or *xue* (pronounced *zhway*). This is a tough concept for Westerners, because it means not only blood in the usual sense of the word—the red stuff in your veins and arteries—but also an invisible substance that flows throughout your body through both your blood vessels and your meridians. In Chinese thinking, xue means not just blood but the Qi within the blood. Qi and xue are so closely intertwined that they can't be separated.

The other crucial substance is *Body Fluids* or *jin ye*, an overall term for all the other liquids in your body, including your saliva, tears, mucus, sweat, and urine. Your Body Fluids moisten and nourish your organs.

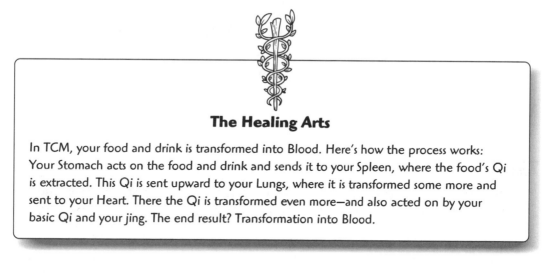

The Healing Arts

In TCM, your food and drink is transformed into Blood. Here's how the process works: Your Stomach acts on the food and drink and sends it to your Spleen, where the food's Qi is extracted. This Qi is sent upward to your Lungs, where it is transformed some more and sent to your Heart. There the Qi is transformed even more—and also acted on by your basic Qi and your jing. The end result? Transformation into Blood.

The Meridians

Remember these? They're the invisible channels your Qi flows through. We already mentioned that there are 12 basic meridians and eight extraordinary ones. Let's get into a bit more detail.

The 12 Regular Meridians

Each of the 12 regular meridians or channels has a corresponding organ (we'll get to organs soon). Half your meridians are Yin channels (corresponding to different Yin organs); the others are Yang channels (corresponding to different Yang organs).

The meridians unify your body and carry Qi and Blood to all parts of you. Because the channels all connect and communicate with each other, a problem with a particular organ can be helped by treating the right connecting channel. And because the 12 regular meridians can easily be reached with needles, blocked Qi can be treated with acupuncture (see Chapter 10, "Acupuncture: Getting Right to the Point").

The Eight Extraordinary Meridians

The eight extraordinary channels act as storage areas for Qi and Blood, sending more to the 12 regular channels as needed. They also move your jing around your body and help the 12 regular channels communicate with each other.

Of the eight extraordinary meridians, the two most important are the Conception Vessel and the Governing Vessel, both found in your torso. That's because only these two channels can be reached with acupuncture needles. The Conception Vessel acts mostly on your Yin, while the Governing Vessel acts mostly on your Yang.

The Zangfu System: Understanding Your Organs

Now let's look at your organs the Chinese way. To do that, you'll have to forget the Western, mechanistic way of looking at your body. In other words, forget the idea that your heart is a pump or your kidneys are like filters. In traditional Chinese medicine, your organs are more like a process.

TCM divides your organs into two main categories: Zang and Fu.

The Zang Organs

In TCM, solid organs are Yin. You have five: your lungs, heart, spleen, liver, and kidneys. Collectively, these organs are called the *Zang organs*. There's also a Zang organ called the *pericardium*, which refers to the area around your heart. For all practical purposes in TCM, your pericardium and heart are the same. The solid Zang organs are part of the process that makes, stores, and controls your Three Treasures, Blood, and Body Fluids.

The Fu Organs

Hollow organs are Yang. You have six of them: your small intestine, large intestine, gall bladder, bladder, stomach, and the *Triple Heater*. Your Triple Heater isn't three baseball games in a row. It's not even a real organ—it's a concept. The Triple Heater is a sort of pathway connecting your organs, but especially your lungs, spleen, and kidneys.

70

In traditional thought, the Triple Heater is imagined as a three-tiered burner: The head and chest are the upper burner, the upper abdomen is the middle burner, and the lower abdomen and pelvic region are the lower burner. Another way to think of the Triple Heater is as the boss of your body, making sure that Qi moves correctly and that your body stays at the right temperature.

The hollow *Fu organs* are part of the process that moves your Three Treasures, Blood, and Body Fluids around your body.

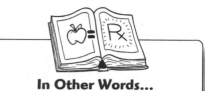

In Other Words...

The **Zang organs** (Yin) are solid organs; **Fu organs** (Yang) are hollow. Just in case everything we've discussed so far is too simple, there's **Extra Fu**. The Extra Fu organs are your brain, uterus (only if you have one), marrow, bones, and blood vessels. For reasons that are way too complicated to go into here, your gall bladder is not only a Fu organ, it's also an Extra Fu organ!

Zangfu in Action

When you put all the elements, meridians, organs, and everything else together, TCM gets really complicated—but also finally starts to make sense.

Here's how it works: Each organ is controlled by one of the 12 meridians and in turn controls some aspect of your body's functions. Each Zang organ is matched with a Fu organ to make six pairs. Each pair is governed by one of the Five Elements (except Fire governs two pairs). Each Yin organ manifests its state of health through an outer organ such as the tongue or eyes; Yin organs also reflect themselves in other body parts, such as the hair or skin.

Got all that? Check the following table to see which organ does what.

Understanding the Zangfu System

Organ	Yin/Yang	Element	Manifested By	Reflected By
Heart	Yin	Fire	Tongue	Face
Small intestine	Yang	Fire	Tongue	Face
Liver	Yin	Wood	Eyes	Nails
Gall bladder	Yang	Wood	Eyes	Nails
Spleen	Yin	Earth	Mouth	Lips
Stomach	Yang	Earth	Mouth	Lips
Lungs	Yin	Metal	Nose	Skin, Body Hair
Large intestine	Yang	Metal	Nose	Skin, Body Hair
Kidneys	Yin	Water	Ear	Skin, Head Hair
Bladder	Yang	Water	Ear	Skin, Head Hair
Pericardium	Yin	Fire	Tongue	Face
Triple Heater	Yang	Fire	Tongue	Face

Organ Functions

In the Western view, your lungs bring in oxygen and remove carbon dioxide. In the Chinese view, things are very different. Your lungs send your Qi and Body Fluids around the outer layers of your body; they also send Qi and Body Fluids to your kidneys and control the passage of water through your body.

The other organs also have different functions in TCM. Here's the breakdown:

➤ **Heart.** Your heart converts Qi from your food into Blood. The heart controls the Blood and blood vessels and is the home of your shen, or spirit.

➤ **Spleen.** In TCM, your spleen is very important for digestion. It controls the movement of the Qi from your food to your heart and lungs. In general, the spleen moves fluids around your body, keeps your Blood in the proper channels, and controls your muscles.

➤ **Liver.** The liver's main role is to control the amount of Blood circulating in your channels. The liver is also really important for the smooth flow of Qi; many illnesses are related to stagnant liver Qi.

➤ **Kidneys.** Your jing is stored in your kidneys, which means they are important for jing functions like growth, reproduction, and development. Your kidneys also produce bones and make Blood.

➤ **Gall bladder.** Your ability to make judgments and decisions is based in your gall bladder. This is also where bile for digestion is made and stored.

➤ **Stomach.** Food goes into your stomach. The Qi is extracted and sent to the spleen; the rest goes on into your small intestine. The role of the stomach is to send the Qi onward.

➤ **Small intestine.** Food from the stomach goes into the small intestine. Impurities are passed on to the large intestine and bladder for removal from the body.

➤ **Large intestine.** Impurities are passed out of the body by the large intestine.

➤ **Bladder.** Waste Body Fluids from the lungs and large and small intestines are removed by the bladder.

➤ **Triple Heater.** All the Water functions of your body are coordinated by the Triple Heater.

As you can see, all the various organs work together. Each has aspects of Yin and Yang, and each is important for some aspect of Qi.

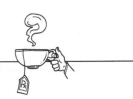

To Your Health!

In traditional Chinese medicine, your gall bladder is responsible for decision-making. What if your gall bladder has to be removed? Will you become indecisive? Not unless you were before the operation—your basic nature remains unchanged. Likewise if you were to have a kidney transplant, lose a leg, need a heart pacemaker, or the like—you'd still be you.

Causes of Disharmony

If you've been counting, you're now up to 12 organs, 12 channels, eight extraordinary channels, Five Elements, three treasures, and a bunch of other stuff. Now you understand how traditional Chinese medicine sees each person as a complicated web of interlocking aspects.

It's also easy to see how imbalances and disharmonies in one organ can have a serious effect on others. But what causes the disharmonies?

TCM answers that question in two ways: internal and external causes.

Disharmony can arise from *internal causes*— another way of saying from emotions such as anger, joy, grief, or fear. Anger, for example, affects the liver and its paired organ, the gall bladder, while grief has an effect on the lungs and large intestine.

External causes of disharmony are found in the climate. There are six factors here, which is why the external causes are sometimes called the Six Evils. The Six Evils can come from outside forces, but they could also come from internal forces. Either way, if one of the Six Evils is affecting you, you're being "invaded" by it.

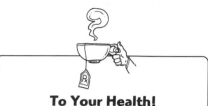

To Your Health!

Anything that keeps your Qi strong and actively flowing—acupuncture, diet, herbs, and other traditional Chinese medicine treatments—will help you cope with internal and external disharmony. And if you do get into disharmony, anything that restores the correct flow of Qi will help restore your internal balance.

The Yin Evils

Yin evils or injuries are caused by cold, dampness, or wind. Cold evil makes you feel cold, of course, but it also causes stiffness, headaches, fatigue, and cramping pains. Dampness evil causes heaviness and soreness, along with lots of fluids, like a runny nose. Dampness evil often comes from a problem with your spleen. Wind evil is generally related to cold or dampness. Wind evil affects the upper part of your body, especially your chest and head. Symptoms include sneezing, coughing, sore throat, and weakness. Disharmony in the liver often causes wind evil.

The Yang Evils

Yang evils are caused by fire or heat, summer heat, or dryness. Fire evil causes heat in the body, like fever or inflammation. It also causes headaches, rashes, and skin problems. Summer heat injury comes from too much heat; symptoms include heavy sweating, high fever, and exhaustion. Dryness evil is connected to fire evil. Symptoms of dryness evil include dry mouth, cracked lips, chest pain, dry cough, and asthma.

Your Lifestyle and Your Health

Outside evils aren't the only underlying causes of poor health, of course. TCM also looks at your lifestyle to find imbalances and excesses. Three lifestyle elements are particularly important:

➤ **Diet.** Too much of the wrong foods can cause bad health. In particular, too much raw food, food that is too spicy, overeating in general, and too much alcohol are bad. And as we'll discuss later in this chapter, changing your diet can be part of your treatment.

➤ **Taxation fatigue.** No, this isn't that tired feeling you get every April when you do your income taxes. In TCM, taxation fatigue means overdoing it, whether by working too hard or playing too hard. Actually, too much of anything—even lying around at the beach sipping lemonade—can cause ill health.

➤ **Sex.** Too much is not enough, you might think, but TCM thinks otherwise. The Chinese aren't prudes, but TCM does recognize that excessive childbearing, for instance, can be harmful to a woman's health. In sex, as in all things, TCM recommends moderation.

The key here is moderation—too much of anything can be as bad as too little.

Diagnosis the Chinese Way

The traditional Chinese approach to understanding your body is very different from what you're used to. So is visiting an Oriental medicine practitioner. That's because the OMP will look at you as an individual and try to understand your unique pattern of health. The OMP will also look for the symptom pattern of your illness.

In traditional Chinese medicine, a doctor uses four basic guidelines to figure out what your problem is and how best to treat it. The process starts with asking, then goes on to looking, hearing and smelling, and pulse-taking and touching. The goal is always to understand the underlying imbalance that is causing your health problem.

Getting to Know You

Whenever you go to any doctor, you're asked a lot of questions about your medical history and your current symptoms. An Oriental medicine practitioner asks you all the usual questions and then some. In TCM, things like how the weather and time of day affect you are important. Your OMP will probably ask you a lot of questions about your digestion, your sleep patterns, and your elimination, as well as other areas, like whether you prefer hot drinks or cold, or if you sweat a lot. The questions might not seem all that relevant, but they all help your doctor build up a picture of you as an individual, not just a bundle of separate symptoms. In particular, your doctor wants to understand your balance of Yin and Yang.

Looking You Over

Your physical appearance tells your doctor a lot about you. He or she will look at your overall appearance—how you stand and move—and also at your hair, your fingernails, your skin, and your tongue. Your appearance and how you present yourself tell a lot about your balance of Yin and Yang, your jing and shen, and your element type.

Sounds Good to Me

An Oriental medicine practitioner will pay attention to the way you sound. Does your voice sound nasal, breathy, hoarse, or loud? Do you have a wet cough, a wheeze, or a dry hack? He or she will also use a stethoscope to listen to your lungs and heart just as any doctor would.

In today's world of frequent bathing, perfumes, and deodorants, smell matters much less in diagnosis. Even so, your OMP may ask you if you have noticed any unusual odors related to your body.

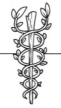

The Healing Arts

How your tongue looks tells your doctor a lot about you—in fact, looking at your tongue is one of the most important parts of the exam. In TCM, the color and shape of your tongue are clues to your interior organs. Each part of the tongue is said to correspond to one of your organs. The very tip of your tongue, for example, corresponds to your heart. The appearance of your tongue is also revealing. If it's dry or red, excess heat could be your problem; if it's pale or has short horizontal cracks, the problem might be not enough Qi.

In a Heartbeat

In traditional Chinese medicine, your *pulse* is the most important diagnostic tool, so your practitioner will spend a lot of time taking it. A Western physician just feels the pulse in your wrist and counts the number of times your heart beats in a minute (about 65 to 75 beats is normal). An Oriental medicine physician takes your pulse in three different places on each wrist. Each pulse position relates to a specific organ in

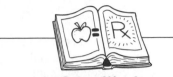

In Other Words...

In traditional Chinese medicine, there are 28 basic **pulse** patterns. Each one reveals something about how your Qi is flowing through your body. If your pulse is rapid, for example, it means you're suffering from internal heat; a slow pulse, on the other hand, means internal cold. A wiry pulse—one that feels taut and stringlike—means liver disharmony from stagnant Qi.

the Zangfu system. The way your pulse feels—its strength, rhythm, rate, and other factors—is also important.

In addition to carefully taking your pulse, your OMP will feel your body, especially along the meridians, to find tender spots. How the pain responds to touch tells which channels and organs are in disharmony. A painful spot that feels better with pressure could mean you have deficient Qi; one that doesn't change could indicate stagnant xue (Blood).

Getting It Together

Using all the information from your examination, your traditional Chinese doctor will have a good understanding of your patterns of disharmony. The next step is to make a diagnosis based on the Eight Principles. Remember our discussion of Yin and Yang? That concept of closely connected polar opposites is the basis of the Eight Principles.

The Eight Principles are really four sets of opposites:

➤ Yin and Yang.

➤ Interior and exterior. Interior is Yin, exterior is Yang.

➤ Cold and hot. Cold is Yin, hot is Yang.

➤ Deficiency and excess. Deficiency is Yin, excess is Yang. Deficiency needs to be tonified; excess needs to be calmed.

One way to detect an imbalance in one of the Eight Principles is to apply its opposite. If, for example, you have a pain that is relieved by cold, excess heat could be the problem.

By applying the Eight Principles to the Zang organs (these are your lungs, heart, spleen, liver, and kidneys), your OMP can decide exactly where your disharmony lies. The problem could be one of deficiency, excess, or stagnation of a Zang organ, caused by an imbalance of Yin and Yang—all of which, in the end, affect the flow of Qi.

Treatment the Chinese Way

The great beauty of Chinese medicine is that it sees you as an individual and looks beyond symptoms to causes. The imbalance that is causing your migraines, for example, could have an entirely different cause than the imbalance that is causing exactly the same symptoms in someone else. The right treatment for you might be completely wrong for someone else.

So, you and your doctor have discovered what sort of imbalance is causing your health problem. Now what?

In general, traditional Chinese medicine follows the basic principle of treatment by applying the opposite. If excess heat is the problem, your treatment will be designed to cool you. If stagnation is the issue, the goal will be to get your Qi moving again. If your Qi is deficient, the goal will be to increase it (in TCM, this is often called *tonifying*).

Whatever the diagnosis ends up being, the treatment generally includes acupuncture and Chinese herbs, often combined with diet changes. Acupuncture and herbs are so important—and so complex—that we've given them separate chapters so we can discuss them more thoroughly. (See Chapter 10 on acupuncture, and Chapter 16, "Ginseng and More: Traditional Chinese Herbs.") As for diet, keep reading.

Eating to Heal

If you love Chinese food (and who doesn't?), you're in luck. Traditional Chinese medicine believes that your diet is central to your health. A balanced diet that avoids excesses helps keep you healthy. If your Qi does get out of balance, diet is a powerful tool for correcting disharmonies and unblocking your energy channels. As you might expect, in Chinese thought, foods have Yin and Yang properties—and lots of other properties as well. Let's take a closer look.

Yin, Yang, and What You Eat

Yin foods are said to be cold; Yang foods are hot. That means Yin foods are cooling or calming while Yang foods are warming and stimulating. Some foods, such as rice and bread, are neutral. Too much of a Yin or Yang food is bad for you. For example, if you eat too much of a Yin food, such as raw vegetables, you put a strain on your Yang, which has to compensate for all that coldness. The season also affects your choice of Yin and Yang foods. During the cold, wet winter, for instance, you would want to eat plenty of Yang foods to counteract the Yin effect of the weather.

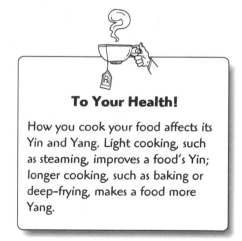

To Your Health!

How you cook your food affects its Yin and Yang. Light cooking, such as steaming, improves a food's Yin; longer cooking, such as baking or deep-frying, makes a food more Yang.

Yin foods include raw fruits and vegetables, ocean fish, milk, and dairy products. Yang foods are all rich, strongly flavored foods, including meat. Flavorings are also Yin and Yang. Among the Yin spices are sugar, salt, soy sauce, coriander, and surprisingly, chili peppers and curry. Yang spices include garlic, ginger, black pepper, basil, and cloves.

The Fives of Foods

In TCM, any food has one of five different kinds of energy; it also has one of five different flavors or tastes. Let's look at energy first.

The energy of a food can be hot, warm, neutral, cool, or cold. Knowing a food's energy helps you balance the Yin and Yang in a meal. To see which foods are which, check out the following table.

The Five Energies in Food

Hot	Warm	Neutral	Cool	Cold
Pepper	Lamb	Beef	Wheat	Shellfish
Cinnamon	Ham	Pork	Tofu	Lettuce
Raw onion	Chicken	Eggs	Cucumber	Bok choy
	Shrimp	Rice	Eggplant	Cauliflower
	Garlic	Corn	Spinach	Banana
	Scallions	Beans	Watercress	Watermelon
	Peach	Carrot	Radish	Salt
	Cherries	Potato	Apple	Tea
	Ginger	Yam	Pear	
	Coriander	Turnip	Lemon	
	Vinegar	Grapes	Strawberries	
	Coffee	Pineapple	Mint	
	Apricot	Plum		
		Olives		

You might notice that some fairly common foods aren't in the table. That's because they're not part of the traditional Chinese diet. You can still eat them, of course—but in moderation.

It's important to know which energy category a food falls into. If you eat too many raw, cold foods, for instance, your Spleen Qi could be damaged, which will harm your digestion. To keep your Qi moving smoothly, you want to select foods that balance each other's energy.

It's also important to balance the flavors of your food. Foods falls into one of five flavor categories: pungent or spicy, sweet, sour, bitter, or salty. (You might remember that we mentioned flavors when we talked about the Five Elements.) Too much of any one flavor—sweet, for instance—can cause disharmony. If you're out of balance, on the other hand, a particular flavor can help the problem.

Here's how the different flavors work:

➤ **Pungent or spicy.** These foods help move your Qi and break up blockages; they also make you sweat. Many spices, such as garlic, ginger, black pepper, cinnamon, fennel, peppermint, and nutmeg, are pungent. Other pungent foods are watercress, radishes, scallions, green peppers, and mustard greens. Pungent foods are often helpful for fevers and the lungs. They're good for getting your Qi circulating and removing blockages.

➤ **Sweet.** In TCM, sweet means that the food aids digestion, and not necessarily that it tastes sugary. Foods that are rich and contain animal fat, such as meat, poultry, and eggs, for instance, are sweet. So are milk, dairy products, wheat, potatoes, beans, carrots, and spinach. Some fruits, like watermelon and bananas, are sweet. Naturally, so are sugar and honey. Sweet foods are said to add to your Qi, help your spleen, relieve internal dryness, and improve your digestion.

➤ **Sour.** Sour foods have a contracting, tightening effect. Citrus fruits are sour, as are grapes, apples, peaches, and olives. In general, sour foods are good for your digestion, particularly if you have diarrhea or nausea. Sour foods are also good for your nervous system and your liver.

➤ **Bitter.** The cool, dry effect of bitter foods releases blockages. Lettuce, cucumbers, asparagus, and celery are bitter foods. So are coffee, tea, vinegar, and pickled foods. Bitter foods help your digestion, especially if you're having trouble with your bowels, and are good for the heart.

➤ **Salty.** Salty foods are said to be softening and to help concentrate your Blood and Body Fluids. They're also good for the kidneys. Ham, pork, shellfish, seaweed, and, of course, salt are salty foods.

A balanced diet—one that balances the flavors and energies of your foods—is always the goal.

Some foods also affect specific Zangfu organs. Dark, bitter greens like watercress, for instance, affect your heart and small intestine. That part of the Chinese approach to diet is a bit too complicated to go into here. If you have a specific health problem, your OMP will recommend foods and food combinations that will help harmonize your Qi and your Zangfu organs.

Qigong: Healthful Energy

When your Qi flows smoothly, you're healthy; when it doesn't, you get sick. To keep their Qi flowing, many people practice *Qigong* exercises. This Chinese approach to exercise strengthens and balances your Qi and removes Qi blockages.

Qigong exercises vary quite a bit, but basically they consist of deep breathing and gentle calisthenics. The best-known approach to Qigong in the West is probably

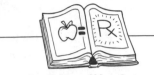

In Other Words...

Qigong is usually translated as "energy cultivation" or "energy development." More loosely, it can be translated as "energy flow." Qigong exercises keep your Qi flowing.

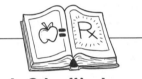

In Other Words...

T'ai chi (sometimes written **taiji**) can be loosely translated as "the supreme ultimate." T'ai chi is a system of gentle, flowing Qigong exercises designed to keep your Qi moving. T'ai chi exercises can be done by anyone, even elderly or handicapped people.

t'ai chi. A system of Qigong exercises done with slow, flowing movements, t'ai chi is based on the concept of the Five Elements we talked about earlier in this chapter. The exercises are done in a graceful sequence that follows the cycle of how the Five Elements transform into each other.

In China and Taiwan today, millions of people start their day in local parks with a session of t'ai chi exercises (your Qi flows best in the early morning). In the U.S., that's a little hard to do. Fortunately, you can do the exercises by yourself anywhere at any time. To learn the basics of t'ai chi, however, you'll need to find a good teacher. T'ai chi has become so popular that many health clubs and Ys now offer classes.

To find a t'ai chi class near you, contact:

> **American Foundation of Traditional Chinese Medicine**
> 505 Beach Street
> San Francisco, CA 94133
> (415) 776-0502

External Qigong

Some Qigong masters claim they can project their Qi out of their bodies and onto other people. If someone is very ill and has very little Qi, for example, a Qigong master can add his Qi to the patient's. This manifestation of the master's *external Qi*, as it is called, is said to help the patient recover. There's not a lot of good evidence for external Qi, and some of the claims made for Qigong masters—that they can leap over buildings, repel attackers with just a flick of their finger, and so on—are just silly.

Can TCM Help You?

Overall, TCM seems to work best for people who have chronic health problems like arthritis, allergies, skin conditions, PMS and menstrual problems, migraines, digestive problems such as irritable bowel syndrome, chronic fatigue, and that "run-down" feeling. Any health problem that causes chronic pain is also often helped by TCM, especially by acupuncture. TCM can also help people who are receiving standard chemotherapy or radiation treatments for cancer. Patients who use Chinese herbs say they can tolerate the side effects of their cancer treatment more easily and recover their

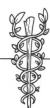

The Healing Arts

A 1998 study at The Johns Hopkins Medical School showed that slow, relaxed t'ai chi exercises lower blood pressure in older adults just as well as moderate aerobic exercise, such as brisk walking. The doctors who did the study were surprised at how well t'ai chi worked, but they shouldn't have been—people in China have known about the benefits of t'ai chi for thousands of years.

Another aspect of t'ai chi is the martial art known as **t'ai chi chuan**, which can be translated as "supreme ultimate fist." T'ai chi chuan offers many physical and spiritual benefits, but in the U.S., it's also seen as a competitive sport.

strength faster. Finally, TCM often works dramatically well for patients who have symptoms that are very real but don't fit into any sort of standard Western diagnosis. Chinese medicine sees the pattern of these symptoms in a different way and takes them seriously, instead of dismissing them as meaningless or caused by depression.

Although some patients get better very quickly once they receive traditional treatment with herbs and acupuncture, in most cases several weeks or even months of treatment are needed. Once your balance of Qi is restored, your Oriental medicine practitioner will recommend ways to keep it that way and avoid future problems.

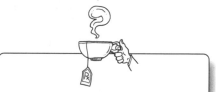

To Your Health!

In 1992 a careful study in England showed that Chinese herbs can be helpful for treating severe eczema (itchy, flaky skin rashes). Patients who took the herbs showed solid improvement within a few weeks and had no side effects.

Finding an Oriental Medicine Practitioner

You've gotten this far, so you know how complex traditional Chinese medicine is. If you want to try it, you need to find a well-trained specialist. This can be a little tricky. Most states have licensing requirements for acupuncturists (see Chapter 10 for more on that), but the license doesn't require any real knowledge of the philosophy behind Chinese medicine or any understanding of using Chinese herbs. Right now the only state to also require a knowledge of Chinese herbs is California.

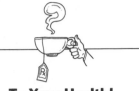

To Your Health!

American-born OMPs should be graduates of one of the 40 or so rigorous training programs in the U.S. that have been accredited by the National Accreditation Commission for Schools and Colleges of Acupuncture and Oriental Medicine. If that's not the case, he or she should have at least 500 hours of formal training in Chinese herbs. Before you visit an OMP, ask about his or her credentials.

At the least, your Oriental medicine practitioner should be a licensed acupuncturist or be certified by the *National Certification Commission for Acupuncture and Oriental Medicine* (NCCAOM). In the U.S., many OMPs were trained as doctors in China or Taiwan. They may not be fully bilingual or bicultural, which could make it hard to communicate well. Also, their medical degrees from Chinese universities aren't usually recognized in other countries, so most aren't licensed to practice medicine.

You probably won't be able to get insurance coverage for traditional Chinese treatment unless it comes from a medical doctor, osteopath, chiropractor, or licensed acupuncturist. Even then, your coverage may pay for acupuncture but not for herbs.

If you don't live in a city with a large Chinese population, you may not be able to find an OMP at all. In that case, you may have to rely on a medical doctor, osteopath, or chiropractor who has studied acupuncture and may know something about Chinese herbs.

To find a qualified practitioner, contact:

> **National Certification Commission for Acupuncture and Oriental Medicine (NCCAOM)**
> 1424 16th Street, NW, Suite 501
> Washington, DC 20073
> Phone: (202) 232-1404
> Fax: (202) 462-6157

This organization can refer you to a well-trained practitioner in your area. So can this group:

> **American Association of Oriental Medicine (AAOM)**
> 433 Front Street
> Catasauqua, PA 18032
> Phone: (610) 266-1433
> Fax: (610) 264-2768
> E-mail: AAOM1@aol.com

More than a thousand practitioners belong to the AAOM.

Disharmony or Misdiagnosis?

Modern Western medicine has a hard time accepting traditional Chinese medicine. Skeptical doctors point out that ideas like Yin, Yang, and Qi are all very interesting, but they don't see how a traditional Chinese doctor can arrive at an accurate diagnosis or prescribe a useful treatment. In some documented cases, the same patient was given different diagnoses by different Chinese doctors—and by Western standards, none were right.

To a Western doctor, a lot of the concepts in TCM are vague, irrational, and have no relation to the way your body actually works. Western doctors have trouble with the idea that TCM can treat problems like heart disease, AIDS, or cancer. They also point out that in TCM there's no germ theory of illness—in other words, according to Chinese medicine, your strep throat comes not from a bacterial infection but from blocked Qi. Given today's scientific knowledge, they feel TCM is hopelessly mired in the past. Western doctors also worry, rightly, that Chinese herbal remedies may contain powerful substances that could be harmful or that might interact badly with any medicine you need to take. Now that some Chinese herbs have been scientifically studied and shown to work, however, Western doctors are becoming a bit more open-minded about them (we'll talk a lot more about that in Chapter 16).

A lot of doctors now even recommend acupuncture for some problems, and they're starting to be more open to the Chinese concepts of prevention, moderation, and balance. Some are also interested in working with Oriental medicine practitioners to combine the best of traditional Chinese medicine with modern medicine.

The Least You Need to Know

➤ In traditional Chinese medicine (TCM), health problems are caused when your flow of Qi (energy) is blocked.

➤ Qi blockages happen when your various body systems get out of balance.

➤ To restore the proper balance and unblock your Qi, your Oriental medicine practitioner (OMP) may recommend acupuncture, Chinese herbs, and dietary changes.

➤ TCM can be helpful for health problems such as chronic pain, menstrual difficulties, arthritis, allergies, skin conditions, digestive problems, and chronic fatigue.

Chapter 7

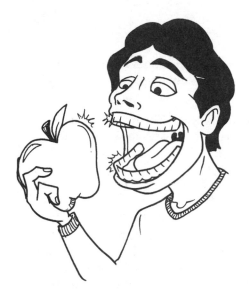

Holistic Dentistry: Sinking Your Teeth into Health

In This Chapter

➤ The holistic approach to dentistry

➤ How holistic dentistry can help common mouth problems

➤ Are your fillings hurting your health?

➤ The holistic way to care for your teeth

Let's face it—almost anything is more fun than spending half an hour sitting in the dentist's chair with someone's hands inside your mouth. Nobody really *likes* going to the dentist, but if you're lucky, all you need are those twice-yearly checkups and cleanings. If you're not that lucky, you could have dental problems that let you get to know your dentist a lot better than you'd like. Either way, taking the holistic approach to your teeth could help you have better dental health.

Open Wide

Holistic dentists see your mouth and teeth as part of your overall good health. Problems in your mouth can have a serious effect on the rest of you—and vice versa. To keep you in good dental health, holistic dentists use natural methods whenever possible. If you're having gum trouble, for instance, a holistic dentist might suggest vitamin supplements, herbs, and homeopathic remedies, along with or instead of traditional treatments. And since a lot of dental problems are caused in part by what you eat, a holistic dentist can give you nutritional advice as well. Some holistic dentists use hypnosis, biofeedback, acupuncture, and meditation techniques to help patients deal with pain without drugs. These techniques are also really helpful for people who are terrified of the dentist.

Some parts of holistic dentistry today are pretty controversial. The mercury filling question, for instance, doesn't have any easy answers. We'll take a look at the different holistic approaches and let you decide for yourself.

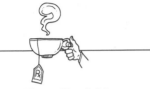

To Your Health!

To keep your mouth in good shape, brush and floss your teeth twice a day. It's pretty simple until you visit the health-food store to buy a natural toothpaste and see all those confusing choices. If you can't find a brand you like, make your own toothpaste. Put a spoonful of baking soda (sodium bicarbonate) into a small dish and add enough hydrogen peroxide to make a paste.

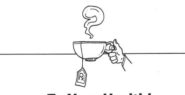

To Your Health!

Here's an easy step toward better dental health: Drink a few cups of tea—black or green—every day, preferably after each meal. Each cup gives you a goodly dose of fluoride along with other decay-preventing compounds.

Holistic Tooth Care

What makes a toothpaste natural? For starters, it doesn't have any sugar or artificial sweeteners in it. Next, it doesn't have any artificial colors or flavorings. It might have herbs said to help the teeth, like bloodroot, bay leaf, or neem, an herb from India. And it may or may not have fluoride in it (we'll get to the fluoride choice a little further on).

We can't really recommend any particular toothpaste brand. Try them until you find one you like. Overall, brushing regularly is more important than which toothpaste you use.

Fluoride: Fighting Tooth Decay

Should you use a toothpaste with *fluoride* in it? What about the fluoride that's added to drinking water in a lot of places? We're not really sure why this is such a controversial question, because the advantages of *fluoridation* are perfectly clear. Fluoride is very valuable for preventing tooth decay and even repairing it in its very earliest stages. Fluoridated drinking water reduces cavities in children by 20 to 40 percent and in adults by 15 to 35 percent—and the effect is even greater if you also use fluoridated toothpaste. Today about 60 percent of the municipalities in the United States add fluoride to their water supplies at the rate of 1 milligram per liter (which is another way of saying one part per million).

Some opponents of fluoridation claim that it causes health problems like cancer, heart disease, kidney disease, and Alzheimer's disease. There's no evidence that this is true. Opponents also claim that fluoride in drinking water causes bone loss and osteoporosis in older adults. In fact, there's solid evidence that people who live in areas with fluoridated water have *less* osteoporosis. And a 1998 study in the prestigious journal *Annals of Internal Medicine* showed that calcium supplements for building bone strength actually work *better* if they're taken with fluoride supplements.

If you live in an area that doesn't fluoridate its water, or if you drink only filtered or bottled water, you're not getting the benefits of fluoride for strong teeth. Talk to your dentist about using fluoridated toothpaste and fluoride mouth rinses.

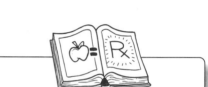

In Other Words...

Fluoridation is the practice of adding tiny amounts of the mineral **fluoride** to municipal water supplies. In small amounts, fluoride strengthens your teeth and protects them against decay.

Gumming Up the Works

If you think a visit to the dentist is bad, just try a visit to the *periodontist*. This specialist in gum disease can make your life really miserable—and expensive—by announcing that you have *gingivitis* or, even worse, *periodontitis*. In the early stages of gingivitis, the usual treatment is brushing and flossing more and maybe using a fluoride mouth rinse. If the problem is further along, your periodontist might have to use those scary-looking dental tools to clean out pockets of infection in the gums around the roots of your teeth. The dentist might enjoy his or her work, but you won't.

Most gum diseases come from not brushing and flossing enough, but holistic dentists believe that other factors are sometimes also at work:

In Other Words...

A **periodontist** is a dentist who specializes in treating gum diseases like **gingivitis**—red, swollen gums that bleed easily—and **periodontitis**—an infection of the bone, connective tissue, and gum supporting your teeth.

➤ **Not enough B vitamins.** Gum disease could mean you're not getting enough of the B vitamins, especially folic acid. If you smoke or use birth-control pills, you might be low on B vitamins. You might also be low if you have a poor diet; older people get low on the Bs because they don't absorb them from their food as well as they used to. Rinsing your mouth with liquid folic acid for one minute twice a day could help. If you can't find liquid folic acid, try emptying an 800 microgram folic acid capsule into a glass of warm water. Stir well.

➤ **Not enough fiber.** The fiber in crunchy or chewy foods like apples, carrots, and whole grains naturally cleans your teeth and stimulates circulation to the gums. Eating more fiber and fewer refined carbohydrates could help heal your gums—so say goodbye to those chocolate chip cookies and eat apples instead. *Bonus*: You'll have a nicer smile *and* lose weight.

➤ **Heavy metal toxicity.** If you have a buildup of dangerous heavy metals like mercury, arsenic, or lead in your system, gum disease could be a sign of it. Your holistic dentist may be able to arrange for testing to see if heavy metals are a problem for you.

No matter what's causing your gum problems, there are natural remedies that can help. Herbalists often suggest swishing an infusion of chamomile, sage, goldenseal, or myrrh around in your mouth. These are antibiotic herbs that can help treat infection. Echinacea, another natural antibiotic, is also a good choice. (See Chapter 15, "Traditional Herbal Medicine," for more information.) Make the infusion (a really strong tea), let it cool, and swish several times until you've used up a cup or so of the liquid. Repeat twice a day.

Some people like using a few drops of antibiotic tea-tree oil or peppermint oil in a cup of warm water as a mouth rinse. If you do this, don't swallow! Essential oils should never be taken internally.

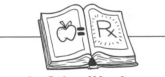

To Your Health!

Take care of gum disease if you get it. Studies show that people with gum disease are more likely to get heart disease.

For mild gingivitis, or for sensitive gums that bleed easily, try *flavonoid* supplements. Flavonoids help strengthen your tiny blood vessels, including the ones in your gums.

Homeopathic remedies that are said to help gum trouble are *mercurius solubilis* and *staphysagria* (sometimes called *stavescare*).

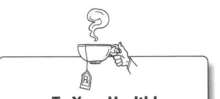

In Other Words...

Flavonoids—also called **bioflavonoids**—are the natural chemical compounds that give fruits and vegetables their bright colors. Among other things, flavonoids strengthen your blood vessels.

Smelling Like a Rose

You go out to dinner with your date and, in a forgetful moment, order onion rings for an appetizer and chicken baked with garlic as your main course. As you dig in, you realize that any chance of romance later on will be done in by your breath. What to do? Easy—when you're done, eat those sprigs of parsley decorating your plate and order peppermint tea with your dessert. For *halitosis* (bad breath) from foods you've eaten, herbs such as parsley, peppermint, fennel seeds, and coriander seeds are very helpful. You could also try one of the natural mouthwashes sold in health-food stores, or you can swish and gargle with strong infusions made from herbs such as eucalyptus, clove, spearmint, sage, peppermint, or thyme—alone or in any combination you like. You could also try a few drops of clove oil, peppermint oil, or tea-tree oil in a cup of warm water. Don't swallow the water! Remember, essential oils should never be taken internally.

Holistic dentists often recommend a product called *Oxyfresh®* for treating bad breath. We can't say whether this works or not, and it is on the pricey side. If nothing else is helping, give it a try.

In Roman times, meals were often rounded off with a few mint sprigs to help the digestion and freshen the breath. After-dinner mints are the modern version of this ancient custom.

The ABCs of TMJ

Here's a jawbreaker of a condition: *temporomandibular joint syndrome*, better known as *TMJ syndrome*. It's a problem of the hinge-like joint that connects your lower jaw to your skull. Sometimes the joint can get out of line, causing jaw pain, a popping or clicking sound when you open your mouth or chew, headaches, and even ringing in the ears.

You might get temporary TMJ from having a dental problem that makes you chew just on one side of your mouth, from arthritis or a problem with a disk in your neck, or just from tension that makes you clench your jaws a lot. In many cases, TMJ goes away by itself in a few months, especially if you try some of these alternative therapies:

➤ **Acupuncture.** This can help, especially if you have TMJ from stress.

➤ **Chiropractic.** If your TMJ comes from a neck problem, chiropractic may be helpful.

➤ **Massage.** Massaging the muscles around the temporomandibular joint can help relax them and relieve discomfort.

Sometimes TMJ is caused by *bruxism*—grinding your teeth when you sleep. If you're a tooth-grinder, your dentist can easily tell just by looking at your teeth—they'll be worn down. Wearing a bite guard at night can be very helpful. Your dentist can make one for you. If the problem isn't too bad, you can try the sort of mouth guard hockey and football players use.

If your TMJ or bruxism is caused by stress, biofeedback has been shown to work well. (We'll talk more about that in Chapter 30, "Use Your Head.")

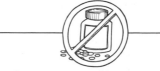

Hazardous to Your Health!

Constant bad breath is usually a sign of gum disease or tooth decay. Sometimes, though, it is a symptom of a more serious problem, like diabetes or kidney disease. Talk to your dentist.

In Other Words...

Temporomandibular joint syndrome, or **TMJ syndrome**, happens when the hinge-like joint that connects your lower jaw to your skull gets out of line for some reason, causing pain, headaches, clicking or popping noises when you chew, and other symptoms. **Bruxism** is the technical term for grinding your teeth in your sleep.

A very common reason for TMJ is bite problems—your teeth don't line up correctly when you bite down. Sometimes it's because they never did—bite problems are one of the main reasons kids have to wear braces. Sometimes it's because you lost a tooth in the past and your teeth have shifted around since then.

To get your teeth to mesh together better, some holistic dentists recommend devices worn in the mouth that are said to move the teeth into a better position. Not all dentists approve of these devices. If they work at all, they could take months to help.

Another approach to treating TMJ is cranial osteopathy (we talked about that back in Chapter 3, "Osteopathy: Boning Up"). This does seem to help, especially for TMJ from stress or injury.

The Mercury Controversy

Are your *mercury amalgam fillings* making you sick? Try asking that question at the annual county dental society dinner and see what happens—you might get a nice brawl going.

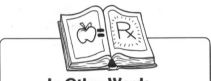

In Other Words...

Mercury amalgam fillings are the "silver" fillings most people have for dental cavities. The mixture, or amalgam, is made of mercury, tin, copper, silver, and sometimes zinc.

Some holistic dentists claim that you absorb dangerous amounts of mercury from mercury amalgam fillings. They say the mercury is the cause of many chronic health problems, including immune system weakness, depression, anxiety, multiple sclerosis, arthritis, mononucleosis, and more. The cure is to remove the mercury fillings and replace them with a "safer" mixture.

There's very little hard evidence that mercury toxicity or toxicity of any sort is caused by fillings or that replacing mercury amalgam fillings has any positive effect on your health. If you have a lot of fillings, replacing them could be a time-consuming, expensive, and painful process. On the other hand, many dentists today now use a nontoxic ceramic composite material instead of amalgam. If you need any new or replacement fillings, you can ask for the composite material.

Finding a Holistic Dentist

There's no national organization for holistic dentists, so you'll probably have to ask around to find someone who uses natural methods whenever possible. Ask other alternative care providers, like your chiropractor, for a recommendation.

Rules, Rules, Rules

If you're lucky enough to have dental insurance, some holistic treatments may be covered. Dental insurance varies a lot, though, so always check first. If you request more expensive composite fillings instead of amalgam for fillings in your back teeth, your insurance may only pay you back for the cost of amalgam. Your insurer probably won't pay for anything related to replacing mercury amalgam fillings (unless they need it) or "biological dentistry." Check first before you start treatments such as cranial osteopathy for TMJ—it's not always covered.

The Critics Bite Back

Critics of some kinds of holistic dentistry have a lot to sink their teeth into. There's very little solid evidence that mercury amalgam fillings are dangerous to your health, but there's a lot to show that they aren't. There's virtually no evidence in favor of "biological dentistry." Some critics also say that most cases of TMJ syndrome get better in a few months just with ibuprofen (Advil®), moist heat, and exercise—they say there's no need for any other treatment.

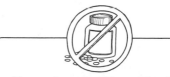

Hazardous to Your Health!

If you can't get a brawl going by bringing up mercury fillings, try "biological dentistry." Some dentists claim that invisible pockets of infection in your jaw bones cause chronic health problems such as arthritis and heart disease. They say the condition is usually caused by teeth that have had root canal treatment. The treatment? Remove the teeth. We suggest that you bite any dentist who recommends this.

On the other hand, a lot of holistic ideas, like vitamin supplements, hypnosis, and cranial osteopathy, have been shown to be helpful and are being adopted by a lot of mainstream dentists. Most mainstream dentists also believe that the newest ceramic composites are as good as mercury amalgam and also look more natural, so they're switching over.

The Least You Need to Know

➤ Holistic dentists believe that natural treatments such as homeopathy and vitamins can be helpful for some dental problems.

➤ Herbal mouth rinses may help minor gum problems.

➤ Herbs such as parsley, peppermint, sage, and tea-tree oil can help stop bad breath.

➤ There's no real evidence that mercury amalgam fillings are harmful to your health.

➤ Jaw pain and headaches from TMJ syndrome often can be helped by natural treatments, such as acupuncture, massage, and biofeedback.

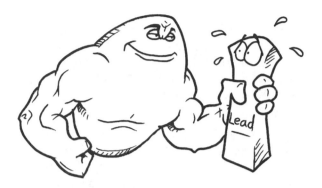

Chapter 8

Chelation: Grabbing for Good Health

In This Chapter

➤ What chelation is and how it works

➤ How chelation may help heart disease

➤ Circulation problems and chelation

➤ Is chelation right for you?

Ah, youth. It's wasted on the young. Wouldn't it be great if you could keep your body youthful and healthy as you grow older? Then you'd have all that hard-earned life experience in a body that could really take advantage of it. Dream on, you say. But what if there really was something that could slow down the aging process and turn back the clock on your aging arteries? Believers in chelation therapy say that's what their treatments do. Are they right? Keep reading.

What's Chelation?

Chelation therapy is a medical approach to *arteriosclerosis* (hardening of the arteries), *atherosclerosis* (narrowing of the arteries from fatty deposits), and other circulation problems. Here's how it works: Chelation (pronounced *key-LAY-shun*) is a chemical process that "captures" metal ions (including lead, iron, calcium, mercury, copper, and zinc) and binds them to an organic molecule. The metal ion is basically handcuffed to the molecule and can't escape. Instead, it passes out of your body in the usual way.

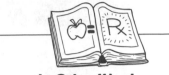

In Other Words...

Chelation therapy is a medical procedure used to remove calcium and metals from the bloodstream. The word chelation (it's pronounced *key-LAY-shun*) comes from the Greek word *chele*, meaning "claw" or "pincer." Chelation works by chemically grabbing hold of the metal ion and hanging on to it so it can't escape and sends it out of your body.

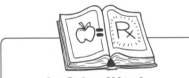

In Other Words...

Fatty deposits on the inside walls of your arteries start out as streaks that gradually become large, hard, calcium-filled deposits called **plaque**. The plaque narrows the artery and reduces the amount of blood that can flow through.

The treatment uses a substance called *EDTA*, which is put into your bloodstream in an *intravenous infusion.* EDTA stands for *ethylene diamine tetra acetic acid* (you can see why everyone uses the abbreviation). A thin needle is inserted into a vein in your arm (that's the intravenous part), and a liquid containing the EDTA (the infusion) slowly drips in. In chelation therapy, the EDTA is the organic molecule. The EDTA leaves your body along with the metal ions it captures.

Believers in chelation therapy say that by capturing calcium in your blood, the EDTA removes calcium from the *plaque*—the fatty deposits—that narrows your arteries. This improves your circulation and gets more oxygen to your cells. Chelation is also said to block the cascade of events that leads to forming the plaque to begin with. In addition, chelation is believed to help hardened arteries become more flexible and to enlarge your small blood vessels. In both cases, your circulation improves, especially to your brain and arms and legs. Chelation also removes buildups of other dangerous metals, like lead, mercury, cadmium, and aluminum, that your body can't metabolize. In fact, the original use of chelation, discovered in the 1930s, was to treat lead poisoning.

Some people also claim that improved circulation from chelation can help lower-back pain, diabetes, high blood pressure, Alzheimer's disease, and arthritis. And by restoring your circulation and making your arteries more flexible, chelation is said to restore youthful vigor.

What a Drip

Chelation therapy is generally painless and easy, but it does take a long time. During a typical treatment, you'll recline in a comfortable lounge chair with a thin intravenous needle in an arm vein near your elbow. The only thing that's mildly uncomfortable about chelation therapy is the needle stick—after that, you don't feel a thing. The EDTA infusion drips in at about one drop a second, so getting the full dose takes about three hours. You can read, talk, listen to music, or just relax during the treatment—you can even get up to go to the bathroom if you need to.

Most of what you get in the infusion is the EDTA, mixed with sterile water. Often some extra B vitamins, vitamin C, and minerals are mixed in to give you an extra boost. The EDTA clears out of your system quickly—usually within 24 hours. Because EDTA removes some zinc from your system, you'll probably be given a zinc supplement. You might also need a supplement of pyridoxine (vitamin B_6). Your doctor will regularly perform some routine blood and urine tests to make sure nothing in your body is getting out of whack as you have the treatments.

Your Chelatin' Heart

The most common reason for trying chelation therapy is to treat heart disease from clogged arteries. When the arteries that nourish your heart are narrowed by plaque, less blood—and the oxygen and nutrients it carries—reaches your heart. The reduced blood flow causes weakness and fatigue and sometimes the severe pain of angina. And if a piece of plaque breaks off or a blood clot forms on it, the blocked artery could get closed off completely. When that happens, you have a heart attack.

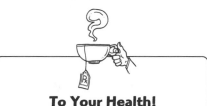

To Your Health!

Believers in chelation therapy say that by cleaning out your arteries and improving your circulation, chelation helps heart disease, intermittent **claudication** (pain and weakness in the legs from poor circulation when walking), dizziness, memory loss, impotence, and fatigue.

Standard medical treatment for blocked heart arteries includes a lot of things that help, like quitting smoking and taking medication that relaxes the artery walls and lowers your blood pressure. If the drugs and lifestyle changes don't help, though, your doctor might recommend *angioplasty*. In this proce-dure, a catheter with a deflated balloon on the tip is threaded through your artery until it reaches the blockage. The balloon then is inflated, which squashes down the plaque and lets more blood through. If angioplasty doesn't work, the next step is *bypass surgery*. In this open-heart operation, veins taken from your leg are grafted onto the clogged arteries to reroute the blood past the blockages.

Doctors who practice chelation therapy point out that angioplasty and bypass surgery are brute-force approaches. Sure, they relieve the immediate problem and could keep you from having a heart attack, but they don't deal with the underlying problem that made the arteries clog up to begin with. That's why a lot of people need repeat angioplasties and find their bypass grafts clogging up with plaque within a few years of the surgery. Chelation, these docs say, is a safer, better ap-

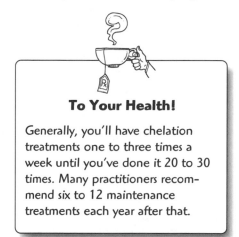

To Your Health!

Generally, you'll have chelation treatments one to three times a week until you've done it 20 to 30 times. Many practitioners recom-mend six to 12 maintenance treatments each year after that.

proach that works, without the risks of invasive procedures. They claim that some-where between 300,000 and 500,000 patients have avoided heart surgery in the past 50 years or so through chelation. In addition, they claim that many patients whose hardened arteries made them have poor circulation in their legs or put them at risk for

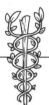

The Healing Arts

There's a big cost difference between chelation and surgery. For heart disease, most chelation therapists recommend 30 treatments over several months. The cost is about $100 a treatment. That adds up, but it's still a heck of a lot cheaper than angioplasty, which runs around $15,000. That's chump change compared to bypass surgery, which typically comes in at around $50,000. Every year in America we spend about $9 billion for about 300,000 coronary artery bypass operations.

a stroke have benefited from chelation to make their arteries more flexible. And if your blood vessels are more flexible, your high blood pressure might come down. Chelation practitioners also claim that, in many cases, patients can reduce the amount of medication they need or even eliminate it altogether.

Is Chelation Right for Me?

We can't say whether chelation will help you. Overall, doctors who do chelation therapy say they get good results about 70 to 80 percent of the time and that chelation has helped many thousands of people avoid heart surgery. The catch is that there isn't a lot of solid evidence to show that patients who choose chelation over surgery do any better in the long run. On the other hand, there's some reasonably good evidence that chelation can help angina symptoms and poor circulation in the legs.

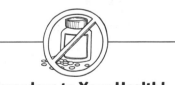

Hazardous to Your Health!

So should you try chelation? Not if your symptoms are so bad that your doctor says you need angioplasty or bypass surgery right away or in the near future.

If you're in the very early stages of heart disease, or if you're starting to have problems with the circulation to your legs, discuss chelation carefully with your doctor. It might be worth trying. Overall, chelation is pretty safe. Literally millions of chelation treatments have been given, with few complications. There's not much to show that the procedure does any harm, even if doesn't help.

There's practically no evidence that chelation will help problems like arthritis, Alzheimer's disease, or diabetes. Some chelation practitioners recommend it as a preventive treatment that helps keep you healthy. As for restoring lost youth, do you really want to go through your teenage years again?

Pregnant women and people with any sort of kidney problems or liver disease should stay away from chelation. If you have congestive heart failure, chelation must be done very carefully to avoid causing problems. It might be best to stay away—talk to your doctor first.

Self–Help Is Key

All the chelation in the world won't help your health problems unless you also take some steps to help yourself. Doctors who do chelation therapy generally take a holistic approach to their patients. They'll spend a lot of time helping you to quit smoking, cut back on alcohol, and change your diet. Because exercise can play a big part in improving heart disease and circulatory problems, your doctor will also help you work out an exercise program that's right for your condition. And because stress also plays a big role in heart disease, your doctor will help you find ways to manage it better.

Finding a Qualified Practitioner

Chelation is not exactly do-it-yourself stuff. You need to find an experienced, well-trained specialist who can help you decide whether chelation is right for you and give it to you safely. To find a doctor near you who's trained in chelation therapy, contact:

> **American College for Advancement in Medicine (ACAM)**
> 23121 Verdugo Drive, Suite 204
> Laguna Hills, CA 92653
> Phone: (800) 532-3688
> Fax: (949) 455-9679

Physicians who belong to ACAM meet high standards for training and are specialists in preventive medicine, including chelation therapy.

Rules, Rules, Rules

Although Medicare or your insurance company will probably pay the whole bill for balloon angioplasty or bypass surgery with no questions asked, there's practically no chance that chelation therapy will be covered. That's because chelation is not medically accepted as a therapy. Some state medical boards are currently trying to ban chelation therapy. Check with ACAM for the status of chelation in your state.

Just Grabbing Your Money?

Conventional doctors tend to be very down on chelation therapy. They point out that there's no published scientific evidence that chelation therapy really makes bypass surgery unnecessary and that nobody really knows the number of patients who have been truly helped by chelation.

Studies of chelation, the conventional doctors say, have been poorly designed. In particular, the studies don't compare people who receive chelation with people who have the same condition and don't get chelation. In the few studies that do, chelation doesn't hold up well. In 1987 a well-designed study in Germany gave some patients real chelation with EDTA and others fake chelation with a placebo. At the end of 20 treatments over three months, neither group of patients showed any improvement in blood flow through their narrowed arteries. A Danish study in 1992 showed that chelation didn't help intermittent claudication any better than a placebo did. The conventional doctors say that any improvement a patient feels is due to making the dietary and lifestyle changes that chelation practitioners recommend, not to the effects of the chelation.

Another thing that really disturbs conventional doctors is that nobody can really say why chelation works—if it does. They also say it's not as safe or complication-free as the believers say—although any fair-minded doctor would have to admit that angioplasty and bypass surgery are much riskier and have much higher chances of complications.

We also have to report that all these medical organizations say chelation doesn't work: the Food and Drug Administration, the American Heart Association, the National Institutes of Health, the National Research Council, the American Medical Association, the Centers for Disease Control and Prevention, the American College of Physicians, the American Academy of Family Physicians, the American College of Cardiology, and the American Osteopathic Association.

The Least You Need to Know

➤ Chelation therapy claims to help heart disease and other problems caused by poor circulation by opening clogged arteries.

➤ Chelation is said to work by removing calcium and heavy metals such as lead and mercury from your bloodstream.

➤ During chelation therapy, an intravenous infusion containing a chemical called EDTA is dripped into your arm.

➤ A typical chelation treatment takes about three hours; most patients need from 10 to 30 treatments.

➤ Believers in chelation therapy say it is a safe and noninvasive alternative to heart bypass surgery.

➤ Chelation therapy is highly controversial and is not considered effective by most doctors and insurance companies.

Chapter 9

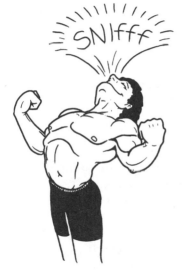

Oxygen Therapy: Airing Out Your Body

In This Chapter

➤ How your body uses oxygen to fight disease

➤ Using hydrogen peroxide therapy to treat cancer and other health problems

➤ How ozone can improve your immune system

➤ Using hyperbaric oxygen to treat brain injuries

Step outside and take a few deep breaths (check the air pollution index first). Feels good, right? That's because you're getting more oxygen—the gas every cell in your body needs to function. Getting too little oxygen is bad for you; so is getting too much. But sometimes just a little bit extra is very good for you. Believers in oxygen therapy say that getting more oxygen into your tissues can help blow away some health problems.

The Air Up There

About 20 percent of the air we breathe is made up of oxygen. Every time you take a breath, you take oxygen into your lungs. From there, the oxygen enters your blood and gets pumped around your body by your heart. But what if for some reason oxygen-rich blood isn't reaching all your tissues? According to the oxygen therapy doctors, that lets dangerous germs and fungi take hold. That's because, although all your cells need oxygen to live, a lot of other kinds of cells, like viruses and bacteria, don't. Even worse, cancer cells don't need oxygen. In fact, they thrive when oxygen levels are low—and it's possible that a shortage of oxygen at the cellular level is what gets cancer started.

Oxygen therapy promoters believe that by increasing the amount of oxygen in your cells, you can treat cancer, infectious illnesses like pneumonia, and chronic health problems like arthritis. In their view, just taking deep breaths isn't anywhere near enough.

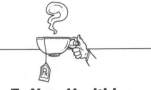

To Your Health!

Oxygen was the first chemical element to be discovered. Joseph Priestly detected oxygen way back in 1773.

You and H₂O₂

Everybody knows the chemical formula for water: it's H_2O. You might have to think back to high-school chemistry class to remember that it means each molecule of water is made up of two hydrogen atoms and one oxygen atom. If you add an oxygen atom to the molecule, then the formula reads H_2O_2, better known as *hydrogen peroxide*.

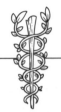

The Healing Arts

Deep breathing is a big part of meditation and yoga (we'll go into that in other chapters). According to recent research, it could soon become a big part of treating heart patients. A 1998 study in the highly regarded British journal *The Lancet* showed that teaching heart patients to breathe at a steady rate of six breaths a minute helped them breathe more slowly and easily, raised their blood-oxygen levels, and helped them be able to exercise more. Interestingly, six breaths a minute is what yoga teachers recommend for breathing exercises.

Hydrogen peroxide is a powerful disinfectant that's used in a lot of cleaning products and antiseptics. Your body naturally makes some hydrogen peroxide—you need it for a lot of normal body functions, including making hormones and the chemical messengers that tell your body what to do.

Hydrogen peroxide kills bacteria, viruses, and other harmful microorganisms. In fact, up until the 1930s, hydrogen peroxide was used both internally and externally to fight germs. With the development of antibiotics, internal hydrogen peroxide went out of style, although it's still something used externally to clean and disinfect cuts and scrapes. It works because hydrogen peroxide reacts with an *enzyme* called *catalase*, found in your blood and body fluids. Catalase splits off an oxygen atom from the hydrogen peroxide molecule, turning it into a molecule of water and a free-floating atom of oxygen. And when that free oxygen atom runs into a bacteria or virus cell, watch out! The cell is slaughtered. In addition to killing germs directly, the oxygen atoms also stimulate your immune system to make natural killer cells that also go after the bad guys.

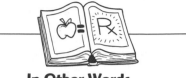

In Other Words...

Enzymes are complex chemical substances your body makes to help speed up chemical reactions in your body. One of the many, many enzymes you make is **catalase**. Its job is to break down hydrogen peroxide into water and an atom of oxygen.

Some alternative doctors today think it's time internal hydrogen peroxide came back into fashion. They claim that the free oxygen atom released by the hydrogen peroxide/catalase reaction can help all sorts of health problems, not just infections. Some even believe hydrogen peroxide can be used to treat serious illnesses such as cancer and AIDS. It's also said to help heart and circulatory problems, lung diseases such as asthma and emphysema, illnesses like flu and herpes, immune disorders such as diabetes and multiple sclerosis, and other problems like migraines. These doctors believe hydrogen peroxide works not just because it kills germs but because it releases extra oxygen into parts of your body that are starving for it.

Getting the Treatment

Don't try this at home, kids. You need a trained doctor to get hydrogen peroxide treatments, better known as *oxidative therapy*. During oxidative therapy, you get an intravenous infusion of very diluted, very pure hydrogen peroxide. The solution drips in slowly and painlessly into a vein in your arm as you lie in a comfortable lounge chair; a treatment usually takes about one to three hours and costs up to about $100. If you have a chronic illness such as angina, you'll probably need one treatment a week for up to 20 weeks. Some patients benefit from fewer treatments, while others might need as many as 50 before they notice any improvement.

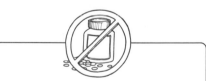

Hazardous to Your Health!

Don't try to swallow hydrogen peroxide from the drugstore. It is too strong and also contains preservatives that are dangerous.

It's also possible to drink a very diluted solution of hydrogen peroxide, but most practitioners don't recommend this—it tastes terrible and makes most patients really nauseous. Some health-food stores carry products that combine diluted hydrogen peroxide with aloe vera and flavorings. Oral hydrogen peroxide is said to be helpful for chronic degenerative diseases like arthritis. If you want to try this approach, talk to your doctor first.

Zone in on Ozone

Let's get back to a little chemistry here. About 20 percent of the air we breathe is made up of oxygen, known chemically as O_2. That little 2 means that oxygen is made of two linked atoms. If you were to add a third atom to oxygen, you'd get *ozone*, known chemically as O_3. That third atom makes ozone less stable than oxygen, so it's more likely to react with other substances around it. When that happens, the third atom zooms off, leaving behind a molecule of oxygen.

In large amounts, ozone isn't so great for you—in fact, it's one of the gasses that makes air quality bad in polluted areas. When it's used as an alternative medical treatment, though, ozone is said to be helpful for getting more oxygen into parts of your body that need it. That could help wounds heal faster and kill harmful germs, including the AIDS virus and the virus that causes hepatitis. It's also been used as an alternative cancer treatment and as a treatment for allergies, colitis, and clogged arteries.

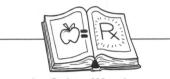

In Other Words...

Ozone is gas made up of three oxygen atoms—chemically speaking, it's O_3. It's found naturally in the air in small amounts, but it is highly reactive and breaks down into oxygen and a free oxygen atom very quickly. If you've ever noticed a sharp odor in the air just after a lightning storm, you've smelled ozone. The electricity in the lightning changes some of the oxygen in the air into ozone.

In the O-Zone

You'll need a trained doctor to get ozone into your body—this isn't for do-it-yourself types. The most common method is to use a needle to withdraw anywhere between 50 and 100 milliliters (only a few ounces) of your blood from a vein in your arm. Ozone is bubbled through the blood, and then it's put back into the vein. It sounds gross, but ozone therapy this way is pretty painless—just close your eyes if you can't stand the sight of blood.

Ozone therapy is extremely controversial. There haven't been a lot of studies to show it works, and you're more likely to have side effects. Although it claims to "cure" AIDS by killing off the HIV virus, there isn't much evidence that it does. Most doctors who do oxidative therapy prefer to use hydrogen peroxide.

Hyperbaric Treatment: It's Not Just Hype

Hyperbaric oxygen therapy (HBOT) has been part of conventional medicine for a long time. For more than a century, it's been used to treat medical problems by giving a patient oxygen at a higher pressure (hyperbaric) than normal. Usually, that means people who have carbon-monoxide poisoning, serious burns, brain injuries, and other major medical problems. It's also been shown to help wounds from surgery heal faster.

Breathing Room

Special oxygen chambers that can be pressurized to levels much higher than the atmosphere are used in HBOT. You lie on a stretcher in the sealed chamber, and oxygen is slowly pumped in until the pressure is about twice the normal pressure. You stay in the chamber, breathing in the pressurized oxygen, for anywhere from 30 minutes to a couple of hours. Then the chamber is slowly depressurized and you can come out.

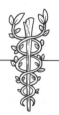

The Healing Arts

A 1998 study in Texas showed that severely brain-injured patients who had a long series of hyperbaric treatments had improved blood flow to specific areas of the brain, as well as improvements in speech and memory. Just breathing extra oxygen at normal pressure doesn't do a thing for your brain, no matter what they say at those trendy "oxygen bars."

Needless to say, HBOT isn't something you can do on your own or even at the doctor's office. HBOT chambers are found only at a few major hospitals and some military hospitals. You'd only be able to use the chamber if you had a good reason. Today there's a lot of research going on about using HBOT for helping stroke patients, people who are having radiation and chemotherapy for cancer, and people with multiple sclerosis or AIDS. In Germany and France, HBOT is already widely used to treat stroke patients. We think it will become more widely used in the United States fairly soon.

Finding a Qualified Practitioner

Oxidative therapy, whether with hydrogen peroxide or ozone, is generally safe, with little risk of complications when it's done by a trained doctor. To find a qualified physician near you, contact:

> **International Bio-Oxidative Medicine (IBOM) Foundation**
> P.O. Box 610767
> Dallas, TX 75261
> Phone: (817) 481-9772

IBOM offers training programs for physicians and supports research on oxidative therapies.

For more information on hyperbaric oxygen therapy, contact:

> **American College of Hyperbaric Medicine (ACHM)**
> P.O. Box 25914-130
> Houston, TX 77265
> Phone: (713) 528-5931
> E-mail: pgapen@aol.com

Doctors in ACHM are trained in the medical uses of hyperbaric oxygen therapy.

Rules, Rules, Rules

Right now, hydrogen peroxide and ozone therapies aren't approved by the FDA. Most insurance companies don't consider them usual and customary medical treatments and won't pay for them. Some states have restrictions on these oxygen therapies or ban them altogether—check with your state medical board or IBOM for the status in your state. Hyperbaric oxygen therapy is fairly uncommon, but the medical reasons for using it are generally understood and accepted by insurance companies. If you're getting it for an approved use, there should be no problem with coverage.

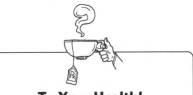

To Your Health!

Do those new oxygenated waters really improve your athletic performance and boost your energy and concentration? Don't believe the hype and company-sponsored "studies." You can't load up on oxygen the way you can on carbos—your body doesn't have anywhere to store it.

A Lot of Hot Air?

Could be. Conventional doctors point out that they stopped using hydrogen peroxide internally for infections because antibiotics work a lot better. They're skeptical that hydrogen peroxide really does anything to get extra oxygen to your tissues. And that extra oxygen atom that's supposed to kill germs is very reactive—it could just as easily damage healthy cells.

Everything the conventional doctors say about hydrogen peroxide they say double about ozone. That's because ozone therapy can have bad side effects and complications, including fainting and heart-rhythm problems. There's also absolutely no evidence that ozone "dissolves" artery-clogging deposits, helps allergies, treats cancer, or "cures" AIDS.

The Least You Need to Know

➤ Your body needs oxygen for normal functions and to keep you healthy.

➤ Oxygen therapy believers say that oxidative therapy—getting more oxygen to your cells—helps treat infections and chronic illnesses.

➤ One popular oxidative therapy is intravenous hydrogen peroxide. When the hydrogen peroxide breaks down in your body, it releases oxygen and water.

➤ Another oxidative therapy is intravenous ozone. As the ozone breaks down in your body, it releases oxygen.

➤ Hyperbaric oxygen therapy—breathing oxygen in a pressurized chamber—is an accepted medical treatment for carbon-monoxide poisoning, bad burns, and other serious problems. It has good potential as a treatment for stroke patients and brain injuries.

Part 3
Acupuncture and Energy

Some alternative treatments are hard for Westerners to grasp. Acupuncture is a good example. How can sticking tiny needles painlessly into your body possibly help anything? The Chinese explanation is that the needles release blocked energy that flows through invisible pathways in your body. Is that really why it works? We can't say, but we can tell you that an expert panel at the National Institutes of Health gave acupuncture the thumbs-up in 1997.

Acupressure, shiatsu, and reflexology all work on the same idea—releasing blocked energy. They're great self-help techniques for relaxation and minor health problems, like a headache or an upset stomach.

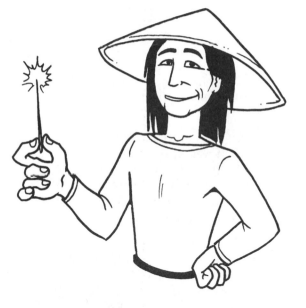

Chapter 10

Acupuncture: Getting Right to the Point

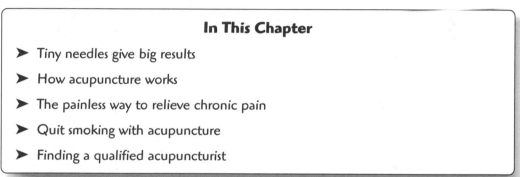

In This Chapter

➤ Tiny needles give big results

➤ How acupuncture works

➤ The painless way to relieve chronic pain

➤ Quit smoking with acupuncture

➤ Finding a qualified acupuncturist

A typical scene at the acupuncturist's office: The nervous first-time patient lies on the examining table, eyes shut, teeth clenched. After a few minutes of this, he asks, "When are you going to put the needles in?" The acupuncturist replies, "I already have."

Is acupuncture really that painless? Yes, usually. Does it really work? Yes, usually. The ancient Chinese art of acupuncture has been around for at least 2,500 years. If the needles really did hurt, or if they really didn't work, don't you think all those Chinese people would have given up on it long ago? In fact, just the opposite is happening. Acupuncture can be so helpful for so many common conditions that today it is widely accepted around the world by the medical community.

An Ancient Art: The History of Acupuncture

Nearly 5,000 years ago, the legendary Yellow Emperor of China is said to have written the first textbook of *acupuncture*. The oldest text we can really be sure about, however, dates back about 2,500 years.

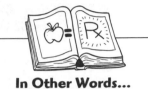

The text that is the basis for acupuncture treatment today dates back to the Ming Dynasty in China (from A.D. 1368–1640). There have been many updates since then, of course, but the basic principles of acupuncture are still the same.

Acupuncture was first introduced to Europe in the late 1600s. By the 1820s, it was widely accepted there and in the United States. By 1916, acupuncture was recommended for the treatment of severe lower-back pain by no less an authority than the great Sir William Osler, considered by many to be the founder of modern scientific medicine.

Even so, for decades, acupuncture went nowhere in the United States, in part because Cold War politics kept America and China far apart. In 1971, however, President Richard Nixon went to China, trailed by a huge entourage of reporters. One of them, James Reston of the *New York Times*, came down with appendicitis on the trip and had emergency surgery at the Anti-Imperialist Hospital in Beijing. Doctors there treated his post-operative pain with acupuncture. When Reston later praised his treatment in his regular column, it caused an explosion of interest in acupuncture.

Acupuncture Today

In 1973, the American Medical Association decided that acupuncture was an experimental medical procedure. Based on that, the Food and Drug Administration (FDA) said that acupuncture needles were experimental medical devices. Both decisions didn't do much to inspire confidence in patients—and they gave insurance companies good reasons not to cover the costs of acupuncture.

Times sure have changed. In 1996, the FDA finally reclassified acupuncture needles as Class II medical devices. In other words, acupuncture needles are now considered to be just like any other respectable medical device, like syringes, and are regulated in the same way. And in 1997, the National Institutes of Health (NIH) brought together a panel of experts to review all the evidence for and against acupuncture. The conclusion? Acupuncture works.

The Concept of Qi

Sure, acupuncture works, but why? The traditional Chinese explanation is that your *Qi*, or vital energy, flows through your *xue* (blood) and through channels in your body called *meridians*. When your meridians are blocked, your Qi backs up and overflows, just like water behind a dam. When acupuncture needles are inserted near the blocked

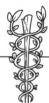

The Healing Arts

In 1979, the *World Health Organization* (WHO) of the United Nations issued a list of 41 conditions that acupuncture can treat. Included in the list are sinusitis, asthma, colitis, migraine, sciatica, low-back pain, osteoarthritis, and tennis elbow.

According to the FDA, in 1993 more than one million people in the United States received up to 12 acupuncture treatments for a total cost of about $500 million. Almost all these patients paid for the treatments themselves.

meridians, the Qi is restored to its normal flow and your symptoms are relieved. (Qi is *the* basic concept of traditional Chinese medicine—it is discussed in detail in Chapter 6, "Traditional Chinese Medicine.")

Unblocking Your Qi

Here's where acupuncture comes in. By inserting the acupuncture needles into the right points along the meridians, the Qi is unblocked, the correct flow of energy is restored, and your symptoms are relieved.

That's the traditional explanation, anyway. According to medical researchers, needling the acupuncture points seems to stimulate your nervous system and make it release *endorphins*, your body's natural painkillers. Acupuncture may also make you release other natural chemicals, such as hormones, that regulate your body and control symptoms such as pain and swelling. There's also evidence that acupuncture can stimulate your immune system.

No matter what causes it, the improved energy flow (or whatever it is) you get from acupuncture stimulates your body's natural healing abilities and puts you on the path to wellness.

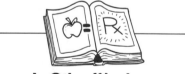

In Other Words...

In traditional Chinese medicine, **Qi** (sometimes spelled *chi* or *q'ui* and pronounced *chee*) is the vital energy of all living things—the source of all movement and change in the universe. It is invisible and flows through your **xue** (blood, pronounced *zhway*) and along a network of 12 **meridians**, or channels, to nourish your tissues. Each meridian is associated with an organ—for example, liver or kidneys.

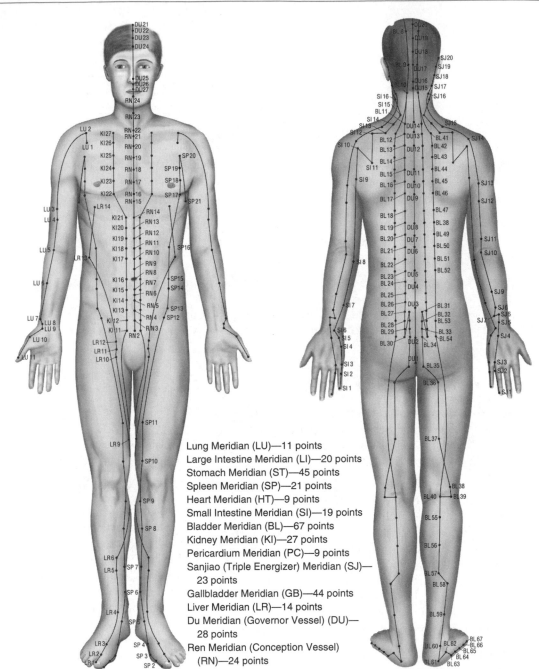

Lung Meridian (LU)—11 points
Large Intestine Meridian (LI)—20 points
Stomach Meridian (ST)—45 points
Spleen Meridian (SP)—21 points
Heart Meridian (HT)—9 points
Small Intestine Meridian (SI)—19 points
Bladder Meridian (BL)—67 points
Kidney Meridian (KI)—27 points
Pericardium Meridian (PC)—9 points
Sanjiao (Triple Energizer) Meridian (SJ)—
    23 points
Gallbladder Meridian (GB)—44 points
Liver Meridian (LR)—14 points
Du Meridian (Governor Vessel) (DU)—
    28 points
Ren Meridian (Conception Vessel)
    (RN)—24 points

Note: The first point of the Ren Meridian (RN 1) cannot be seen in this figure. It is located between the scrotum and the anus in men, and between the posterior commissure of the labia and the anus in women.

The major acupuncture meridians and points of the front and back. Additional meridians run down your sides, on your head, and on your ears.

I Really Hate Needles

Hey, nobody *likes* needles, but acupuncture needles aren't the same as the hypodermic needles your doctor uses to give you a shot or to draw blood. Hypodermics are hollow, with sharp, beveled edges and points—no wonder they hurt when they go in. Acupuncture needles are solid and very thin. You could easily put several inside a typical hypodermic. When a skilled acupuncturist inserts the needles, you generally feel just a tiny prick or sting—and many people don't feel anything at all. The pain lasts for just a few seconds during insertion. Once the needle is in place, you shouldn't feel it at all. There's almost never any bruising or bleeding from acupuncture needles.

The needles usually go in just a little way below your skin, although in some cases they are inserted deeper. Acupuncture needles vary in length from about half an inch to three inches long. Usually the shorter needles are used in bony places where your skin is thin, like your knee; longer needles are used in fleshier spots, like your thigh. (We'll talk about finding a qualified practitioner later in this chapter.)

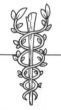

The Healing Arts

In ancient times, acupuncture needles were made of bamboo or bone. Some people today believe that needles made of gold or silver have extra power, but ordinary stainless steel seems to work just fine. You don't need to worry about infection. Today acupuncture is done with sterile stainless steel needles. The needles come in sealed packages and are thrown away immediately after use. Certified acupuncture practitioners have been carefully trained in sterile needle techniques.

The whole art and science of acupuncture lies in deciding where to insert the needles to unblock the Qi. There are more than 2,000 acupuncture points all over your body, so picking the right ones makes a difference. To decide which points to use, your acupuncturist will gently press on the part of your body where the Qi is blocked— usually the same part that hurts. The tender spots are called *ashi* points. Based on your symptoms and where the ashi points are, the acupuncturist will then decide where to insert the needles.

113

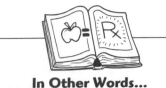

In Other Words...

Ashi points are tender spots on your body. The word comes from the Chinese words meaning "approximately right there" or "that's it." (That's why in the old movies, the Chinese detective Charlie Chan always says "Ah, so" when he stumbles across a clue.)

Generally, the needles are placed on or near where your pain is and are left in place for about 20 to 30 minutes. If your knee hurts, for example, the acupuncturist might insert up to 10 or 12 needles in and around your knee. But the meridian for your knee extends all the way down your leg to your toes. In traditional Chinese medicine, the *distal end* of the meridian—the point farthest from the pain point—must also be needled. For knee pain, then, the acupuncturist might also insert a few needles in your ankle. For back pain, the acupuncturist might put the needles into the muscles of your back and also into your ear.

What a Stimulating Idea

Once the needles are in place, they need to be stimulated to break up the obstruction in the meridian and to get the Qi flowing again. In Chinese, point stimulation is called *deQi*; in English, it's usually called *needling*.

Needling is usually done simply by twirling the needles; sometimes the needle is moved gently in and out.

Traditional acupuncturists sometimes use *moxibustion*. A small cone made from dried *moxa* leaves is placed on top of a special acupuncture needle that has a coil of copper wire wound around the top. The moxa is very carefully set on fire. The heat from the burning moxa flows down the needle. The heat is very gentle and doesn't burn you. Instead of burning moxa on a needle, your acupuncturist may use a moxa stick instead, holding it about an inch above the acupuncture point for a few minutes.

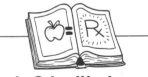

In Other Words...

DeQi (pronounced *deh chee*) is the Chinese term for stimulating the acupuncture needles once they are in place. Literally translated, it means "acquiring the Qi." **Needling**, as it is called in English, breaks up the obstruction in the meridian and lets the Qi flow smoothly again.

Today many practitioners use a device that applies a very mild electric current to the needles. Electroacupuncture is very safe—the electricity involved is no more than that from a flashlight battery. Recently some acupuncturists have been using ultrasound or very low-power laser beams to stimulate the needles, with good results. In fact, sometimes mild electrical stimulation is applied directly to the acupuncture points without using needles.

No matter what technique is used, needling produces a mild, painless sensation in the area. Most people describe the feeling as a tingling, bursting, or numbing sensation; sometimes it travels up and down the meridian. Once the needling stops, the sensation stops as well.

Can Acupuncture Help You?

The chances are pretty good that acupuncture can help you, especially if you have a health problem that causes chronic pain. Careful studies have shown that acupuncture helps chronic pain about 70 percent of the time. That's at least as good as standard pain drugs—and without the side effects.

The NIH Consensus Statement of 1997 points to two areas where acupuncture really works:

➤ Nausea, especially from chemotherapy, surgical anesthesia, and morning sickness.

➤ Dental pain, especially pain from dental surgery such as extractions.

In both cases, careful studies have shown that acupuncture is just as effective as other treatments, including drugs, but has no side effects. The NIH also says that acupuncture may be useful for treating painful muscle and skeletal problems, such as fibromyalgia, lower-back pain, and post-operative pain, and may actually be safer than the current standard treatments.

According to the NIH, acupuncture may also help these problems, especially when it's combined with standard remedies:

➤ **Osteoarthritis.** In one study of patients with severe knee arthritis, 80 percent said that acupuncture gave them lasting relief from pain and stiffness. Of the 29 patients in the study scheduled for knee-replacement surgery, seven decided against it after receiving acupuncture treatment.

➤ **Asthma and other lung problems.** Studies in Scotland show that acupuncture helps people with asthma feel better overall and need less medication. That's good, because most asthma medications have nasty side effects. The less of them you need, the better.

➤ **Headaches, including migraines.** There aren't a lot of good studies here, but many migraine patients say they have fewer severe headaches if they get regular acupuncture treatments.

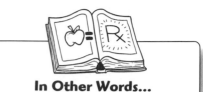

In Other Words...

To stimulate the needles, traditional acupuncturists use **moxibustion**, or heat from burning a small cone of dried **moxa** leaves on the end of the needle. Also known as **mugwort** (*artemisia vulgaris*), moxa is a traditional Chinese herb said to help promote healing.

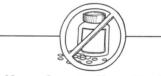

Hazardous to Your Health!

Do not use acupuncture to treat pain of unknown origin. You could delay the diagnosis and treatment of a serious underlying problem.

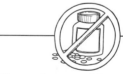

Hazardous to Your Health!

Do not stop taking your prescribed medicines while you have acupuncture treatment. If you feel that acupuncture has relieved your symptoms, discuss changing your medication with your doctor. Never stop taking your medication, and never change the dosage on your own.

115

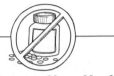

Hazardous to Your Health!

Even mild asthma is a serious health problem, because it can suddenly get much worse. If you already take medicine for asthma (even nonprescription drugs), don't stop. Talk to your doctor about changing your drugs after you have tried acupuncture.

The NIH report didn't cover some of the other problems often helped by acupuncture. Based on practical experience, however, acupuncture can be very helpful for painful nerve conditions caused by diabetes and other problems. It can also help high blood pressure, sinusitis, ringing in the ears, jaw pain, joint pain, and many other chronic conditions, especially when it's used along with standard medical treatments. Women who have severe menstrual pain have benefited from acupuncture. And some careful studies show that paralyzed stroke patients are helped by acupuncture. When acupuncture is combined with standard stroke treatment, it is effective more than 80 percent of the time.

A 1998 study showed that acupuncture reduced or even eliminated symptoms of depression in two-thirds of the patients—in other words, acupuncture worked as well as psychotherapy or antidepressant drugs.

In general, acupuncture is very helpful for physical problems related to stress. Everyone gets occasional tension headaches, but if you get them all the time, or if stress throws your digestion completely out of whack, gives you back pain, makes your asthma worse, gives you insomnia, or consistently affects you in some other physical way, you're a good candidate for acupuncture.

Acupuncture and Addiction

Today more than 300 rehab clinics across the United States use acupuncture to help people addicted to drugs and alcohol. In some cases, patients receive daily treatment for up to an hour at a time. Acupuncture doesn't cure addiction, of course, but studies show that it helps patients stay in treatment and increases their chances of becoming drug-free. Some studies claim that patients who go through rehab with acupuncture are less likely to get arrested again on a drug charge than patients who do rehab without acupuncture.

Finding Help

Acupuncture is such a fruitful area in treating addiction that there are two professional organizations devoted to it:

> **The American College of Addictionality and Compulsive Disorders**
> 5990 Bird Road
> Miami, FL 33155
> Phone: (305) 661-3474

This organization offers board certification for doctors.

National Acupuncture Detoxification Association (NADA)
3320 N Street NW, Suite 275
Washington, DC 20007
Phone: (888) 765-6232
Fax: (805) 969-6051

NADA offers literature to the general public, along with training and certification.

Stick It in Your Ear

Ear acupuncture, or auriculotherapyrapy, was developed in the 1950s by a French physician named Paul Nogier. That makes it a mere infant compared to the long history of traditional acupuncture, but auriculotherapy has been eagerly accepted by many practitioners. That's because it works really, really well for people who want to quit smoking.

The idea behind auriculotherapy is that points on your outer ear correspond to acupuncture points elsewhere on your body. By massaging or needling these points in combination with traditional acupuncture, your Qi gets an extra boost.

Kicking Butts

If you've decided to stop smoking, ear acupuncture can help you make the break. The acupuncturist will probably insert some needles into traditional points on your body, especially the *tim mee* point on your wrist. A tiny needle called a press needle or staple will also be inserted into your ear, taped into place, and left in (sometimes traditional acupuncturists use tiny seeds instead of press needles). For the next week, you'll be told to press on the needle every time you want a cigarette. The urge to smoke will pass quickly and you'll have fewer nicotine withdrawal symptoms. You'll probably need at least five sessions to stop smoking for good.

To Your Health!

You've tried—and tried and tried—to quit smoking. If other methods have failed for you, acupuncture could be the one that works. Acupuncture is completely drug-free. Unlike those expensive nicotine patches, acupuncture seems to work by reducing your desire for tobacco, not by substituting one nicotine delivery system for another.

Animal Acupuncture

Even animals can be helped by acupuncture. It's particularly valuable for older dogs, who often have arthritis in their hips or spine. Acupuncture can relieve the pain and put the wag back in their tails. Lots of horse trainers now use acupuncture to treat their valuable animals without drugs. It has even been used on dolphins!

To find a veterinarian near you who is trained in animal acupuncture, contact:

International Veterinary Acupuncture Society
2140 Conestoga Road
Chester Springs, PA 19425
Phone: (215) 827-7245

What to Expect from Your Treatment

Your first visit to an acupuncturist could easily take an hour. That's because he or she needs to understand your problem thoroughly before deciding where to place the needles. You'll be asked a lot of frank questions about your condition and your lifestyle. Some of the questions might seem a little weird—like how the wind affects your symptoms—and you might also be asked to stick out your tongue so the acupuncturist can examine it. The acupuncturist will also take your pulse the traditional Chinese way (check Chapter 6 for more information). This is all part of traditional Chinese medicine and helps the acupuncturist plan your treatment. After your first visit, your next visits will probably be shorter, usually just 20 or 30 minutes.

When you go for acupuncture, wear loose, comfortable clothes. You may need to remove some of your clothing, so wear clean underwear! Don't have a big meal, drink alcohol, exercise heavily, or have sex for at least two hours before your appointment. Leave off perfume, makeup, deodorants, and aftershave lotion; you'll also be asked to remove your watch and jewelry during the treatment.

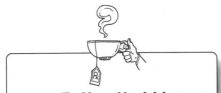

To Your Health!

A lot of patients are surprised by how relaxing acupuncture treatment is. In part, that's because of the unhurried setting and personal attention you get. Mostly, though, it's because unblocking your Qi has an overall calming effect. Try to arrange your schedule so that you can take it easy for a couple of hours after your treatment.

To get the full benefits of acupuncture, you'll probably need up to 10 weekly treatments. After your first treatment, you may actually feel worse, not better. Not to worry—this is a good sign that shows the treatment is starting to work. You'll probably start feeling a lot better after the second or third treatment. Then you'll get a little better after each of the next treatments, until after 10 or so treatments, you've made as much progress as you're likely to. To keep your symptoms from returning, most practitioners suggest having a maintenance treatment every few months.

Is It Working Yet?

Chances are good that acupuncture will help you, but there are some people who just don't respond. In fact, some well-regarded acupuncture researchers are among the 20 percent or so who aren't affected. Don't give up too soon, though. Stick with it for at least three or four sessions before you decide that it isn't working.

In general, acupuncture isn't used on babies, children, acutely ill people, or the very elderly. If you're pregnant or think you might be, be sure to tell the acupuncturist. Acupuncture can help morning sickness, but there are some points that should not be needled on pregnant women.

Finding a Qualified Practitioner

Today there are more than 7,000 highly trained acupuncturists across the country. Most are also qualified as medical doctors, osteopaths, or chiropractors; some have been trained in acupuncture as part of their overall training in traditional Chinese medicine. At a minimum, select someone who meets your state's licensing requirements and is also certified by the National Certification Commission for Acupuncture and Oriental Medicine (NCCAOM). To be certified by this group, an acupuncturist must have three years of formal training, either 4,000 hours of apprenticeship or four years of professional practice, and pass a tough exam. (Confusingly, until recently the NCCAOM was called NCCA, for National Commission for the Certification of Acupuncturists. You may still run across the old name in some materials.) As of 1998, all but three states that regulate acupuncture require NCCAOM certification. For more information and to find a qualified acupuncturist near you, contact:

> **National Certification Commission for Acupuncture**
> **and Oriental Medicine (NCCAOM)**
> 11 Canal Center Plaza
> Suite 300
> Alexandria, VA 22314
> Phone: (703) 548-9004
> Fax: (703) 548-9079
> E-mail: info@nccaom.org

Acupuncturists without medical training should always have the appropriate state licenses. The initials C.A. after a practitioner's name stand for *certified acupuncturist*; L.Ac. stands for *licensed acupuncturist*; Dipl.Ac. stands for *diplomate of acupuncture*. All are recognized degrees indicating solid training in the field, but the most common is L.Ac. The initials O.M.D., for *Oriental medical doctor*, and Ph.D., for *doctor of philosophy*, aren't recognized for the practice of acupuncture in the United States.

Another good way to find practitioners near you is to check with local pain clinics—ask your doctor or check with the American Academy of Pain Management (see Chapter 2, "Myths and Realities," and Appendix C, "National Organizations," for more information). If you have doubts about a practitioner, contact your state medical board.

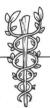

The Healing Arts

Amazingly, in most states a medical doctor can do acupuncture without any formal training in it at all. Most medical doctors seriously interested in acupuncture, however, belong to the American Academy of Medical Acupuncture. To be accepted, a physician must have at least 200 hours of training in acupuncture. For more information and to find a medical acupuncturist near you, contact:

American Academy of Medical Acupuncture
5820 Wilshire Boulevard, Suite 500
Los Angeles, CA 90036
Phone: (213) 937-5514
Fax: (213) 937-0059

Rules, Rules, Rules

The regulatory picture for acupuncture varies considerably from state to state. As of 1998, 36 states and the District of Columbia have laws or regulations controlling acupuncture. In California, for instance, practitioners must have extensive training and experience and must also pass a state examination—unless they're already physicians, in which case they can do acupuncture with no training at all. In some states, like Georgia, only physicians can practice acupuncture; in others, like Illinois, your doctor has to refer you to an acupuncturist. In a lot of states, an acupuncturist must work under the supervision of an M.D.—but here, too, the M.D. doesn't have to have any training. A few states, like Idaho, haven't gotten around to regulating acupuncture yet.

Not all health insurance policies cover acupuncture right now, so you may end up paying for your treatments yourself. To avoid an unpleasant surprise later on, check with your insurance company before you get started. Acupuncture sessions generally cost between $45 and $100.

Puncturing Acupuncture Claims

More and more doctors today grudgingly accept that acupuncture can sometimes help patients who have chronic pain, but they seriously question the whole concept of meridians full of flowing Qi and the idea that acupuncture can help problems aside from pain. They say acupuncture has no scientific basis and point out that even the

NIH panel sidestepped the Qi issue and couldn't really say how acupuncture works. It is true that acupuncture doesn't help everyone and that results are inconsistent from patient to patient. It's also true that some acupuncture studies aren't as well-designed as they should be. Even worse, some acupuncturists have made claims that don't hold up very well. Acupuncture doesn't treat AIDS (although it can help relieve some symptoms), for example, or cure cataracts or deafness. Claims of surgery being done in China with only acupuncture for anesthesia don't hold up either—it turns out that in almost all cases, drugs were also used. Some patients have been injured by improper placement of acupuncture needles or have had bad reactions, such as fainting. These cases are very rare, however, especially considering the number of acupuncture treatments—between nine and 12 million—given in the United States yearly.

The Least You Need to Know

➤ An ancient Chinese healing technique, acupuncture is now widely accepted by the medical community.

➤ Acupuncture is done by inserting very fine needles into selected points of the body to release blocked Qi, or energy.

➤ Acupuncture is virtually painless. It's very safe and has no side effects.

➤ Nausea and chronic pain respond very well to acupuncture treatment.

➤ Acupuncture is also an effective treatment for many other conditions, including asthma, nerve pain, lower-back pain, arthritis, and physical problems such as severe tension headaches caused by stress.

Chapter 11

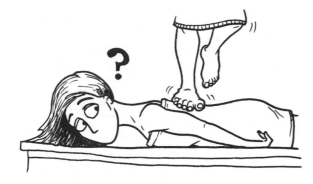

Acupressure and Shiatsu: Press On!

The last time you banged your funny bone, you probably yelped loudly and then swore colorfully. After that, you probably rubbed the spot. We don't know if the yelping and swearing helped much, but the rubbing made your aching elbow feel better. When something hurts, rubbing or pressing on it is your natural response. Take that one step further, and you have acupressure—the hands-on healing art of using pressure to relieve pain. It's a great way to let your fingers do the walking on the road to better health.

Needles Made Needless

We explained the ancient Chinese practice of *acupuncture* back in Chapter 10, "Acupuncture: Getting Right to the Point." *Acupressure* is probably even more ancient. That's because acupressure—the Chinese practice of pressing on specific *meridian* points to restore the proper flow of *Qi*—doesn't use needles of any sort. All you need for acupressure are your hands.

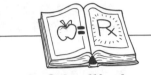

In Other Words...

Acupuncture is the insertion of very fine needles into selected parts of the skin to relieve pain and other symptoms of illness or injury. Your **Qi**, or life energy, flows through invisible pathways or channels in your body called **meridians**. **Acupressure** uses gentle but firm hand or finger pressure on points along the meridians.

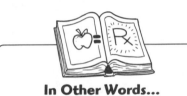

In Other Words...

An **acupoint** is a shorthand way of saying an **acupressure point**—a specific point along an acupressure meridian.

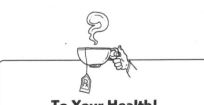

To Your Health!

All sorts of acupressure balls, bars, rollers, and other devices can be found in health-food stores and back-health stores. Do you need them? Probably not—most people find that a tennis or golf ball works just fine.

Acupuncture uses needles to stimulate specific points along your meridians to help specific symptoms. Acupressure uses gentle but firm pressure from your fingers and hands on the same points. The goal is still the same: To remove blocks in your meridians and restore the normal flow of your Qi. The difference is who's in charge. With acupressure, you're holding your health in your own two hands.

Acupressure works for many of the same health problems that acupuncture is recommended for. Because you can do acupressure on yourself, it's particularly good for stress-related problems like tension headaches, neck and back pain, depression, anxiety, and insomnia. It's also very effective for a variety of other problems, such as nausea, motion sickness, constipation, allergies, menstrual discomfort, and muscle aches.

Putting Your Finger on It

The basic techniques of acupressure are easy to learn. To massage an *acupoint*, you can use your thumb or a finger, or a knuckle, or the palm of your hand—whatever feels best. Most people use the thumb or middle finger, since these are the strongest.

To massage the acupoint, apply steady, firm, but gentle pressure directly on the point for about 30 seconds. Over the next 30 seconds or so, steadily press harder, then hold that pressure on the point for one to three minutes. Release the pressure steadily over the next 30 seconds and then move on to the next point.

For areas you can't reach yourself, such as your back, try lying on a golf or tennis ball.

You can press hard on large muscles and fleshy areas, but go easy on sensitive areas like your abdomen and face and on bony areas like your skull.

Your fingertip is a lot broader than an acupuncture needle, so you can't be as precise about exactly which point you're stimulating. Fortunately, that doesn't matter much. Acupressure works even if you're only close to the point. In general, if you're within an area about the size of the circle you make when you join your thumb and forefinger, you're close enough. On the other hand, if you're not getting any relief from pressing on a point, move your finger a little and try again.

No matter what you do, always remember one thing: Be firm. Press hard enough to make the acupoint hurt, but only in a pleasurable way. If the pressure stops feeling good and just plain hurts, ease up. A lot of acupressure is instinctive—do what feels best to you.

First Aid at Your Fingertips

There are hundreds of acupoints along your meridians, just as there are for acupuncture. We can't go into all the meridians and acupoints here—it would take another book—but we can give you some basic pointers (get it?) for helping some common minor problems:

➤ **Nausea.** This little acupressure trick is worth the cost of this book. To relieve nausea, turn your arm palm up. See those creases on your wrist? Put your thumb on the middle of your wrist two finger-widths up from the creases. Press firmly and hold for one to three minutes. Repeat again three to five times, then switch over to your other arm and do it all over again. It's amazingly effective for nausea, especially from indigestion, morning sickness, and motion sickness.

➤ **Indigestion, heartburn, constipation.** In traditional Chinese medicine, all these ailments are related to the stomach meridian. To relieve them with acupressure, sit in a hard chair with your legs bent. Measure down four finger widths along your shinbone from just below your kneecap. Place your thumb or finger just outside the shinbone at that point—you've found the right place if you feel the muscle move when you flex your foot. Press firmly for one to three minutes, then switch legs. Repeat up to three times on each leg.

➤ **Headache.** Here's another amazing acupressure trick. For a headache, pinch the web between your thumb and forefinger with the thumb and forefinger of your other hand. Squeeze for a minute, then repeat on the other hand. Repeat up to

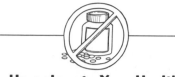

Hazardous to Your Health!

Don't use acupressure on an open wound, a swollen area, a bruise, a varicose vein, or any sort of lump. You could make the problem worse. Don't use acupressure on the abdominal area if you are pregnant.

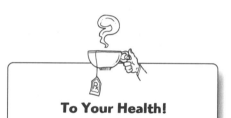

To Your Health!

If you get motion sickness, try acupressure wristbands. A wide elastic band holds a round bead tightly against the wrist acupoint. Put a band on each wrist about half an hour before your start your trip. Some women say the bands help prevent morning sickness—try sleeping with them on. You can get acupressure wristbands at drugstores and health-food stores.

125

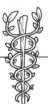

The Healing Arts

Does the mere thought of getting on a boat or airplane make your stomach queasy? Does car-sickness keep you from going on long trips? Doctors often recommend over-the-counter drugs such as dimenhydrinate (Dramamine®) or scopalamine (Transderm-Scop®) for motion sickness. Just reading the long list of who shouldn't take these drugs and their possible side effects is enough to turn your stomach. For a trouble-free trip, try the drug-free, cost-free acupressure method instead.

three times on each hand. For some reason, this works especially well for sinus headaches. If the hand trick doesn't do it, try this one: Place a finger or thumb on each side of your spine at the base of your skull. Press firmly for one minute, then relax for one minute. Repeat twice more.

➤ **Menstrual cramps.** Two acupressure points help relieve menstrual cramps. To find the first, sit in a hard chair with your legs bent. On the inside of your leg, measure up four finger widths from the top of your ankle. Press firmly on the point just inside your shinbone. Hold for one to three minutes, then do it again on the other leg. Repeat up to three times on each leg.

You can also apply acupressure to any area of your body that feels tight, tense, or achy. Gently prod the whole area with your fingertips until you pinpoint the painful spot, then apply acupressure for a few minutes. Repeat as needed, waiting a few minutes between each time.

Shiatsu: Acupressure the Japanese Way

The basic principles of traditional Chinese medicine, including acupressure, arrived in Japan about 1,500 years ago. The Japanese quickly accepted many of the ideas but gave them their own unique twist. Mostly, they used them in the Japanese form of therapeutic massage called *anma*.

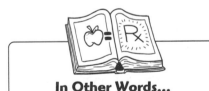

In Other Words...

Anma is an ancient form of traditional Oriental massage still practiced in Japan today. **Shiatsu** (also sometimes written *shiatzu*) is the Japanese version of acupressure. The name comes from the Japanese words *shi*, meaning "finger," and *atsu*, meaning "pressure." The acupoints themselves are called **tsubos** in Japanese.

For centuries, anma in Japan was mostly a traditional healing and relaxation treatment that used some acupressure techniques. Early in the 20th century, Japanese doctors trained in Western medicine began to combine anma with their scientific knowledge. The result was *shiatsu*, a combination therapy that literally means "finger pressure."

In its basics, shiatsu is very much like acupressure. In shiatsu, Qi (or life energy) is called *ki*. Shiatsu therapists decide where your ki is *jitsu* (overactive) or *kyo* (underactive) and then use acupressure and massage techniques to remove the blockages causing the imbalance.

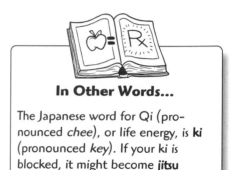

In Other Words...

The Japanese word for Qi (pronounced *chee*), or life energy, is **ki** (pronounced *key*). If your ki is blocked, it might become **jitsu** (overactive) or **kyo** (underactive).

To restore your flow of ki, shiatsu uses the same concept of meridians found in traditional Chinese medicine (see Chapter 6 for a detailed explanation). Rather than applying pressure just to specific points, however, shiatsu treats the whole meridian. That makes it a lot more vigorous than acupressure. In addition to using their fingers and thumbs, shiatsu practitioners also use their elbows, knees, and even feet to apply pressure all along the meridian. The pressure on each point is firm and rhythmic but brief, lasting only about 10 to 30 seconds. So that they can apply the maximum pressure, shiatsu therapists usually have you lie on the floor on a mat.

Like acupressure, shiatsu can be used for self-treatment, or you can visit a practitioner who can treat you and show you how to do some techniques at home.

Schools of Shiatsu Thought

The basic shiatsu concepts are used in several different methods, each slightly different from each other. Here's the rundown:

➤ **Do-in.** Pronounced *dough in*, this popular form of shiatsu is the do-it-yourself version designed to encourage overall health. It encourages the flow of ki through massaging acupressure points combined with stretching and breathing exercises. To learn how do-in works, it's best to take a class.

➤ **Jin shin.** There are several different styles of jin shin shiatsu, but the basic idea is to combine gentle finger pressure on acupoints with simple meditation techniques and deep breathing exercises. You can take classes to learn how to do it. Popular styles include jin shin do and jin shin jyutsu.

➤ **Zen shiatsu.** This is the most traditional form of shiatsu. It's based on the jitsu/kyo idea of ki flow along the entire meridian. This is not a home technique—you'll need to find a shiatsu therapist.

➤ **Barefoot shiatsu.** Some shiatsu practitioners believe that the only way to really get pressure on those points is to do it with their feet. It sounds a little kinky, but the therapists say it works.

Any shiatsu therapist can teach you some basic self-help techniques. You can also try to find a shiatsu class in your area. These are often taught at martial arts schools or alternative health centers—you might even find one at your local Y. Local massage therapists and chiropractors may be able to refer you to reputable shiatsu instructors and classes. The American Oriental Bodywork Therapy Association (see below) may be able to help you find a nearby class.

Finding a Qualified Practitioner

Many acupuncturists also offer acupressure. To find a qualified acupressure practitioner in your area, contact:

> **National Certification Commission for Acupuncture**
> **and Oriental Medicine (NCCAOM)**
> 11 Canal Center Plaza, Suite 300
> Alexandria, VA 22314
> Phone: (703) 548-9004
> Fax: (703) 548-9079
> E-mail: info@nccaom.org

This organization can refer you to a well-trained acupressure practitioner in your area. So can this group:

> **American Association of Oriental Medicine (AAOM)**
> 433 Front Street
> Catasauqua, PA 18032
> Phone: (610) 266-1433
> Fax: (610) 264-2768
> E-mail: aaom1@aol.com

To find a shiatsu therapist in your area, contact:

> **American Oriental Bodywork Therapy Association (AOBTA)**
> Glendale Executive Campus, Suite 510
> 1000 White Horse Road
> Voorhees, NJ 08043
> Phone: (609) 782-1616
> Fax: (609) 782-1653
> E-mail: AOBTA@prodigy.net

To be accepted as a certified practitioner in the AOBTA, therapists have to complete a 500-hour course taught by an AOBTA-certified instructor.

Rules, Rules, Rules

Because acupressure is basically another aspect of acupuncture, it can be done by anyone licensed to do acupuncture in your state. If you get acupressure treatments from a licensed acupuncturist, your insurance company may cover you—see Chapter 10 on acupuncture for more on this.

Right now shiatsu is another story. Although it's been officially recognized as a therapy in Japan since 1964, it barely registers on American regulatory radar screens. When it does, it comes up as a form of massage, which may or may not be regulated in your state (see Chapter 22, "Massage: There's the Rub," for more on this). If your policy covers massage therapy, you might be able to get reimbursement for shiatsu treatments, but only if the therapist is properly licensed for doing massage in your state.

Pressure as Placebo?

Not too many Western doctors buy into the traditional Chinese medicine concepts of Qi and meridians. They do know, however, that some acupressure techniques, like wristbands for motion sickness, really seem to work for their patients. The overall medical opinion seems to be that the techniques are harmless and may be helpful for relieving stress and minor aches and pains.

The Least You Need to Know

➤ Acupressure uses the same basic principles as acupuncture but substitutes finger pressure for needles.

➤ Acupressure applies gentle finger pressure to specific points of the body to help relieve pain and discomfort.

➤ Acupressure is a useful self-help treatment for minor problems such as nausea, motion sickness, indigestion, and headaches.

➤ Shiatsu is the Japanese version of acupressure. It's more vigorous than acupressure and also uses some massage techniques.

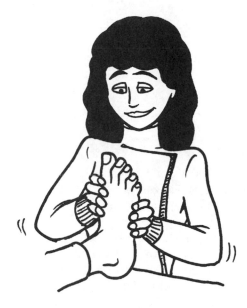

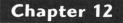

Chapter 12

Reflexology: Rubbing It In

In This Chapter

➤ How reflexology points on your feet and hands relate to other parts of your body

➤ Using reflexology to relieve PMS, insomnia, chronic pain, and other conditions

➤ How reflexology can help stimulate your body's natural healing power

➤ Relaxing with do-it-yourself reflexology

We have this theory about why some women get a reputation for being a little difficult to work with. It doesn't have anything to do with the struggle to compete in a male-dominated business environment. It has nothing to do with post-feminist ideology. It's because their feet hurt from wearing stylish but uncomfortable shoes. And anyone whose feet hurt—male or female—is automatically in a bad mood.

Fortunately for all of us, there are two easy solutions to the foot problem. First, wear good, low-heeled shoes that fit properly. Next, pay a visit to a reflexologist.

The Foot Bone's Connected to the...

Reflexology does help aching feet, but that's not its real purpose. The goal of reflexology is to help your overall health. That's because reflexology practitioners believe that

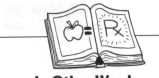

In Other Words...

Reflexology is a form of touch therapy that uses pressure on specific points of the feet (and also hands) to affect other parts of the body. Every part of your body has a corresponding **reflex point** on your feet and hands. Massaging the points releases energy blocks and stimulates your natural healing powers.

every part of your body has a matching *reflex point* at a very specific spot on your feet. By massaging the correct reflex points, the corresponding organ or body part is helped as well.

Entering the Zone Theory

Reflexology began back in 1915, when an American physician named William H. Fitzgerald noticed that when he pressed hard on certain points on someone's hands or feet, other parts of the person's body were numbed—to the point that he could insert a needle painlessly. Dr. Fitzgerald divided the human body into 10 vertical zones, five on each side of an imaginary center line running down the middle of the body. Each of the five zones on each side corresponds with the fingers and toes. The zone theory says that all zones are of equal width and extend through your body from front to back. All the parts of the body within the zone are linked to each other by energy flows. Because they're linked, anything that affects the energy flow at one point will affect the entire zone.

Dr. Fitzgerald's zone theory had a certain amount of popularity, but it didn't really single out the foot reflexes. That came in the 1930s, when a physical therapist named Eunice Ingham spent years mapping out how specific reflex points on the feet related to the zones. Today Eunice Ingham (1879–1974) is regarded as the true founder of modern reflexology. In the early 1960s, reflexology was introduced to England and then the rest of Europe. Today it is extremely popular overseas and is used even in hospitals and clinics. Reflexology is the number one alternative health therapy in Denmark.

Any sort of foot rub feels great, and reflexology does too. It's not just a massage, though—reflexology is more of a healing technique. By restoring the energy balance in

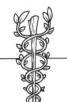

The Healing Arts

Your foot has 28 bones, 114 ligaments, 20 muscles, and more than 7,000 nerve endings. Your hand also has 28 bones. In fact, just over half the bones in your body are found in your hands and feet (you have 206 bones altogether).

your zones, reflexology is said to speed healing, eliminate toxins, and energize you. It's especially helpful for chronic pain and migraines, stress-related problems like tension headaches and insomnia, and other health problems like eczema, back pain, constipation, PMS, and menstrual discomfort.

The Reflexology Points

How does pressing on particular points on your feet help the rest of your body? Reflexology theory says that tiny crystals of calcium and uric acid, which are waste products of your body, accumulate around the reflex point. Pressing on the point breaks up the crystals, restores the energy flow in the zone, and improves circulation to the area.

In reflexology, your feet are a mirror of your body. As you can see from the foot diagrams on the following pages, the points on your feet that correspond with other parts of your body are quite specific. Your right foot matches up with the organs on the right side of your body; ditto for the left foot and left side.

In general, here's how the correspondences work:

➤ Your toes correspond to your head and neck. Think of your big toes as two halves of your head. Reflex points in your toes relate to your brain, teeth, neck vertebrae, sinuses, nose, mouth, and ears.

➤ The ball of your foot corresponds to your chest area. Reflex points here relate to your lungs, heart, esophagus, throat, and diaphragm as well as your thyroid and thymus glands.

➤ The arch of your foot corresponds to your abdominal area. The reflex points in the upper part of the arch (closer to your toes) relate to organs above your waist, including your liver, gall bladder, stomach, pancreas, spleen, and kidneys.

➤ The reflex points in the lower part of your foot's arch (closer to the heel) relate to organs below your waist, including your small intestine, appendix, large intestine, kidneys, and bladder.

➤ Your heel corresponds to your pelvic area. Reflex points here relate specifically to the nerves of the lower back.

➤ Your ankle corresponds to your reproductive organs. The reflex points here relate to your ovaries, womb, and genitals; or to your prostate and genitals.

➤ The inside part of your foot, running along the side of your foot from your big toe almost to your heel, relates to reflex points on your spine.

➤ The outer part of your foot, running along the side of your foot from your little toe almost to your heel, relates to reflex points on your joints, such as your knee, hip, elbow, and shoulder.

➤ The top of your foot corresponds to reflex points for your circulation and breasts.

1. Brain
2. Sinuses/outer ear
3. Sinuses/inner ear/eye
4. Temple
5. Pineal/hypothalamus
6. Pituitary
7. Side of neck
8. Cervical Spine (C1–C7)
9. Shoulder/arm
10. Neck/helper to eye, inner ear, eustachian tube
11. Neck/thyroid/parathyroid/tonsils
12. Bronchial/thyroid helper
13. Chest/lung
14. Heart
15. Esophagus
16. Thoracic spine (T1–T12)
17. Diaphragm
18. Solar plexus
19. Liver
20. Gallbladder
21. Stomach
22. Spleen
23. Adrenals
24. Pancreas
25. Kidney
26. Waist line
27. Ureter tube
28. Bladder
29. Duodenum
30. Small intestine
31. Appendix
32. Ileocecal valve
33. Ascending colon
34. Hepatic flexure
35. Transverse colon
36. Splenic flexure
37. Descending colon
38. Sigmoid colon
39. Lumbar spine (L1–L5)
40. Sacral spine
41. Coccyx
42. Sciatic nerve

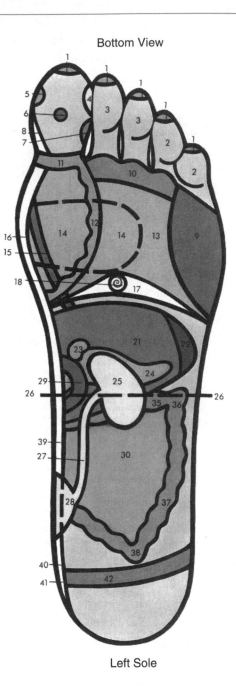

Bottom View

Left Sole

The reflex points of your feet, bottom (this page) and top (next page). Additional points are found on the sides of the feet. Charts courtesy Laura Norman, Laura Norman and Associates, (800-FEET-FIRST).

Top View

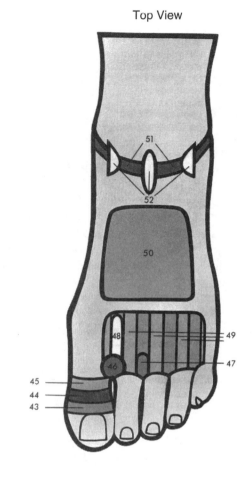

43. Upper jaw/teeth/gums
44. Lower jaw/teeth/gums
45. Neck/throat/tonsils/thyroid/
    parathyroid
46. Vocal cords
47. Inner ear helper
48. Lymph breast/chest
49. Chest/breast/mammary glands
50. Mid-back
51. Fallopian tubes/vas deferens/
    seminal vesicle
52. Lymph/groin

When a reflexology therapist presses on the points of your feet, some points may feel sore or tender. A basic principle of reflexology is the greater the tenderness, the greater the imbalance. A tender point needs more work to release the energy in the zone and restore you to balance.

Thumbs Up: Reflexology Techniques

If there's one thing a reflexology therapist needs, it's powerful thumbs. A lot of the pressure on the reflex points is applied using the thumb alone, or sometimes the thumb and index finger. No matter

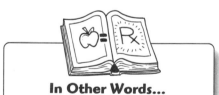

In Other Words...

Applying pressure to a reflex point is called **working the point**. According to reflexology theory, massaging the point breasks up tiny crystals of accumulated waste products, improves the circulation to the area, and restores the proper flow of energy in the zone.

how it's done, applying pressure to the reflex point is known as *working the point.*

We're going to describe the ways to work a reflex point from the point of view of doing it to someone else's feet.

Thumb and Thumber

The most basic technique in reflexology is *thumb walking.* When you do this, you "walk" your thumb along the reflex points, inching it along and pressing firmly on each point. To do the thumb walk, use your left hand (assuming you're right-handed—if you're left-handed, reverse the instructions) to gently hold the patient's foot steady. Next, lightly wrap your right hand around the foot, with your fingers against the top of the patient's foot and your thumb along the sole. Extend your thumb almost but not quite all the way and put gentle, steady pressure on the reflex point, using the tip or edge of the first joint. To "walk" your thumb, bend it slightly at the first joint, move it forward just a bit to the next reflex point, and then apply pressure again—sometimes this technique is said to take "bites" of the foot. As a general rule, you work each point at least four times before moving on to the next. Sensitive areas need more working. Finger walking is done much like thumb walking, except you use your index finger.

Thumb and finger walking take a bit of practice. When you first start, your thumb and index finger may quickly get tired and sore. Use your whole arm, not just your finger joint, when you do the walking technique. As you practice, you'll build up strength.

Pressure Techniques

Once you've mastered thumb walking, you can move on to the different ways of applying pressure:

➤ **Pressing on a point.** The most basic reflexology pressure technique. Press down firmly against the point, then release.

➤ **Rotating on a point.** Place your thumb lightly onto the reflex point and hold it in place. With your other hand, gently grasp the top of the foot and rotate the foot slightly down and forward against your thumb—in other words, instead of moving your thumb in a circular way to put pressure on the point, you're rotating the foot to do the same thing.

➤ **Hook and back up on a point.** This is a good technique for working small points and points on the toes. Place your thumb on the point and press gently. Pull your thumb back a bit, still applying gentle pressure. Your thumb should stay in place, not slide off.

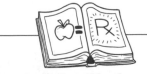

In Other Words...

Thumb walking is the most basic reflexology technique. Using your thumb, apply steady, gentle pressure to the reflex point. Then move your thumb slightly forward to the next point and apply pressure again. By applying pressure to different reflex points on your feet and hands, you affect related parts of the body.

The different pressing techniques are used to work reflex points that are sensitive. We don't have the space to go into which techniques should be used when. In general, using the thumb walk is good for fleshier areas, like the sides and balls of the feet, while the other techniques are used on bonier areas, like the toes, or for points that are quite small, like the ones for the adrenal glands.

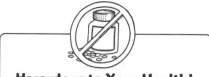

Hazardous to Your Health!

Watch out for foot problems such as corns, blisters, and the like, and stay away from those areas.

Hurting Good

Reflexology uses steady, firm, but gentle pressure on the points. Press just hard enough to make the points hurt, but only in a pleasurable way. If the person you're working on feels discomfort, ease up. You can use more pressure on fleshier areas like the ball of the foot, but be gentler on bony areas like the toes and the tops of the feet.

Amazing Feets: Do-It-Yourself Reflexology

You can easily give yourself a relaxing foot rub and work some of the reflexology points at the same time. Find a comfortable place to sit—on the floor, on the couch, or wherever you can reach your feet easily. Start by thumb walking up and down one foot from toes to heel, then switch to the other foot. Go back to the first foot and massage it again, this time working any points that seem sore and any specific reflex points that relate to any health problems you might have. Repeat on the other foot. Total time for all this? Just 10 minutes or so.

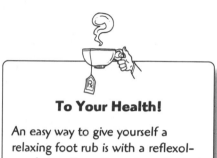

To Your Health!

An easy way to give yourself a relaxing foot rub is with a reflexology foot roller—all you have to do is move your bare feet over the roller. You can buy inexpensive foot rollers in health-food stores; they're also sold in many personal care catalogs.

Hands-Down Winner: Hand Reflexology

Your hands have reflex points just as your feet do. Reflexology therapists believe that the feet are far more sensitive and in greater need of reflexology. That stands to reason—after all, you squeeze your feet into shoes and then walk around on them all day long. According to reflexologists, that plus gravity make the toxins settle in your feet. They consider hand reflexology more of a self-care technique.

The various reflex points on your hands are pretty close to where they are on your feet. The basic techniques of working the points are the same. Because the points on your hands are smaller and closer together, you may want to use your index finger more than your thumb to work them. You might find it easier to use a golf ball to work some of the hand points, especially the ones on the fingertips.

Handy Reflexology Techniques

In the middle of a busy day at the office, it's not so easy to take off your shoes and socks (much less your pantyhose) and give yourself a reflexology treatment. Here's where hand reflexology comes to the rescue. You can do it anywhere, anytime, and it takes just a couple of minutes. Even better, you can use it to help relieve some minor problems, like a headache or upset stomach, quickly and unobtrusively. Who wants to be seen chewing an antacid in the middle of a business meeting? Use these hand techniques instead:

➤ **Headache.** Work the head, eye, and ear points. These points are on your fingers, including your fingertips, so use finger walking or a golf ball for best results.

➤ **Upset stomach.** For indigestion, try working the stomach and intestines points. These points are on the palms of your hands—use thumb walking.

➤ **Stress.** Reflexology is great for dealing with stress. Try this one if your day is getting worse by the minute: First, take a few minutes to give yourself an overall reflexology treatment on both hands. Then thumb walk up and down a few times on the spine reflexes, which are on the outer edge of your thumb, from just below the nail down to your wrist.

You may have to practice a bit to find the exact points. By working the general area of the reflex point, you'll probably find it and feel the benefits.

Finding a Qualified Practitioner

Right now, there's no national standard or certification program for professional reflexologists. Many alternative healthcare professionals have taken courses in reflexology and have a certificate to prove it, but it's really just a piece of paper that says they know the basics. Some training programs are better than others. Here are three that are said to be top-notch:

International Institute of Reflexology
5640 First Avenue North
St. Petersburg, FL 33733-2642
Phone: (813) 343-4811

Laura Norman and Associates, Reflexology Center
41 Park Avenue, Suite 8A
New York, NY 10016
Phone: (800) FEET-FIRST

Reflexology Research
P.O. Box 35820
Albuquerque, NM 87176-5820
Phone: (888) 777-9911
Fax: (505) 344-0246
E-mail: footC@aol.com

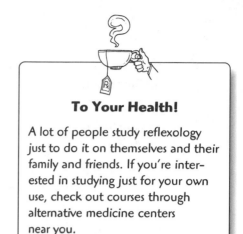

To Your Health!

A lot of people study reflexology just to do it on themselves and their family and friends. If you're interested in studying just for your own use, check out courses through alternative medicine centers near you.

To find a qualified reflexologist in your area, you'll have to ask around. Check your Yellow Pages and with local chiropractors, alternative health centers, and the bulletin board at your local health-food store.

A typical reflexology session lasts for 30 minutes to an hour. Reflexologists generally charge by the session. The rates vary quite a bit; half an hour could cost anywhere from about $20 on up to $50 or more. Hour-long sessions cost more. There's really no way to tell how helpful reflexology will be for you or how many sessions you might want to have. Reflexologists usually suggest weekly sessions, but it's really up to you.

Rules, Rules, Rules

Reflexology isn't recognized as a usual medical treatment in the United States, so you may end up footing the bill (aren't we witty?) yourself. The exception might be if the reflexology is done by a licensed medical professional in another area, like a chiropractor, acupuncturist, naturopath, or massage therapist (if your policy covers their services). Check with your insurance company to be sure.

Right now reflexology isn't a separately licensed profession, and the certificates given by training programs don't have any legal status. In some states, reflexology still seems to be below the watchdog radar screens and there are no rules. In other states, you need to have a massage license to do reflexology. In part, that's because some unscrupulous characters say they offer "foot massages" when they really offer sex for sale. To find out where your state stands, contact the state medical licensing board.

Reflexology or Foot Rub?

Medical types scoff at the idea of zones and reflex points, saying there's no proof that they even exist. The few serious studies of reflexology haven't shown that it does anything more than massage your feet. A nice foot rub is always relaxing and pleasurable, but from a medical standpoint, it has no therapeutic value.

The Least You Need to Know

➤ Reflexology is a touch therapy that uses pressure on specific points on the feet and sometimes hands to remove energy blockages and restore balance to the body.

➤ Specific reflex points on your feet and hands correspond to specific parts of your body. By pressing on the points, reflexology helps related health problems.

➤ Reflexology is very helpful for problems such as chronic pain, eczema, back pain, and PMS. It is also very helpful for stress-related problems like tension headaches and insomnia.

➤ Do-it-yourself foot and hand reflexology can help relieve minor problems like indigestion and headaches and is also good for overall relaxation.

Part 4
Homeopathy and Herbs

How can a tiny dose of something that's a poison in big doses help you? See our chapter on homeopathy—one of the safest and easiest alternative treatments—for the answer. Flower essences, a form of homeopathy, are growing (get it?) in popularity— they're a wonderful way to deal with problem emotions.

Traditional herbal medicine uses the healing herbs of Europe and the Americas to treat health problems the gentle, natural way—inexpensively and without the side effects and chance of addiction of prescription drugs. For a more sophisticated approach to herbal medicine—but one you need a trained herbalist to use—try traditional Chinese herbs. A typical Chinese herbal remedy uses at least six different herbs!

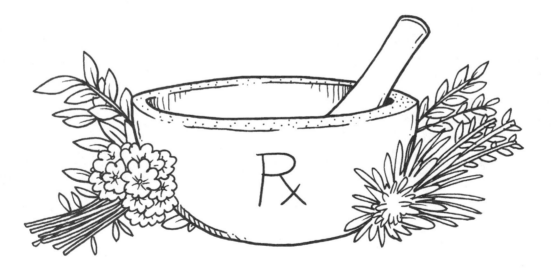

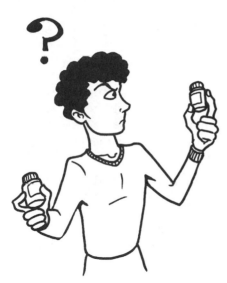

Homeopathy: Let Like Cure Like

In This Chapter

➤ The history and theory of homeopathic medicine

➤ How homeopathy helps allergies, chronic illness, pain, and other problems

➤ The top homeopathic remedies

➤ Your homeopathic constitutional type

➤ Your homeopathic medicine kit

Two hundred years ago, medical treatments were pretty awful. The doctors of the time believed that the more drastic the remedy, the better it worked. At the very least, they gave you medicines that tasted just awful. If that didn't work, they bled pints of blood from your veins, gave you powerful drugs made from mercury and lead that caused severe vomiting and diarrhea, or rubbed on ointments that blistered your skin. They never bothered with little details like washing their hands or sterilizing their instruments. They managed to kill a lot of their patients. Those who survived usually got better in spite of their doctor, not because of him.

Dr. Hahnemann's Experiments

Medical treatment in the late 18th century was so awful that a well-known German doctor named Samuel Hahnemann gave up on it and devoted himself to research instead. In the 1790s, Dr. Hahnemann was doing an experiment on himself with a drug called cinchona (what we today call *quinine*) that was used to treat malaria. When he took the drug, he got the same sort of fever that someone with malaria gets. When he stopped taking the drug, the fever stopped as well. Hahnemann reasoned that if taking a big dose of cinchona gave a healthy person the same symptoms as malaria, someone who really had malaria might benefit from a small dose. The idea was that the small dose would stimulate the sick person's body to fight the disease.

Dr. Hahnemann tested his breakthrough idea on himself, a process he called a *proving*. He then tested it on some friends and family members. Over the next six years, Hahnemann went on to do many more provings with other common medicines of the time, like belladonna.

Based on the provings, Hahnemann went on to test his remedies on sick people. He studied their symptoms and treated them with the remedy that most closely matched. The idea was that the drug, by closely mimicking the symptoms of the disease, would somehow cancel it out.

Hahnemann called his new medical system *homeopathy*, meaning "similar suffering." Homeopathy is a powerful method for stimulating your body's own healing process. Homeopathy is based on three essential principles.

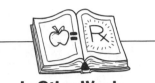

In Other Words...

Homeopathy is a holistic medical system that uses very, very tiny doses of drugs to produce symptoms similar to the illness. The remedies stimulate your natural healing powers. The word comes from the Greek *homeo*, meaning "similar" or "the same," and *pathy*, meaning "suffering" or "illness." **Provings** are the tests Dr. Hahnemann did to discover the effects of various drugs.

The Law of Similars

The most fundamental idea in homeopathy is "like cures like." (If you want to impress your friends, say it in Latin: *Similia simibilus curentur*.) A remedy that produces the same symptoms as the illness counteracts it and cancels it out. In homeopathic theory, this is known as the *Law of Similars*.

Less Is More

Drugs like arsenic are poisonous, so Dr. Hahnemann used them in very, very small doses. In addition, he prepared the remedy by *succussing* it—repeatedly shaking it vigorously and banging it down on a hard surface. Succussing the remedy is said to release the energy in the drug.

To his surprise, Hahnemann found that the more dilute the drug was, the more potent it was and the better it worked. In homeopathy, then, *potency* means the dilution of the remedy. Paradoxically, the more dilute the remedy is, the more potent it is. In homeopathic theory, this is known as the *Law of Infinitesimal Doses*.

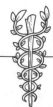

The Healing Arts

The concept of like cures like is the basis of vaccination. By giving you a very tiny amount of the disease organism—the polio virus, for example—the vaccine stimulates your body to create the antibodies that make you immune. Like cures like is also the basis for allergy shots. By giving you small amounts of what you're allergic to, the shot desensitizes you to it.

Treat the Patient

Most important of all, Dr. Hahnemann believed that you had to treat the patient, not the disease. Every patient is unique, so every illness is unique as well. A remedy that works for one patient might have no effect on another, even if their illnesses are similar. If that sounds familiar, it's because it comes up in every chapter of this book—it's the basis of all holistic medicine. As we'll discuss a little further on, Dr. Hahnemann believed that every person has a constitutional type that matches up with one of the most common homeopathic remedies.

Tiny Doses, Big Results

Today homeopathy is more popular than ever—sales of homeopathic remedies in the United States top over $200 million a year. A major reason is that the remedies are safe and nontoxic, with no side effects. They can be used by anyone, even babies and the elderly, and it's impossible to overdose on them. The remedies can be used by themselves to treat minor problems. For more serious medical problems, homeopathic remedies can complement standard treatments.

Homeopathy can be used to treat almost anything, but it seems to be particularly effective for chronic conditions and mysterious ailments that don't respond well to the usual medical treatments. Here's a rundown:

➤ **Allergies.** Many patients claim that homeopathic remedies have helped their allergies, especially hay fever.

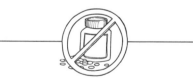

Hazardous to Your Health!

Do not use homeopathic remedies to treat a medical emergency. If you need to take medicine for a health problem, don't stop. Homeopathic remedies are safe to use with any medication you may need.

➤ **Skin problems.** Rashes, eczema, and psoriasis are often helped by homeopathic remedies.

➤ **Headaches.** All sorts of headaches, including migraines and tension headaches, can be helped with homeopathy.

➤ **PMS.** A lot of women say homeopathy helps relieve premenstrual symptoms, especially fatigue and irritability.

➤ **Colds and flu.** Homeopathic remedies help relieve the annoying symptoms of a cold or flu and may help you get over it faster.

➤ **Stress.** Stress symptoms, like insomnia, irritability, and depression, respond well to homeopathic remedies.

➤ **Chronic fatigue syndrome.** Some CFS patients say homeopathic remedies help.

Another good reason for homeopathy's popularity today is that you can often treat yourself. If you've matched up your ailment with the right remedy, you'll feel better. And if you've goofed, no problem—the remedy won't necessarily work, but it won't hurt you. Be careful about this, though. Taking the wrong remedy might cause additional symptoms over time. In general, if a remedy doesn't help within a couple of days, it's the wrong one. Try something else.

How Remedies Are Made

To make a homeopathic remedy, the manufacturer starts with the basic plant or mineral (or sometimes animal). In general, plant and animal raw materials are finely chopped and then soaked in a mixture of about 80 percent pure alcohol and 20 percent pure water for several weeks. Minerals are ground very finely and soaked in the alcohol mixture.

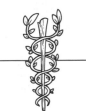

The Healing Arts

A homeopathic remedy with 3c potency contains one drop of the remedy for one million drops of the alcohol/water mixture. That's not very much. After the mother tincture has been diluted beyond 12c, it probably doesn't contain even one molecule of the original material. The remedies are said to work anyway. Why? Because of the succussing, say the homeopaths, the liquid "remembers" the energy pattern of the remedy. That's enough to make your own healing mechanisms kick in.

To make the remedy, the solids are strained out. What's left is the alcoholic liquid, called the *mother tincture*. The next step is to dilute the mother tincture with a mixture of alcohol and water. Homeopaths use two different dilution scales:

➤ **The decimal scale.** In this scale, the dilution is one in 10, or 1:10. In other words, for every drop of the tincture, nine drops of an alcohol/water mixture are added. Homeopaths use the abbreviation *x* to indicate a remedy made using the decimal scale.

➤ **The centesimal scale.** Remedies made using this scale are diluted to one in 100, or 1:100. For every drop of the tincture, 99 drops of an alcohol/water mixture are added. The abbreviation *c* is used to indicate that the centesimal scale was used.

After each dilution is made, the mixture is succussed (shaken vigorously). Then one drop of the mixture is added to the next dilution (either decimal or centesimal), and the mixture is succussed again. At the least, homeopathic remedies are diluted three times. The number of dilutions and the scale used are written on the label after the remedy name. So a label that reads *Aconite 3c* means that it has been diluted and succussed three times.

The usual remedy strengths for home use are 6c and 12c; 30c, the most potent strength, generally is used only by professionals.

Once the mother tincture is dilute enough, it can be bottled to be used in liquid form, or it can be made into pills. A few drops of the remedy are added to tiny lactose (milk sugar) pills; the pills are sometimes also swirled around in the dilution for a few seconds as well.

Basic Homeopathic Remedies

In his lifetime, Dr. Hahnemann did about 100 provings. Since then, other researchers have added more homeopathic remedies, to the point that today there are well over 1,000. In practice, though, only about 30 are commonly used, while another 100 or so are minor remedies used occasionally. Homeopaths disagree as to exactly which are the top 30 remedies, but we think the following table is a good starting point.

We can't go into the details of all the remedies here. That would take volumes—and even professional homeopaths refer to standard reference books called *repertories* or *materia medica*. (Up-to-date practitioners use computerized databases.) There are many, many outstanding books about

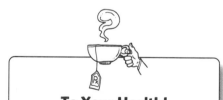

To Your Health!

Homeopathic remedies are usually taken as pills, but you can get them as liquids, powders, and granules. Whichever form you choose, keep the remedy tightly sealed in a cool, dark place away from direct sunlight.

homeopathy at any good bookstore. We recommend two by Dana Ullman, one of the leading homeopaths in the United States: *Discovering Homeopathy* and *Everybody's Guide to Homeopathic Medicines*.

Thirty Most Common Homeopathic Remedies

Remedy	Uses
Aconite	Sudden infections, fear, shock, burning pain
Allium	Burning pain, hay fever, colds, earaches
Apis	Burning pain, insect stings, fever, rashes
Argent. nit.	Anxiety, fear, digestive upsets from sweet foods
Arnica	Bruises, pain, shock, sore muscles, sprains
Arsen. alb.	Anxiety, fear, digestive upsets, burning pain helped by heat
Belladonna	High fever, migraines, flu
Bryonia	Coughs, flu, severe headaches, swollen joints
Calc. carb.	Bone and joint pain, fear, anxiety
Cantharis	Burns, stings, bladder problems
Ferrum phos.	Fever, coughs, colds, headaches, earaches
Gelsemium	Headaches, fever, eyestrain, colds, flu, phobias
Graphites	Skin problems, rashes, eczema, stomach ulcers
Hypericum	Nerve pain, shooting pains, back pain, wounds
Ignatia	Emotional problems, headaches, coughs
Ipecac	Nausea, vomiting
Kali bich.	Heavy colds, sinus problems, joint pain
Lachesis	Circulatory problems, PMS, menopause
Ledum	Cuts, scrapes, prevents wound infection
Lycopodium	Digestive upsets, kidney problems, bladder problems, prostate enlargement
Merc. sol.	Sore throat, laryngitis, mouth sores, gum disease
Nux vomica	Insomnia, digestive upsets, colds, flu
Natrum mur.	Grief, colds, wet coughs, gum disease
Phos.	Fear, anxiety, digestive upsets, circulatory problems, respiratory problems, burning pain
Pulsatilla	Digestive upsets from rich food, depression, gynecological problems, sinusitis
Rhus tox.	Poison ivy, rashes, eczema, arthritis
Ruta grav.	Bruises, muscle aches, sciatica
Sepia	Gynecological problems, PMS, menopause, exhaustion
Silica	Skin problems, frequent infections
Sulfur	Skin problems, eczema, stress, gynecological problems, digestive upsets

Homeopaths usually refer to remedies by their abbreviations. To help you understand the abbreviations for the major remedies and what they stand for, we've done another chart. And don't worry about taking a remedy that has snake venom, mercury, or other poisonous substances in it. The remedies are so dilute that you could take hundreds of pills at once and still not be harmed.

Homeopathic Abbreviations

Abbreviation	Stands For
Aconite	*Aconitum napellus* (monkshood)
Allium	*Allium cepa* (onion)
Apis	*Apis mellifica* (honeybee)
Argent. nit.	*Argentum nitricum* (silver nitrate)
Arnica	*Arnica montana* (sneezewort)
Arsen. alb.	*arsenicum album* (arsenic)
Belladonna	*Atropa belladonna* (deadly nightshade)
Bryonia	*Bryonia alba* (bryony root)
Calc. carb.	*calcarea carbonica* (calcium carbonate)
Cantharis	*Cantharis vesicatoria* (Spanish fly)
Ferrum phos.	*ferrum phosphoricum* (iron phosphate)
Gelsemium	*Gelsemium sempervirens* (yellow jasmine)
Graphites	graphite
Hypericum	*Hypericum perforatum* (St. John's wort)
Ignatia	*Ignatia amara* (Ignatia plant seeds)
Ipecac	*Cephaelis ipecacuanha* (ipecac root)
Kali bich.	*kali bichromium* (potassium bichromate)
Lachesis	*Lachesis mutus* (bushmaster snake venom)
Ledum	*Ledum palustre* (wild rosemary)
Lycopodium	*Lycopodium clavatum* (club moss)
Merc. sol.	*mercurius solubilis* (mercury)
Nux vomica	*Strychnos nux-vomica* (Quaker buttons)
Natrum. mur.	*natrum muriaticum* (rock salt)
Phos.	phosphorus
Pulsatilla	*Pulsatilla nigricans* (wind flower)
Rhus tox.	*Rhus toxicodendron* (poison ivy)
Ruta grav.	*Ruta graveolens* (rue)
Sepia	*Sepia officinalis* (cuttlefish)
Silica	*silicea terra* (quartz)
Sulfur	sulfur

Taking Your Medicine

Experienced homeopaths recommend matching your symptoms to the remedy as closely as possible and using only one remedy at a time. To get the most from your remedy, follow these guidelines:

➤ Don't touch the remedy with your hands. For liquids, use the dropper to put a drop on your tongue. For pills, use a teaspoon to put a pill directly on your tongue.

➤ Take the remedy by itself, without food or water. Wait at least half an hour after eating before taking it.

➤ Avoid coffee, mint, and spicy foods while you're taking a homeopathic remedy. Also stay away from perfumes and scented products.

➤ Homeopathic remedies can be used along with herbal treatments and even medical drugs.

➤ Doses vary considerably, depending on the problem. Often the dose is one pill three times a day, but for acute problems like migraines, the dose might be one pill every half hour for up to six or 10 doses.

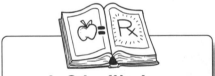

In Other Words...

An **aggravation** is a temporary worsening of your symptoms from taking a homeopathic remedy. Aggravations happen when your body's healing powers start working. They make you feel worse for a few hours, but after that, you'll probably start to feel a lot better.

Homeopathic remedies should be taken only as needed and for the shortest possible time. Stop taking them as soon as you feel better.

Sometimes taking a homeopathic remedy seems to make your symptoms worse for a few hours or even a day. This is called an *aggravation*, and it's perfectly normal, according to homeopathic theory. The aggravation is actually a sign that your body's natural healing mechanisms are being activated. If you have an aggravation, stop taking the remedy and let your body do its work. Start taking the remedy again if the symptoms come back.

If your problem doesn't improve or go away within a few days, or if gets worse, it's possible you're taking the wrong remedy. It's also possible that you need standard medical attention—call your doctor, especially if you have a chronic health problem like heart disease or diabetes.

A Mixed Bag: Using Homeopathic Formulas

Although homeopaths suggest taking only one remedy at a time, that's not always a practical approach. You might not be able to diagnose the problem or pinpoint your symptoms that well. That's why combination remedies are useful for some problems.

There are many different formulas from a lot of different manufacturers, and new products come out all the time. The formulas vary—read the labels, then try them and see if they help you.

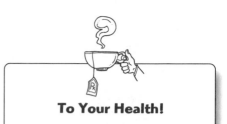

Tissue Salts

Back in the 1870s, Dr. Wilhelm Schussler, a German physician, decided that many health problems were caused by a lack of certain minerals in the body. Schussler believed that each deficiency had a particular set of symptoms. He took the homeopathic approach to treating the deficiency, using tiny amounts of 12 different biochemic tissue salts, or *Schussler salts*, as they came to be called. In addition to the individual salts, Schussler recommended some specific combinations of several salts for some problems.

To Your Health!

The most popular cold and flu medicine used in France today is a homeopathic remedy called **Oscillococcinum**. It's becoming very popular here as well. It works best if you start taking it as soon as symptoms begin. **Calms Forte** is a popular homeopathic tranquilizer. It's said to relieve tension and insomnia.

He gave the combinations imaginative names like *Combination H* and *Combination R*. Check your health-food store for Schussler salts. Directions on how to use them are on the label; information about Schussler salts is found in all good books on homeopathy.

Constitutional Issues

In homeopathic theory, your *constitutional type* is very important. That's because each constitutional type has a different weak area and reacts differently to illness. If you are an argent. nit. type, for example, you tend to get stomach upsets and generally feel better when cool. If you're an ignatia type, you tend to get depressed and usually feel better when warm. Each type might respond differently to the same homeopathic remedy.

To choose the right remedy for your health problem then, you need to know which constitutional type you are. The types are based on your physical makeup and also your personality and temperament—even things like the foods you like to eat and the things you fear are taken into account. Since every one of the 100 or so major homeopathic remedies has a matching constitutional type, we can't go into all of them here, but we can take a closer look at the two examples we've already given: argent. nit. and ignatia.

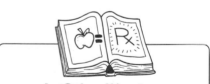

In Other Words...

In homeopathic theory, everybody has a **constitutional type** that matches up with a homeopathic remedy. Your constitutional type is based on your body type, your personality, and your basic temperament.

Argent. nit.

Appearance	Pale complexion, premature wrinkles, deep-set eyes
Personality	Extroverted, emotional, tends to worry a lot
Foods	Likes salty and sweet foods; upset by cold foods
Fears	Heights, failure, being late
Better	Cool, fresh air
Worse	Warmth, at night, under stress
Weak areas	Nerves, stomach, intestines, eyes, left side of body

Ignatia

Appearance	Thin, dark-haired, usually women
Personality	Sensitive, high-strung, perfectionist, moody
Foods	Likes sour foods, dairy, bread; dislikes sweet foods, fruit, alcohol
Fears	Emotional hurt, losing control, crowds
Better	Warmth, eating, changing position
Worse	Cold, stress, touching
Weak areas	Mind, nervous system

Constitutional types aren't exact—hardly anyone is strictly one type, and there's often some overlap. Whatever your type, you'll generally respond well to that homeopathic remedy. In other words, if you're a silica type, taking silica will usually help you. If you're more of an overlap sort, you'll respond well to all the remedies that are right for your types.

Your Homeopathic First-Aid Kit

To deal with minor, everyday health problems like insect bites, heartburn, colds, and the like, you need only about 10 homeopathic remedies. Let's take a closer look:

Aconite	For fevers, colds, and flu; also useful for panic attacks.
Apis	This one's actually made from bees. It soothes insect bites and stings and also helps hives and rashes.

Arnica	In cream form, arnica soothes sore muscles, bumps, and bruises—but don't use it on broken skin. Probably the most popular homeopathic remedy among athletes.
Arsenicum	Helpful for nausea, vomiting, and diarrhea.
Belladonna	Good for sore throats, headaches, earaches, and fevers.
Carbo. veg.	Helpful for heartburn, gas, bloating, and stomach upsets, especially from overeating.
Hypericum	In cream or ointment form, hypericum relieves pain and infection in cuts, scrapes, stings, and so on. Taken internally, it's helpful for nerve pain and backaches.
Nux vomica	Very helpful for motion sickness; also good for hangovers.
Ruta	Relieves pain from joint and muscle sprains and strains.
Rhus tox	Take for poison ivy rashes, sprains, and strains.

For emergency or first-aid use, homeopathic remedies are usually taken frequently. To treat motion sickness with nux vomica, for instance, you would take one 6c pill every 15 minutes, for up to 10 doses. Homeopathic first-aid kits for home use are sold in health-food stores. They usually contain anywhere from 10 to 30 remedies, along with a reference chart or booklet.

Homeopathy for Your Pet

Any animal—your dog, your cat, your horse, your bird, even your hamster—can be treated homeopathically. Homeopathy has become very popular for treating valuable horses and show dogs, because any drug that might affect their performance is forbidden at racecourses and show rings. According to veterinary homeopaths, homeopathic remedies can help chronic problems like itchy skin, arthritis, and poor digestion. They're also helpful for some behavior problems and for preventing motion sickness.

Finding Homeopathic Remedies

Homeopathic remedies have become so popular that today you can find at least some in any drugstore. For a wider selection and a broader range of manufacturers, try a well-stocked health-food store. Homeopathic remedies and kits are sold through dozens of mail-order catalogs. You can also purchase remedies straight from the manufacturers. Some major suppliers in the United States follow:

Boiron
Six Campus Boulevard
Newton Square, PA 19073
Phone: (800) BLU-TUBE

Capitol Drugs, Inc.
8578 Santa Monica Boulevard
West Hollywood, CA 90069
Phone: (800) 858-8833

Dolisos America, Inc.
3014 Rigel Avenue
Las Vegas, NV 89102
Phone: (800) 365-4767

Hickey Chemists
888 Second Avenue
New York, NY 10017
Phone: (800) 724-5566

Nature's Way Products
10 Mountain Springs Parkway
Springville, UT 84663
Phone: (801) 489-1520

Finding a Qualified Homeopath

Who exactly is qualified to practice homeopathy is a little confusing. Strictly speaking, only someone who's medically trained can offer homeopathy as a medical treatment. In fact, a lot of open-minded medical doctors, osteopaths, chiropractors, acupuncturists, nurse practitioners, and dentists now use homeopathy in their treatments. The problem is that there really isn't a good national training standard. Some practitioners just go to a few weekend seminars or even do a home-study course, while others study homeopathy seriously for years. No diploma or certificate alone from any school or program is recognized as a license to practice homeopathy in the United States.

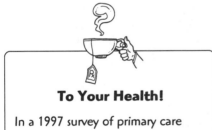

To Your Health!

In a 1997 survey of primary care doctors belonging to the American Medical Association, nearly half were interested in getting trained in homeopathy.

To help you sort it out, we've listed major independent organizations that set a high standard for their members. All require their members to complete a minimum number of training hours and to pass an exam.

To become certified as a homeopathic specialist, medical doctors can take a stiff exam sponsored by:

American Board of Homeotherapeutics
801 North Fairfax Street, Suite 306
Alexandria, VA 22314
Phone: (703) 548-7790
Fax: (703) 548-7792

Doctors who pass the test can put the letters D.Ht., meaning Diplomate in Homeotherapeutics, after their name.

Naturopathic physicians can take a certifying exam given by:

Homeopathic Academy of Naturopathic Physicians
12132 SE Foster Place
Portland, OR 97266
Phone: (503) 761-3298
Fax: (503) 762-1929
E-mail: hanp@igc.apc.org

Many well-trained homeopaths aren't medically trained. To find a qualified homeopath—medically trained or not—near you, contact the main national organization:

National Center for Homeopathy
801 North Fairfax Street, Suite 306
Alexandria, VA 22314
Phone: (703) 548-7790
Fax: (703) 548-7792
E-mail: nchinfo@igc.apc.org

You can also get a referral to a homeopath near you from:

International Foundation for Homeopathy
2366 Eastlake Avenue East, Suite 325
Seattle, WA 98102
Phone: (425) 776-4147
Fax: (425) 776-1499

The Council for Homeopathic Certification offers a certificate to anyone who passes its tough exam. The certificate doesn't have any legal status, but it does show that someone has a fairly high level of homeopathic knowledge. People who've passed the exam can put the letters C.C.H., for Certified in Classical Homeopathy, after their name. For more information, contact:

Council for Homeopathic Certification
1199 Sanchez Street
San Francisco, CA 94114
Phone: (415) 789-7677

The National Board of Homeopathic Examiners is a certifying organization for graduates of accredited homeopathic training programs. Again, the certificate doesn't have any legal status. For more information, contact:

National Board of Homeopathic Examiners
5663 NW 29th Street
Margate, FL 33063
Phone: (954) 420-0669

Not all experienced homeopaths belong to national organizations. A good way to find someone in your area is to ask for referrals from local alternative health practitioners; you can also check the Yellow Pages and with your local health-food store.

Learning More

Once you start learning about homeopathy, it can be hard to stop—it's a very complex, very interesting subject. Right now there are at least eight homeopathic colleges or institutes across the United States offering training courses. If homeopathy intrigues you but you don't want to take formal courses, you can look into a study group or a home-study course. The National Center for Homeopathy (see the preceding section) can help you find a training program or study group in your area. For an outstanding collection of books and resource materials on homeopathy and for information on correspondence courses, contact:

Homeopathic Educational Services
2124 Kittredge Street
Berkeley, CA 94704
Phone: (510) 649-0294
Fax: (510) 649-1955
E-mail: mail@homeopathic.com

A Visit to the Homeopath

When you visit a professional homeopath, the first step is to determine your constitutional type. That usually means a long discussion—an hour or more—about your basic personality, your food preferences, your fears, and general characteristics, like when you feel best and worst over the course of the day. You'll also be asked to describe your symptoms in great detail. Professional homeopaths usually prefer to prescribe just one remedy at a time, so they'll want to be sure of your homeopathic constitution. The main remedy will be the one that most closely matches your overall constitution. You'll probably need some follow-up visits that will be shorter, taking maybe 15 or 30 minutes.

Because your first visit will be a long one, the charge may be a bit higher. Homeopaths who are licensed medical professionals charge just as any professional does. A typical first visit could cost anywhere from $100 to $300. Follow-up visits cost less. The remedies themselves are very inexpensive, rarely costing more than $10 and usually less.

Rules, Rules, Rules

In a lot of countries, like India, Germany, and France, homeopathy is very popular and is widely used, even in hospitals. In England, homeopathy has been covered by the national health system since 1950. The situation is very different in the United States. Although homeopathy is getting more popular all the time, relatively few health-care professionals use it. The remedies themselves are regulated by the FDA just as vitamins and herbs are, but they're not considered drugs, and the FDA has no position on how effective they are.

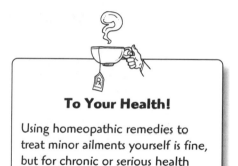

To Your Health!

Using homeopathic remedies to treat minor ailments yourself is fine, but for chronic or serious health problems, we suggest the advice of a professional homeopath.

The licensing picture is pretty confusing. As we've already mentioned, there are a lot of organizations that offer some sort of certification, but that's not the same as being licensed to practice homeopathy. Technically speaking, someone who prescribes homeopathic remedies to another person is practicing medicine and needs to be licensed in some way. But how do you license someone who recommends over-the-counter remedies? In a lot of states, only medically licensed professionals like medical doctors, osteopaths, naturopathic physicians, chiropractors, and acupuncturists can formally practice homeopathy. In some states, other licensed healthcare professionals, like physician's assistants and registered nurses, can prescribe homeopathic remedies. The laws vary quite a bit from state to state though, so check with your state medical board first.

Your health insurance company will probably cover homeopathy if it's provided by a licensed medical doctor, osteopath, chiropractor, acupuncturist, or naturopath. If it's provided by anyone who's not a licensed professional, you're probably not covered. Because homeopathic remedies are sold over the counter without a prescription, they're not usually covered by insurance.

To Your Health!

Three states do have homeopathic licensing laws: Arizona, Connecticut, and Nevada. Any physician practicing homeopathy in those states has to be licensed by the state homeopathy licensing board.

Some unscrupulous practitioners use "electrodiagnosis" with impressive-looking devices that are said to measure energy imbalances. Stay away—these devices are fraudulent.

Is Anything Really There?

Most homeopathic remedies contain no detectable amounts of the active ingredients. That certainly makes it hard to prove that the remedies have any effect at all. Scientists, physicians, and other health practitioners point out that since the remedies don't actually have anything in them, any benefit you get is strictly a placebo effect—you think it's helping you, so it does. Homeopaths counter by saying the liquid in the tincture used to make the remedy "remembers" the energy pattern and somehow transmits this to you when you take the remedy. They claim that this idea was proven in a scientific study by a French homeopath named Jacques Benveniste back in 1988. There are two problems with this idea, though. First, how does the lactose pill "remember" the energy after the water evaporates? Second, nobody—not even other homeopaths—has ever been able to reproduce the results Benveniste claimed in the 1988 study.

Homeopathic believers often say that scientific studies show that homeopathy works. They cite a handful of scientific papers that have appeared in prestigious medical journals such as *The Lancet* over the years. Unfortunately, these studies have since been shown to be seriously flawed—they proved nothing. And in 1996, an expert panel assembled by the Commission of the European Communities looked at 184 recent studies of homeopathy and decided that only 17 were truly scientific and objective. In some—but far from all—of the 17 studies, homeopathic remedies seemed to work better than a placebo or no treatment at all, but there just wasn't enough good evidence to say that homeopathy was effective.

On the other hand, in 1997 researchers at the National Institutes of Health's Office of Alternative Medicine looked at 89 different studies that used homeopathic remedies. They threw out the badly designed studies and looked again at the 26 that were left. When the results of the 26 studies were combined, homeopathic remedies turned out to be 1.6 times as effective as a placebo. Even so, the researchers concluded that there's still not enough research to explain why homeopathy works.

The Least You Need to Know

➤ Dr. Samuel Hahnemann discovered the basic principles of homeopathy nearly two hundred years ago.

➤ The fundamental idea in homeopathy is *like cures like.* A substance that causes symptoms similar to the health problem may also help it.

➤ Homeopathic remedies contain very, very tiny amounts of the minerals, herbs, or other substances used to make them. Paradoxically, the more dilute the remedy is, the better it works.

➤ Homeopathic remedies are often very helpful for chronic problems such as headaches, hay fever, fatigue, stress, skin problems, PMS, and pain.

➤ You can easily treat occasional problems yourself with the most popular homeo-pathic remedies. For more serious or chronic problems, check with a professional homeopath. Many naturopathic physicians, acupuncturists, and chiropractors are trained in homeopathy.

➤ You can easily find homeopathic remedies in health-food stores and many drugstores. The remedies are safe, with no side effects, and can be taken by children, pets, and the elderly.

Chapter 14

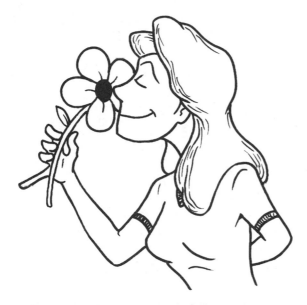

Flower Remedies

> **In This Chapter**
>
> ➤ The philosophy of flower remedies
>
> ➤ How negative emotions may cause illness
>
> ➤ Using flower remedies to resolve inner conflict
>
> ➤ Flower remedies and emotional emergencies

You spend a delightful spring morning walking through fields and woods full of wildflowers in bloom. To enjoy the flowers more, you sniff them, touch them, maybe even pick a few to carry with you. When your walk's over, you feel great—relaxed, energetic, optimistic. Why? Fresh air, sunshine, and a little exercise probably have a lot to do with it, but the real emotional boost may have come from the flowers. By touching them, you absorbed some of their healing energy—the healing energy found in flower remedies.

Dr. Bach's Discovery

In the late 1920s, Edward Bach (pronounced *batch*), a doctor and homeopath in England, realized that many of his patients had harmful, negative emotions that later led to illness. It was a good insight, but there was just one problem: How could he help his patients get rid of the negative emotions using simple, natural methods? One day, while walking in a meadow, Dr. Bach noticed how the dewdrops on the flower petals sparkled in the sunlight. He realized that each dewdrop, heated by the sun, would absorb the healing essence of the plant.

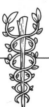

The Healing Arts

Edward Bach, M.B., B.S., M.R.C.S., L.R.C.P., Ph.D. (1886–1937), was a medical doctor, homeopath, and bacteriologist. As a doctor, he knew the connection between his patients' emotions and their health. In the 1930s, after extensive research, he identified 38 flowering plants, trees, and special waters that had a positive effect on emotions and stress. Dr. Bach believed his flower remedies helped remove the negative emotions that keep people from healing.

Taking this insight to the next level, Dr. Bach began to explore the healing properties of a wide variety of plants. He discovered 37 different flowering plants and trees that each have their own positive effects on the underlying emotions and psychological stress that can lead to bad health. In addition, Dr. Bach discovered Rock Water, made with water from a natural spring said to have healing properties. He also formulated his Rescue Remedy, a mixture of five different essences for use in stressful situations.

Each essence treats not physical symptoms but the underlying negative emotions that are the root cause of the problem. The essences can be used for prevention, when you're feeling under stress, or as part of your treatment for illness. They help relieve the psychological problems, such as depression, that come along with physical illness and slow your recovery.

The Flower Essences

Each of the 38 Bach Flower Essences is for a particular negative emotional state—someone who's despondent and discouraged, for instance, might try Gentian. Taking the essence is said to help transform the negative emotion into a positive one. According to Dr. Bach, negative emotions cause disease; positive emotions fight disease. To see which essences affect different emotional states, check out Table 14.1.

Table 14.1   The Flower Essences

Bach Flower Remedy	State of Mind
Agrimony	Hiding worries behind a brave face, concealing problems
Aspen	Apprehension and vague fears for no known reason

Bach Flower Remedy	State of Mind
Beech	Critical and intolerant of others, unable and unwilling to make allowances
Centaury	Weak-willed, exploited or imposed upon, anxious to please
Cerato	Those who doubt their own judgment, seek confirmation of others
Cherry Plum	Uncontrolled, irrational thoughts and rages
Chestnut Bud	Refuses to learn by experience, continually repeats same mistakes
Chicory	Possessive, self-centered, clinging and overprotective, especially of loved ones
Clematis	Inattentive, dreamy, absent-minded, mental escapist
Crab Apple	Feelings of self-disgust, shame, or uncleanness
Elm	Overwhelmed by responsibility
Gentian	Despondency due to past disappointments
Gorse	Pessimism, despair, hopelessness
Heather	Talkative, obsessed with your own troubles, self-absorbed
Holly	Hatred, envy, jealousy, suspicion
Honeysuckle	Living in the past, nostalgia, homesickness
Hornbeam	"Monday morning" feeling, procrastination
Impatiens	Impatience, irritability
Larch	Lack of self-confidence, feelings of inferiority, fear of failure
Mimulus	Fear of known things, shyness, timidity
Mustard	"Dark cloud" that descends, making you sad for no known reason
Oak	Normally strong, but losing the strength to fight illness or adversity
Olive	Fatigued, drained of energy
Pine	Guilt feelings and self-reproachful
Red Chestnut	Obsessed by care and concern for others
Rock Rose	Suddenly alarmed, scared, panicky, experiences nightmares
Rock Water	Narrow-minded, self-denying
Scleranthus	Uncertainty, indecision, vacillation, mood swings
Star of Bethlehem	Shock, grief
Sweet Chestnut	Utter dejection, bleak outlook

continues

Table 14.1   The Flower Essences   (continued)

Bach Flower Remedy	State of Mind
Vervain	Overenthusiasm, fanaticism, argumentative
Vine	Dominating, inflexible, tyrannical, arrogant
Walnut	Adjusting to transition or change—for example, puberty, menopause, divorce, or new surroundings
Water Violet	Proud, reserved, aloof, enjoys being alone
White Chestnut	Persistent, unwanted thoughts, preoccupation with worry
Wild Oat	Dissatisfaction, lack of motivation
Wild Rose	Resignation, apathy
Willow	Resentment, bitterness, "poor old me!"
Rescue Remedy	For people in emergency stress situations

Dr. Bach grouped the essences into seven categories, based on fundamental conflicts and emotional states:

Fear
Aspen
Cherry Plum
Mimulus
Red Chestnut
Rock Rose

Uncertainty
Cerato
Gentian
Gorse
Hornbeam
Scleranthus
Wild Oat

Insufficient interest in present circumstances
Chestnut Bud
Clematis
Honeysuckle
Olive
White Chestnut

Loneliness
Heather
Impatiens
Water Violet

Oversensitivity to ideas and influences
Agrimony
Centaury
Holly
Walnut

Despondency or despair
Crab Apple
Elm
Larch
Oak
Star of Bethlehem
Sweet Chestnut
Willow

Overconcern for the welfare of others
Beech
Chicory
Rock Water
Vervain
Vine

Within each group, specific essences cover the different aspects of the conflict. For example, in the Fear group, Aspen helps you deal with fears of unknown origin, while Rock Rose helps you deal with terror and nightmares.

Choosing Essences

Which essence is right for you? That's a more complicated question than you might think. You'll probably benefit from combining more than one essence together. Generally speaking, you can combine up to six or seven essences and get the benefits of all of them at once. To figure out which essences will help you the most, use the questionnaire provided in Table 14.2. Look at the questions honestly and check the ones you feel strongly apply to you at this moment. If you answer yes to all the questions in any one group, that essence should definitely be part of your personal formula. Remember, though, that the formula is right for you now. As things change in your life, you might need to make adjustments. Go back to the questionnaire every now and then and make changes in your formula if you need to. And if you pick the wrong essence, don't worry—it just won't have any effect on you.

Table 14.2 The Right Flower Essences for You

Agrimony

____ Do you find yourself hiding your worries behind a cheerful, smiling face in an attempt to conceal your pain from others?

____ Are you distressed by arguments and quarrels, often "giving in" to avoid any conflict?

____ When you feel life's pressures weighing you down, do you often turn to drugs, alcohol, or other outside influences to help you cope?

Aspen

____ Do you have feelings of apprehension, anticipation, or uneasiness with no known cause?

____ Do you worry that something bad may happen but you're not sure what?

____ Do you awaken with a sense of fear and anxiety of what the day will bring?

Beech

____ Are you annoyed by the habits and shortcomings of others?

____ Do you find yourself being overly critical and intolerant, usually looking for what someone has done wrong and not right?

____ Do you prefer to work or be alone because the seemingly foolishness of others irritates you?

continues

Table 14.2   The Right Flower Essences for You   (continued)

Centaury

____ Are you unable to say no to those who constantly impose on your good nature?

____ Do you tend to be timid and shy, easily influenced by those stronger in nature than yourself?

____ Do you often deny your own needs in order to please others?

Cerato

____ Do you constantly question your own decisions and judgment?

____ Are you often seeking advice and confirmation from other people, mistrusting your own wisdom?

____ Do you change direction often, first going one way, then another because you lack the confidence in yourself to stick with one direction?

Cherry Plum

____ Do you fear losing control of yourself?

____ Are you afraid of hurting yourself or others?

____ Do you have a tendency to act irrationally and violently, exploding into unexplained fits of rage and anger?

Chestnut Bud

____ Do you find yourself making the same mistakes over and over again, such as choosing the wrong type of partner or staying in a job you dislike?

____ Do you fail to learn from your experiences?

____ Does it take you longer to advance in your life because you are slow to learn from past mistakes?

Chicory

____ Are you possessive and manipulative of those you care for?

____ Do you need to be needed?

____ Do you feel unloved and unappreciated by your loved ones "after all you've done for them"?

Clematis

____ Do you often feel spacey and out of touch with the "real world"?

____ Do you find yourself preoccupied and dreamy, unable to concentrate for any length of time?

____ Are you drowsy and listless, sleeping more often than necessary?

Crab Apple

____ Are you obsessed with cleanliness?

____ Are you embarrassed and ashamed of yourself physically, finding yourself unattractive?

____ Do you tend to concentrate on small physical conditions, such as pimples or marks, neglecting more serious problems?

Elm

____ Are you often overwhelmed by your responsibilities?

____ Do you feel inadequate when it comes to dealing with the tasks ahead of you?

____ Do you become depressed and exhausted when faced with your everyday commitments?

Gentian

____ Do you become discouraged and depressed when things go wrong?

____ Are you easily disheartened when faced with difficult situations?

____ Does your pessimistic attitude prevent you from making an effort to accomplish something?

Gorse

____ Do you feel despondent and hopeless, at the end of your rope both mentally and physically?

____ Do you lack confidence that things will get better in your life and therefore make no effort to improve your circumstances?

____ Do you believe that nothing can be done to relieve your pain and suffering?

Heather

____ Are you totally self-absorbed, concerned only about yourself and your own problems and ailments?

____ Do you talk incessantly, not interested in what anyone else has to say?

____ Do you dislike being alone, always seeking the companionship of others?

Holly

____ Are you full of jealousy and hate?

____ Do you mistrust others' intentions, feeling that people have "ulterior motives"?

____ Do you feel great anger toward other people?

continues

Table 14.2   The Right Flower Essences for You   (continued)

Honeysuckle

_____ Do you find yourself living in the past, nostalgic and homesick for the "way it was"?

_____ Are you unable to change present circumstances because you are always looking back and never forward?

_____ Are you dissatisfied with your accomplishments?

Hornbeam

_____ Do you often feel too tired to face the day ahead?

_____ Do you feel overworked or bored with your life?

_____ Do you lack enthusiasm and therefore tend to procrastinate?

Impatiens

_____ Are you impatient and irritable with others who seem to do things too slowly for you?

_____ Do you prefer to work alone?

_____ Do you feel a sense of urgency in everything you do, always rushing to get through things?

Larch

_____ Do you lack self-confidence?

_____ Do you feel inferior and often become discouraged?

_____ Are you so sure that you will fail and therefore do not even attempt things?

Mimulus

_____ Do you have fears of known things—for example, illness, death, pain, heights, darkness, the dentist, and so on?

_____ Are you shy, overly sensitive, and often afraid?

_____ When you are confronted with a frightening situation, do you become too paralyzed to act?

Mustard

_____ Do you feel deep gloom that seems to quickly descend for no apparent reason and lifts just as suddenly?

_____ Do you feel your moods swinging back and forth?

_____ Do you feel depressed without knowing why?

Oak

____ Are you exhausted but feel the need to struggle on against all odds?

____ Do you have a strong sense of duty and dependability, carrying on no matter what obstacles stand in your way?

____ Do you neglect your own needs in order to complete a task?

Olive

____ Do you feel utterly and completely exhausted, both physically and mentally?

____ Are you totally drained of all energy with no reserves left, finding it difficult to carry on?

____ Is everything an effort; does your life lack zest?

Pine

____ Are you full of guilt and self-reproach?

____ Do you blame yourself for everything that goes wrong, including the mistakes of others?

____ Do you set overly high standards for yourself, never satisfied with your achievements?

Red Chestnut

____ Are you excessively concerned and worried for your loved ones?

____ Do you constantly worry that harm may come to those you care for?

____ Are you distressed and disturbed by other people's problems?

Rock Rose

____ Do you feel terror and panic?

____ Do you become helpless and frozen in the face of your fear?

____ Do you suffer from nightmares?

Rock Water

____ Are you inflexible in your approach to life, always striving for perfection?

____ Are you so rigid in your ideals that you deny yourself the simple pleasures of life?

____ Are you *overly* concerned with diet, exercise, work, and spiritual disciplines?

continues

Table 14.2 The Right Flower Essences for You (continued)

Scleranthus

_____ Do you find it difficult to decide when faced with a choice of two possibilities?

_____ Do you lack concentration, always fidgety and nervous?

_____ Do your moods change from one extreme to another: joy to sadness, optimism to pessimism, laughing to crying?

Star of Bethlehem

_____ Have you suffered a shock in your life, such as an accident, loss of a loved one, terrible news, or illness?

_____ Are you numbed or withdrawn as a result of recent traumatic events in your life?

_____ Have you suffered a loss or grief that you have never recovered from?

Sweet Chestnut

_____ Do you suffer from extreme mental anguish?

_____ Do you feel that you have reached the limits of what you could possibly endure?

_____ Do you feel as though the future holds nothing for you?

Vervain

_____ Do you feel tense and highly strung?

_____ Do you have strong opinions, and only yours are the right ones?

_____ Is your overenthusiasm almost to the point of being fanatical?

Vine

_____ Do you tend to be domineering and overbearing?

_____ Do you feel the need to always be right?

_____ Are you inflexible and feel you know more than anyone else?

Walnut

_____ Are you experiencing any change in your life—a move, new job, loss of a loved one, new relationship, divorce, puberty, menopause, or giving up an addiction?

_____ Are you distracted by outside influences?

_____ Do you need to make a break from strong forces or attachments in your life that may be holding you back?

Water Violet

___ Do you appear to others to be aloof and overly proud?

___ Do you have a tendency to be withdrawn and prefer to be alone when faced with too many external distractions?

___ Do you bear your grief and sorrow in silence?

White Chestnut

___ Do you find your head full of persistent, unwanted thoughts that prevent concentration?

___ Do you relive unhappy events or arguments over and over again?

___ Are you unable to sleep at times because your mind seems to be cluttered with mental arguments that go around and around?

Wild Oat

___ Do you find yourself in a complete state of uncertainty over major life decisions?

___ Are you displeased with your lifestyle and feel dissatisfied with your achievements?

___ Do you have ambition but feel that life is passing you by?

Wild Rose

___ Are you apathetic and resigned to whatever may happen in your life?

___ Do you have the attitude, "I will just live with it"?

___ Do you lack the motivation to improve the quality of your life?

Willow

___ Do you feel resentful and bitter?

___ Do you have difficulty forgiving and forgetting?

___ Do you feel that life is unfair and find yourself taking less and less interest in the things you used to enjoy?

Source: Reproduced courtesy of Nelson Bach USA, Ltd., and the Original Bach Flower Essences.

Getting to the Essence

Dr. Bach developed a method for making essences from freshly picked wildflowers using only pure water. To this day, his methods are followed at The Bach Centre at Mount Vernon in England. The process begins with making a *mother tincture* that is the basis for the essences. The plants are picked, placed in glass bowls, and left in the sunshine for three to four hours. The flowers then are removed. The mother tincture is

Dr. Bach's cottage in the English countryside, known as Mount Vernon, is now The Bach Centre. Photo courtesy of Nelson Bach USA, Ltd.

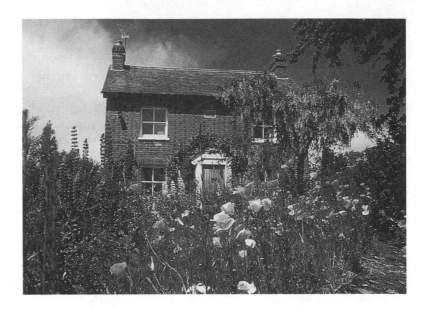

the liquid left in the bowl. Twenty of the Bach flower remedies use mother tinctures made with sunshine; the other mother tinctures are made by boiling the plant parts.

The mother tinctures then are brought to the bottling plant, where they are diluted to the standard homeopathic strength of one in 240, or one part in 100,000, or 5*x* (refer to Chapter 13, "Homeopathy: Let Like Cure Like," for more on what all these numbers mean).

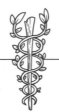

The Healing Arts

While researching his flower remedies, Dr. Bach lived in a cottage in Oxfordshire in the English countryside. His home, called Mount Vernon, is now The Bach Centre, a foundation that continues to produce Dr. Bach's remedies and promote his principles and teachings. The plants used to make the remedies are harvested from the same places Dr. Bach gathered the flowers he used. The mother tinctures for the Bach Flower Essences are still prepared there exactly as Dr. Bach himself prepared them.

Most flower essences, no matter who makes them, are sold in 5 ml stock bottles made of brown or amber glass.

Using Flower Essences

Whether you use just one flower essence or several in combination, taking them is simple. Just put two drops of whatever single essence or combination you choose into a small cup of water or juice, stir gently, and sip it down; repeat at least four times a day. If you prefer, you can take the essences directly by putting four drops on your tongue at least four times a day. Another method is to put four drops of each essence into about 6 ounces of pure spring water. Stir gently and sip the mixture down over the course of the day.

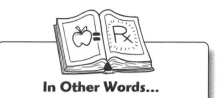

In Other Words...

A **mother tincture** is the mixture of water, herbs, and sometimes alcohol that is the basis for any homeopathic remedy.

To make up a batch of your personal formula, fill a 1-ounce (30 ml) brown or amber glass dropper bottle (often called a dose bottle) three-quarters full with pure spring water. Add two drops of each essence to the water. The mixture will stay fresh for three weeks. You can add a teaspoon of brandy or apple cider vinegar as a preservative if you want. Light is bad for the remedies, so store them in a cool, dark place.

In some cases, such as sudden depression or Monday-morning blues, taking the remedies should help you feel a lot better almost at once. Often, though, the remedies work slowly and gently over several days or even weeks. Once you notice an improvement in your physical or mental state, taper off or stop taking the remedy.

If you don't feel you're improving, maybe it's time to rethink your choices. Perhaps you need different essences or a different combination.

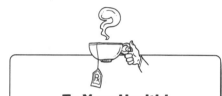

To Your Health!

If for some reason you don't want to put flower essences on your tongue, moisten your lips, wrists, or temples with them instead.

No matter how you take the flower essences, be sure to use them as soon as you get up in the morning and again before you go to sleep.

Dr. Bach to the Rescue

Dr. Bach created an emergency formula called Rescue Remedy. It has five essences in it: Cherry Plum, Clematis, Impatiens, Rock Rose, and Star of Bethlehem. The idea behind Rescue Remedy is that it helps you stay balanced as you go through a difficult period. You might want to take it if you've just received some bad news, for instance, or if you're about to go into a stressful situation, like an exam or a job interview.

In an emergency, the usual dosage for Rescue Remedy is four drops in a small glass of water or other liquid. Sip it down and repeat if necessary. You can also take the drops directly from the bottle by putting four drops on your tongue. All the flower essences are preserved with brandy, so if you don't want the alcohol, dilute the drops in liquid. Rescue Remedy is also available as a cream.

Other Flower Remedies

Since Dr. Bach's time, other researchers have developed their own flower remedies. They're all based on Dr. Bach's basic concept, but they use different flowers and plants from different regions of the world, including California, Australia, and the Himalayas. Would Dr. Bach approve? We think so. The good doctor died tragically young—he would surely have gone on studying more flowers and adding to his own formulas had he lived longer.

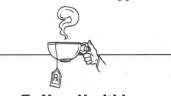

To Your Health!

In the United States, Bach flower remedies are sold under the brand names Bach Flower Essences, Healing Herbs, and Ellon. Another popular flower essence brand is Quintessentials, produced by the Flower Essence Society.

Modern researchers have added many more flower remedies—and more conditions that they claim the remedies help. Research by the Flower Essence Society, for example, has discovered more than 100 North American flower remedies. They're helpful for a wide range of problems that Dr. Bach never had a chance to solve. For example, Golden Yarrow helps you deal with performance anxiety.

Some people believe that gem essences, made by placing precious and semiprecious jewels in spring water, are helpful. They claim that gem essences work on the same principles as flower essences.

Essence Advisors

The whole beauty of the flower remedies is that they're do-it-yourself—you decide what's best for you. The system is basically very simple, and the essences themselves are harmless. They won't interact with any drugs you need to take. You cannot overdose on an essence or become dependent. And if you take the wrong one for you, nothing bad happens.

A lot of homeopaths, naturopaths, and other practitioners use flower remedies to help their patients understand and deal with the underlying emotions that cause their physical problems. The Nelson Bach Company offers weekend seminars for people interested in learning more about flower remedies and Dr. Bach's philosophy. There's also an education program for people who want to include flower remedies in their health practice or become registered Bach Practitioners. For more information, contact:

Nelson Bach USA, Ltd.
Wilmington Technology Park
100 Research Drive
Wilmington, MA 01887-4406
Phone: (800) 334-0843
Fax: (978) 988-0233
E-mail: webmaster@nelsonbach.com

The Flower Essence Society also offers seminars and a certification program. For more information, contact:

Flower Essence Society
P.O. Box 459
Nevada City, CA 95959
Phone: (800) 736-9222
Fax: (530) 265-0584
E-mail: info@flowersociety.org

Courses at the Flower Essence Society incorporate the basic teachings of Dr. Bach and provide instruction in using the Bach remedies along with North American flower essences.

Essences of Nothing?

There are many anecdotes (often called case studies) about the value of flower remedies, but there's no scientific evidence for them. Chemical analyses of flower essences show only alcohol and spring water. There's even less to say about gem essences. Doctors generally dismiss flower essences as harmless and say that any improvement you might show by using them is really caused by your natural healing processes or by any conventional treatment you're also getting.

The Least You Need to Know

➤ Flower essences are homeopathic remedies that claim to counteract the negative emotions that cause illness.

➤ The original concept of flower essences was developed by Dr. Edward Bach in the 1930s.

➤ There are 38 Bach flower remedies. Each remedy treats a specific negative emotion. Dr. Bach's Rescue Remedy mixture contains five flower essences and is meant to be used in times of stress.

➤ Since Dr. Bach's time, additional flower remedies and uses for them have been discovered.

➤ Most people use a personal combination of several different remedies to help their own emotional and physical problems.

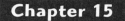

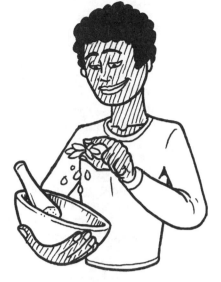

Chapter 15

Traditional Herbal Medicine

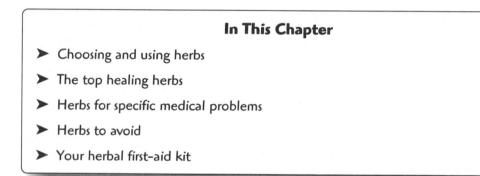

In This Chapter

➤ Choosing and using herbs

➤ The top healing herbs

➤ Herbs for specific medical problems

➤ Herbs to avoid

➤ Your herbal first-aid kit

Who was the family physician you saw most often when you were growing up? Dr. Mom, of course, assisted perhaps by Dr. Grandma. And when Dr. Mom prescribed peppermint tea or flat ginger ale for your upset stomach, she was carrying on a very, very long tradition of herbal healing by women. Her herbal home remedies worked, and not just because they came with a hug. Why? Because herbs—plant parts such as leaves or roots—have natural healing powers that can help a whole range of ailments ranging from the common cold to heart disease and other serious medical problems. Over thousands of years, we've discovered through practical experience which herbs work best for which medical problems. In fact, herbs work so well that the active ingredients in about a quarter of all prescription drugs used today come directly from plants.

Healing with Herbs

Humans have been using *herbs* as medicine for thousands of years. Traditional Chinese herbal medicine, for example, is at least five thousand years old (and it's so detailed that we don't have room for it here—see Chapter 16, "Ginseng and More: Traditional Chinese Herbs"). Ancient Egyptian doctors were writing down their herbal prescriptions more than four thousand years ago. And over two thousand years ago, Hippocrates, the father of modern medicine, was recording his favorite herbs. Through millenniums of trial, error, and careful observation, the herbs that work have been discovered, along with the best ways to use them and the conditions they help the most.

Over the centuries, as Western medicine became more scientific and more male-dominated, traditional herbal medicine was only kept alive by folklore and the hands of local healers (usually women). Considering how harsh and useless many standard medical treatments were even well into the 20th century, it's not surprising that in the 1830s an important movement back to herbal medicine arose in the United States. Known as *eclecticism*, this system was a form of scientific herbalism. Eclectic physicians used a standard medical approach to diagnosis, but then they treated the illness with herbs, including those drawn from Native American lore. Eclecticism remained quite popular for decades, but

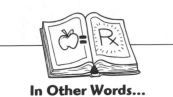

In Other Words...

Technically speaking, an **herb** is a fleshy, annual plant that grows from a seed. The word comes from the Latin word *herba*, meaning "grass" (that's why grazing animals like cows are called **herbivores**). Practically speaking, an herb is any sort of plant part used for cooking or medicine—roots, stems, leaves, seeds, fruits, and even bark.

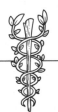

The Healing Arts

In the 1500s, the great Swiss physician Paracelsus was the first Western doctor to use opium as a painkiller. He also came up with the idea that herbs that look like a particular part of the body would be good for treating diseases that affect that part. So, for instance, Paracelsus thought the herb eyebright, whose leaves look like bloodshot eyes, could help eye problems. It doesn't, but he did have a few lucky guesses, and the *Doctrine of Signatures*, as this idea came to be called, is with us today. Except as an interesting bit of medical history, though, the Doctrine of Signatures is worthless.

by the beginning of the 20th century, eclectic physicians were gone from the medical scene. The herbs they had used were forgotten or replaced by drugs.

But today, even with all our modern drugs, more and more people are turning back to herbs to help their health. Why? One very good reason is that herbs are almost always gentler and safer than drugs. They have fewer side effects and interactions with other medications. You'd have to work hard to overdose on a healing herb, and it's almost impossible to get addicted to one. And the fact is, for many minor health problems (and even some not-so-minor ones), herbal remedies work as well as if not better than standard prescription or even nonprescription drugs.

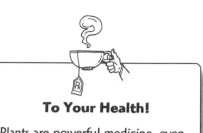

To Your Health!

Plants are powerful medicine, even against serious diseases like cancer. The drugs vincristine and vinblastine, used to treat leukemia, are made from a plant in the periwinkle family. And tamoxifen, a drug that treats breast and ovarian cancer, is made from the Pacific yew.

Using Herbs

Safe, natural herbs can help with life's little aches and pains and minor illnesses. They can even help with some bigger health problems. We'll get into some specific examples later in this chapter, but before we do that, we need to explain the different ways you can take your herbs.

Herbal Drinks

Lots of herbs can be made into *teas*, *infusions*, or *decoctions* that you drink down. Generally speaking, if the herb is a leaf or flower—like peppermint or chamomile—it will make a good tea or infusion. If the herb is a root, bark, or seed, you'll need to make a decoction.

If you want to try raspberry-leaf tea, be sure to buy exactly that at the health-food store—don't buy raspberry-flavored black tea or herbal mixes that contain only a small amount of raspberry leaves or raspberry flavoring.

To make an herbal tea: Use one prepared tea bag or a teaspoon or so of the herb in a tea ball or infuser for each cup of water. Pour boiling water over the herb and let the tea steep for a few minutes before drinking it.

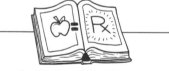

In Other Words...

Tea: Steep a small amount of an herb in boiling water for a few minutes. **Infusion**: Steep a larger amount of an herb in boiling water for 10 to 20 minutes. **Decoction**: Combine herb with cold water in a small pot, bring to a boil, and simmer for 10 to 20 minutes. Teas and infusions are usually made with leafy or flowery herbs; decoctions are made with roots or barks.

Herbal teas are very mild—they're pleasant to drink, but they don't have much medicinal power. To get the real value from an herb, you need to make an *infusion*. Start with a heaping tablespoon of the herb (about the equivalent of three prepared tea bags) for each cup of water. Pour boiling water over the herb and let the infusion steep for at least 10 minutes (20 is better).

To make a *decoction*, put about a tablespoon of the herb for each cup of cold water into a small pot. Bring the water to a boil, then lower the heat and simmer gently for 10 to 20 minutes.

Teas, infusions, and decoctions don't keep well—drink them as soon as they're ready. A spoonful of sugar, honey, or maple syrup helps cover up the nasty bitter flavor many herbs have. Mixing the decoction with fruit juice is another good way to disguise the taste.

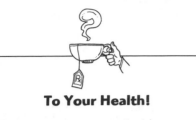

To Your Health!

Drying concentrates an herb's healing compounds. If you're using fresh herbs to make your infusion or decoction, use about twice as much.

Tinctures

A *tincture* is an herbal extract made with alcohol instead of water. The advantage of tinctures is that they're more concentrated, so you can take less, and they keep well, so you're not always boiling up brews when it's time to take your dose. You can make your own tinctures using vodka (never use rubbing alcohol or wood alcohol!), but it's a fair amount of work spread over several weeks. We suggest buying high-quality herbal tinctures from your health-food store. You can even get nonalcoholic versions made with vinegar.

Because tinctures are so concentrated, a typical dose might be anywhere from just 5 or 10 drops to a teaspoon or two. Tinctures taste pretty strong. If you can't stand the taste straight, try mixing the tincture into fruit juice.

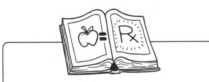

In Other Words...

A **tincture** is made by soaking an herb in pure grain alcohol instead of water. Tinctures are more concentrated than infusions or decoctions. They're convenient and keep well. If you don't want to use a product that contains alcohol, look for tinctures made with vinegar instead.

Capsules

A lot of herbs taste just terrible. There's a reason for that. Plants can't run away, so they protect themselves from critters that want to eat them by tasting awful. It's just good luck when the same bitter or pungent chemicals that protect the plant happen to also be helpful to humans.

Instead of forcing down a foul-tasting infusion, you can swallow the dried, powdered herb in a gelatin capsule. Capsules are very convenient, and they also let you control your dose pretty accurately. Many medicinal herbs are now available in capsules from reputable manufacturers. If you like doing it yourself, you can buy 00-size capsules very inexpensively and fill them yourself.

If you follow religious dietary laws or don't eat animal products, read the label carefully when you buy herbs in capsules. Many but not all manufacturers now use vegetable cellulose to make the capsules.

External Herbs

Sometimes the best way to use an herb is externally—as a *compress* on a skin rash, for instance. To make a compress, soak a clean washcloth in a cooled infusion or decoction, wring it out lightly, and place it on the spot for 20 minutes or so. Repeat as needed.

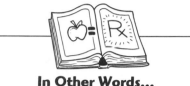

In Other Words...

A **compress** is a cloth soaked in an herbal infusion or decoction and placed directly on the skin. (In older herb books, a compress is sometimes called a **fomentation**.) A **poultice** is a small amount of an herb soaked in water and placed directly on the skin.

A *poultice* is a small amount of an herb put directly on the skin. To make a poultice, soak a handful of the herb in hot water until it's softened. Squeeze out the moisture and place the herb on the skin. Hold it in place with a wet washcloth for about 20 minutes.

You can make an herbal ointment by mixing a few drops of a tincture into a tablespoon or so of any unscented hand cream.

Choosing Herbs

When it comes to herbs, quality counts—you want your herbs to have as much of their active ingredients as possible. Buy your herbs from a well-stocked, reputable health-food store. If you buy a prepared herbal product such as a tincture or tea bag, choose a reliable manufacturer. If you prefer to buy your herbs in bulk, look for herbs that are aromatic and have good color—skip any herbs that are faded, dusty, crushed, or have a musty or "off" smell. Skip herbs that seem to have a lot of *chaff* (bits of stems and the like) mixed in. And of course, don't buy any herbs that have bugs in them!

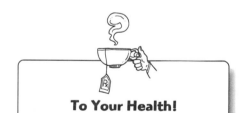

To Your Health!

Light and moisture are the enemies of herbs. Store your herbs in brown glass containers with tightly fitting lids. Keep the jars in a cool, dry, dark place—the fridge is good. Most herbs will keep for about a year if you store them properly.

Getting the Herbs You Want

Selling herbs is a business just like any other business. And just like any other business, sometimes the people who sell herbs aren't completely honest with their customers. The biggest problem for herb consumers is being sure that what you're paying for is really what you're getting. Sometimes herbs are mislabeled—accidentally through ignorance or purposely through greed. The popular herb goldenseal, for instance, is quite expensive. Some unscrupulous producers have substituted bloodroot, an herb that looks like goldenseal but is a powerful laxative. More commonly, an herb is labeled only with its common name, not its two-part scientific name. Since some herbs have several different common names, you can't always be sure of what you're getting.

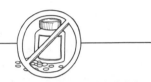

Hazardous to Your Health!

Collecting herbs in the wild—**wildcrafting**—is a lot of fun, but be absolutely sure you know what you're gathering. It's easy to confuse a safe plant with one that could kill you. Wild parsley resembles three other dangerous plants: water hemlock, poison hemlock, and fool's parsley. Burdock root resembles the root of deadly nightshade—confusing the two is a mistake you don't want to make.

Be an informed consumer, buy only from reputable dealers, and don't buy the herb if you have any doubts.

If you don't live near a large health-food store, you might prefer the reasonable prices and large selection of a mail-order herb company. Here are three firms that have good reputations for high quality:

Herb Pharm
P.O. Box 116
Williams, OR 97544
Phone: (800) 348-4372

Nature's Herbs
1010 46th Street
Emeryville, CA 94608
Phone: (510) 601-0700

Nature's Way
10 Mountain Springs Parkway
Springville, UT 84663
Phone: (800) 962-8873

Standardized Herbs

The strength of an herb depends on a lot of factors, including how fresh it is, how long you steep it, and even where it was grown and when it was picked. That means you can't really be sure of the dose you're getting. But when you need a prescription drug, you want to take exactly the dose your doctor prescribes. Why should herbs be any different? More and more herbs today are available in *standardized* capsules or tablets. The herbs have been slightly processed to make sure that every dose in every capsule contains the same amount of the most important active ingredients. Standardized herbs are a bit more expensive, but we recommend them to make sure you're getting exactly what you want. Some reliable manufacturers include Solgar, Nature's Way, and Twin Labs.

Herbal Cautions

How can something as natural as an herb be harmful? Well, there's a reason some plants have names like deadly nightshade and poison hemlock. To avoid problems, follow these rules for using herbs:

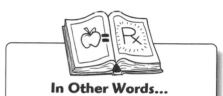

In Other Words...

Standardized herbs have been lightly processed to make sure each dose has the same basic amount of major active ingredients.

➤ Use an herb only if you are positive that you know what it is and what it does.

➤ When in doubt, don't use the herb!

➤ Use only the recommended amount of an herb. If you want to take a larger dose, build up to it gradually.

➤ Don't take an herb for a long period of time. If the problem you're taking the herb for doesn't get better or go away in a few days or gets worse, stop taking the herb and see your doctor as soon as possible.

➤ If you have a chronic medical problem such as heart disease, asthma, emphysema, or the like, talk to your doctor about herbal remedies before you try them. The herbs could interact badly with any drugs you take.

➤ Never take an herbal remedy instead of a drug—even a nonprescription drug—prescribed by your doctor.

➤ Stop using an herb if you get an upset stomach, diarrhea, headache, skin rash, hives, or other unpleasant symptoms within two hours of taking it.

➤ Don't give herbal remedies to children under two.

➤ Don't give full-strength herbal remedies to people over 65; use lower doses.

➤ Don't use herbal remedies if you're pregnant or think you might be.

Most of all, use your common sense. It's better to be too cautious than really sorry.

The Herbal Hit Parade

Six herbs top the herbal hit parade: garlic, ginger, ginkgo, ginseng, goldenseal, and echinacea. Why do five of the six begin with the letter G? We have no idea.

Each of these six herbs has a long, long tradition of use for a wide range of problems. Garlic, number one on the worldwide hit parade, is used medicinally in just about every culture on earth. Ginger originally came from India and China, but it's been used in Western herbal medicine for centuries. Ginkgo and ginseng come originally from ancient China. Their use in the West is more recent. Goldenseal and echinacea are homegrown herbs that were well known to the Native Americans.

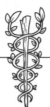

The Healing Arts

Sales of herbal remedies have been taking off in the United States in recent years. According to *Nutrition Business Journal*, in 1995 echinacea sales were $180 million; in 1997 they had jumped 72 percent to $310 million. In the same period, sales of ginko biloba jumped 50 percent, from $160 million to $240 million, and garlic sales went up 33 percent, from $150 million to $200 million. Sales of St. John's wort skyrocketed from a minor $10 million in 1995 to $200 million in 1997, an increase of 1,900 percent.

Garlic for Good Health

You can ward off a vampire with garlic—and you might also be able to ward off infections, heart disease, stroke, high blood pressure, and cancer. Let's take a closer look at the world's most popular herbal remedy:

➤ **Garlic as an antibiotic.** Garlic contains allicin, a compound that's a powerful antibiotic—and also kills fungi. Eating a lot of garlic can help prevent colds, flu, and bronchitis—and not just because other people stay away from your garlic breath. Actually, you get garlic breath because the germ-killing allicin and other compounds in garlic pass out of your body through your lungs—exactly the right place to find those cold and flu viruses. To treat a cold, swallow two to four finely chopped garlic cloves three times a day.

➤ **Garlic as a fungicide.** Garlic kills the annoying fungus that causes athlete's foot. Crush some garlic cloves and use them in a footbath with warm water. Garlic's also an effective treatment for vaginal yeast infections. Don't apply the garlic to the area, though—eat three or four cloves three times a day.

➤ **Garlic as a heart helper.** Garlic thins your blood, which can help prevent the blood clots that cause heart attacks. If you're at risk of a heart attack, many doctors recommend taking one aspirin tablet a day to thin your blood. Three or four cloves of garlic have the same effect. A study in 1998 showed that garlic helps keep your aorta (the main artery leading from your heart) flexible—which could help prevent a heart attack.

➤ **Garlic for high blood pressure.** Garlic helps to lower your blood pressure if it's too high. It doesn't take much—just one clove a day could do the trick. And keeping your blood pressure down cuts your chances of a heart attack or stroke.

➤ **Garlic for cancer prevention.** Garlic has at least 15 different substances that could help prevent or treat cancer. There's a lot of research going on in this area, especially since large studies in China and Italy have shown that people who eat a lot of garlic are less likely to get stomach cancer. A 1997 study showed that garlic can bring prostate cancer to a screeching halt—at least in the test tube. Stay tuned for big developments here.

The best and cheapest way to get your garlic is to eat finely chopped raw cloves. Mixed with honey, they're surprisingly easy to swallow. Large amounts of garlic can upset your stomach, though, and they sure don't do much for your breath. If you want your social life to be more than the monthly meeting of the Garlic Lover's Club, try commercial garlic capsules or liquids made with odorless aged garlic extract—you get the benefits without the bad breath. We like the Kyolic® and Kwai® brands.

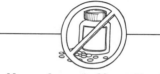

Hazardous to Your Health!

If you're taking medicine such as warfarin (Coumadin®) to thin your blood, talk to your doctor before you try large amounts of garlic.

Ginger It Up

More than four thousand years ago, the ancient Greeks ate ginger wrapped in a piece of bread after a big meal to prevent indigestion. (A bit of that old remedy survives today when you have gingerbread for dessert.) Those old Greeks knew a thing or two: The best use of ginger is for relieving nausea, especially when it comes from motion sickness. In many cases, ginger actually works better than over-the-counter motion-sickness remedies such as dimenhydrinate (Dramamine®)—without the side effects. Many women report that ginger really works on their morning sickness—again, without side effects or possible harm to the unborn baby. That's because ginger works in your stomach, not on your nervous system.

Ginger seems to work best against motion sickness if you take it about 20 minutes before the trip starts. For morning sickness, try taking ginger before going to bed and again as soon as you get up. The form of the ginger doesn't matter very much. You could try half a teaspoon of ground ginger mixed with water or in a capsule, or a cup of ginger tea. Or, you could eat a small piece of fresh gingerroot or even a few pieces of candied ginger.

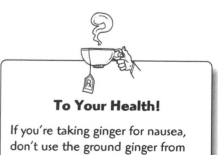

To Your Health!

If you're taking ginger for nausea, don't use the ground ginger from the spice rack—go for the fresh root or get capsules or tea bags at your health-food store.

In traditional Asian medicine, ginger is widely used for just about any medical problem. Ginger tea is indeed a good appetite stimulant and can relieve heartburn and gas. It also helps clear your stuffy head if you have a cold. There's some evidence that ginger can help lower your cholesterol, but not enough to make any sort of recommendation. The Chinese say ginger helps reduce the swelling, pain, and stiffness of arthritis and aids circulation, but there's no evidence to back this up.

Ginkgo: What's Really Old Is New

Ginkgo biloba trees were thriving back when dinosaurs roamed the earth 200 million years ago in the Jurassic era. The dinosaurs are gone, but the ginkgo tree lives on—the oldest tree species on earth.

Gingko leaves are chock full of amazing compounds that improve your blood circulation by relaxing and dilating your blood vessels. The improved circulation is especially helpful to your brain, ears, and extremities. When your blood circulates better, your cells get more oxygen and nutrients and their waste products get carried away more efficiently.

Let's take a closer look at what ginkgo can do:

➤ **Helping cerebrovascular insufficiency.** Poor blood flow to the brain, or cerebrovascular insufficiency, can lead to memory problems (especially in the elderly), hearing problems, dizziness, and dementia. Ginkgo can help by improving blood flow to the brain. For the same reason, ginkgo may help people with Alzheimer's disease.

➤ **Helping peripheratory circulation problems.** People with circulatory problems, such as cold fingers and toes and impotence, may also be helped by ginkgo. Again, that's because ginkgo improves the blood flow to your extremities.

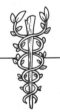

The Healing Arts

You've probably seen ginkgo biloba trees, with their distinctive fan-shaped leaves, lining the sidewalks in big cities. Ginkgo trees, also called maidenhair trees, thrive in cities because they're amazingly resistant to air pollution. They're also very long-lived—there are living ginkgo trees that may be more than a thousand years old. Ginkgos make nice ornamental trees for your property—the leaves turn a beautiful yellow in the fall. Ginkgos, like some other trees and shrubs, can be male or female. The trees sold in nurseries are males; female ginkgo trees produce a nasty-smelling fruit.

➤ **Helping asthma.** Ginkgo is also sometimes helpful for people with asthma. Taking it regularly can help prevent attacks and make them less severe when they do happen.

➤ **Coping with stress.** A lot of people like to take gingko to help them deal with stress, especially stress from overwork. Studies show that gingko does help lift your mood and reduce anxiety. Unlike tranquilizing drugs, it also helps you feel more alert with no side effects.

➤ **Improving alertness.** Ginkgo is often recommended to help concentration and memory and to make you feel more alert. That's why it's popular with students and anyone whose work requires a lot of concentration. And unlike caffeine, ginkgo doesn't keep you from sleeping.

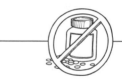

Hazardous to Your Health!

Even mild asthma is a serious health problem, because it can suddenly get much worse. If you already take medicine for asthma—even nonprescription drugs, don't stop. Talk to your doctor about taking ginkgo or any other herb or nutritional supplement before you try it.

Ginkgo is one of the best-studied and safest herbal remedies in the world. It's safe to use even in very large doses, and there don't seem to be any long-term side effects. Ginkgo is so popular and safe that it's the most widely prescribed drug in Germany and is said to be the best-selling natural healthcare product in all of Europe. Worldwide, sales of ginkgo extract top $1 billion.

The best way to take ginkgo is as standardized *ginkgo biloba extract* (GBE), which contains 24 percent flavoglycosides and 6 percent ginkgolides. Flavoglycosides and ginkgolides are complex chemical compounds that are the active ingredients in ginkgo. Ginkgo is available in pills, capsules, tinctures, or extracts at any health-food store—even a lot of drugstores now carry ginkgo. We don't recommend making your own tea from the leaves—it's awful.

The usual dose for GBE tablets or capsules is 40 to 60 mg two to three times a day. Ginkgo usually takes a few weeks to kick in, although some people feel it sooner and others need to take it for a few months before they notice any improvement.

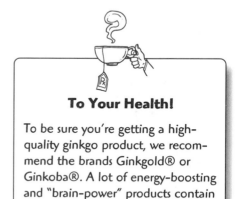

To Your Health!

To be sure you're getting a high-quality ginkgo product, we recommend the brands Ginkgold® or Ginkoba®. A lot of energy-boosting and "brain-power" products contain ginkgo along with other ingredients. Try them and see if they work for you.

Ginseng: The Chinese Secret

Ginseng is one of the world's most popular herbal remedies. In traditional Chinese medicine, it's used for just about everything. Ginseng is said to help your memory, give you energy, slow down the aging process, boost your immune system, improve your love life, and lower your cholesterol. Is ginseng really as magic as some people claim? Keep reading. There's so much to say about this amazing root, and it's so important to traditional Chinese herbal medicine, that we gave it its own long section in Chapter 16.

Goldenseal: Natural Antibiotic

The root of a plant related to buttercups and peonies, goldenseal (*Hydrastis canadensis*) is a powerful antibiotic that should be used with caution. Native Americans used the liquid from pounded goldenseal roots to treat eye irritations, cuts and scrapes, intestinal ailments, and minor infections. Pretty soon European settlers were also using goldenseal, or *hydrastis*, as they sometimes called it, as a sort of cure-all for infections and anything else that ailed them.

By the late 1800s, goldenseal had gotten so popular and was used in so many patent medicines that it started to get very scarce in the wild. To this day, it's hard to find naturally. It's also hard to grow, which is why goldenseal is very expensive today. Is it worth the money? Maybe. Goldenseal contains berberine and hydrastine, chemical compounds that really do slaughter bacteria. (The same chemicals are found in the herbs Oregon grape and barberry; they can be used as low-cost substitutes for goldenseal.)

The Indians were right when they treated digestive problems such as infectious diarrhea with goldenseal. It's also likely that goldenseal gives your immune system a boost, although it's not a really big boost. The mild antibiotic activity is helpful for mouth irritations—try using a goldenseal infusion as a mouthwash for a few days.

Goldenseal is sometimes recommended for women who have very heavy menstrual flows. We can't say if this works. Some of Dr. Pressman's patients have had good results, but others didn't get any benefit. Try it—cautiously—and see, but only if you're positive you're not pregnant.

Berberine in goldenseal can lower your blood pressure, but hydrastine can raise it—a sort of chemical whipsawing that could be bad for you. Don't use goldenseal if you have high blood pressure, glaucoma, diabetes, heart disease, or a history of stroke.

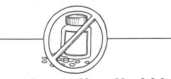

Hazardous to Your Health!

Do not use goldenseal if you are pregnant. Do not use goldenseal if you have had a stroke, or if you have high blood pressure, glaucoma, diabetes, or heart disease.

Goldenseal suddenly got a lot more popular in the 1970s when a rumor went around that taking it masks traces of illegal drug use in urine tests. It doesn't.

A Spoonful of Sugar Makes the Goldenseal Go Down

To make a goldenseal infusion, use ¹/₂ to 1 teaspoon of the ground root per cup of boiling water. Don't drink more than 2 cups a day, and don't use it for more than a few days. Goldenseal is very bitter—to make it drinkable, you'll probably have to add sugar, honey, or fruit juice. Because of the taste, most people prefer to use a tincture. Take up to 1 teaspoon no more than twice a day, and don't use it for more than a few days.

As we mentioned earlier in this chapter, goldenseal is one of those pricey herbs that can tempt people to cheat. If your dose of goldenseal gives you diarrhea, makes you nauseous or causes vomiting, or if you get dizzy or very thirsty, you've probably taken bloodroot. Stop using it immediately. When you feel better, complain to the store where you bought it.

Echinacea: The Indians' Antibiotic

Echinacea was first discovered centuries ago by the Native Americans of the central plains. They, and the settlers who learned from them, used echinacea root as a sort of general cure-all, especially for infections. The Indians were on to something. As recent research has shown, taking echinacea can give your immune system a boost that helps you fight off illness. A lot of people swear by echinacea for preventing colds and flu or helping you get over them faster. Echinacea is also often helpful for other illnesses, like bronchitis, yeast infections, and bladder infections. There's also some good evidence that it can help prevent infections in cancer patients who are getting radiation therapy.

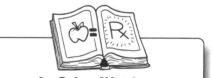

In Other Words...

Echinacea (*Echinacea angustifolia* and *E. purpurea*) is also sometimes called **purple coneflower**. It's pronounced *eh-kin-AY-sha*. The name comes from the Greek word for "hedgehog"—that's because the central cone part of the flower is prickly.

Echinacea seems to work best if you take it at the very first sniffle or other symptom. We suggest using a commercial tincture—there are a number of reliable brands. The usual dose is 1 teaspoon one to three times daily. Don't worry if taking it makes your tongue tingle or even a little numb— it's harmless and goes away quickly. Skip echinacea capsules and tea made from powdered root—you won't get as much of the active ingredients, and besides, the tea tastes terrible.

In Other Words...

Salicin, a chemical found in willow bark, and salicylic acid, the purified version of salicin, get their names from the Latin name for the willow family, *Salix*. The word **aspirin** comes from the Latin name for meadowsweet, *Spiraea*.

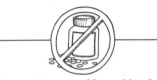

Hazardous to Your Health!

Do not give willow bark or meadowsweet to children under the age of 16 who have a cold, flu, or chicken pox. Pregnant women should not use these herbs.

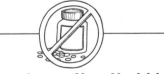

Hazardous to Your Health!

If you're pregnant, talk to your doctor before you try any herbs.

Herbal Aspirin

"Take two aspirin and call me in the morning," your doctor may say. What he or she is really saying is "Use one of the oldest herbal remedies known—it'll help so much you probably won't need me." Willow bark, especially the bark of the white willow, contains *salicin*, which is the active ingredient in *aspirin*. Salicin is a powerful pain reliever and fever reducer. It's been manufactured artificially for just over a century—the first commercial aspirin tablets were introduced in 1899.

Frankly, there's not much that willow bark or meadowsweet can do that an aspirin tablet can't do better. Relatively speaking, there just isn't that much salicin in meadowsweet. Willow bark has more, but it's still a lot less than an aspirin, plus you have to make it into a really bitter-tasting decoction. In their favor, meadowsweet and willow bark are less likely to upset your stomach or cause other aspirin side effects, like ringing in the ears. Even so, don't take more than 3 cups of willow bark or meadowsweet tea in a day. Try it for headaches, mild fevers, muscle pain, and arthritis.

Herbs for Women

For every women's health problem there must be 20 herbs that are said to help. Not all of them do, of course, but a number of herbs truly are useful for things like PMS, menstrual cramps, bladder infections, and breast-feeding problems. We made up a table showing the most useful herbs for various problems, but we can't give any dosages or recommendations. Which herb and how much you take depend a lot on your individual pattern of symptoms. In general, follow the directions on the container and be cautious. And if you're pregnant, talk to your doctor before you try any herbs.

Herbs for Women

Problem	Herbs That Help
Bladder infection (cystitis)	bearberry (*uva-ursi*)
	birch leaves
	blueberry
	cranberry
	echinacea
Breast-feeding problems	anise
	chasteberry (*Vitex*)
	echinacea
	fennel
	fenugreek
	garlic
Menopause	angelica (*dong quai*)
	black cohosh root
	chasteberry
Menstru l cramps	black haw (crampbark)
	raspberry leaves
	valerian
Morning sickness	ginger
	peppermint
Premenstrual syndrome (PMS)	angelica
	chasteberry
	valerian
Vaginitis	garlic
	goldenseal
	tea-tree oil
Yeast infections	bearberry (*uva-ursi*)
	blueberry
	cranberry
	echinacea
	garlic
	goldenseal

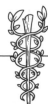

The Healing Arts

Wild yam root (*Dioscorea villosa*) was used by the Native Americans to help during childbirth. Later, the first birth-control pills were made from a substance found in the roots, but there's a word for women who think taking wild yam prevents pregnancy: Mommy. Because wild yam root has small amounts of natural hormones in it, some women claim that a skin cream containing it helps relieve menopause symptoms such as hot flashes and vaginal dryness. If your menopause symptoms are very mild, you might want to try this instead of taking hormone replacement pills. Rub the cream into the skin on your abdomen twice a day.

Herbs for Men

Okay guys, listen up. There's two herbs you need to know about:

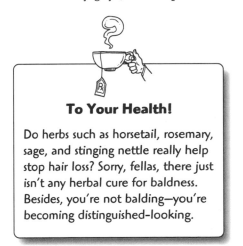

To Your Health!

Do herbs such as horsetail, rosemary, sage, and stinging nettle really help stop hair loss? Sorry, fellas, there just isn't any herbal cure for baldness. Besides, you're not balding—you're becoming distinguished-looking.

➤ **Yohimbé.** An African herb, yohimbé can help impotence problems by increasing the blood flow to the penis. The active ingredient, yohimbine, is approved by the FDA for use in prescription drugs to treat impotence. The drugs (Yocon® and Yohimex®) work reasonably well without bad side effects. There are a lot of over-the-counter preparations containing yohimbé designed for helping out a romantic evening, but we advise against them. Raw yohimbé can have nasty side effects, including trembling, rapid heartbeat, and a dangerous jump in your blood pressure.

➤ **Saw palmetto.** The berries of the saw palmetto (*Serenoa repens*), also known as sabal, are great news for men with *benign prostate hyperplasia* (BPH, also known as *prostate enlargement*). Saw palmetto can help relieve the annoying symptoms of BPH, such as frequent urination, as well as if not better than expensive prescription drugs such as finasteride (Proscar®), and without the side effects. In Germany, several good studies have shown that saw palmetto works and it is widely prescribed there. Here in the United States, saw palmetto can only be sold as a nutritional supplement in the health-food store.

Ginkgo can be very helpful for erection problems caused by poor circulation. Two other herbs are said to help BPH symptoms: stinging nettle and another African herb, pygeum.

Herbs for the Digestion

Treating minor digestive upsets is probably the most common use of herbs. Problems like nausea, vomiting, heartburn, gas, diarrhea, and constipation respond pretty well to herbs, if you know which ones to use for what—check out the following table. The herbs listed usually work best if you make them into infusions and sip them down.

Herbs for Digestive Problems

Problem	Herbs That Help
Appetite loss	gentian
	ginseng
Constipation	flax seeds
	psyllium seeds (flea seeds)
	slippery elm bark
Diarrhea	black tea
	dried blueberries
	goldenseal
	raspberry leaves
Gallstones	dandelion
	devil's claw
	gentian
	milk thistle
	turmeric
Gas (flatulence)	anise seed
	caraway seeds
	chamomile
	dill seed
	fennel seeds
	ginger
	peppermint

continues

Herbs for Digestive Problems   (continued)

Problem	Herbs That Help
Heartburn	chamomile
	dill seed
	gentian
	peppermint
Nausea	chamomile
	ginger
	peppermint

Everyone gets occasional digestive upsets, but use your common sense about treating them. What you think is just bad heartburn, for instance, could actually be a heart attack or gall bladder trouble. Severe diarrhea in children and the elderly can be fatal. If your digestive problem doesn't clear up quickly, with or without herbs, call your doctor.

Letting Loose: Herbal Laxatives

A typical health-food store has a whole shelf full of herbal remedies for constipation. Watch out—a lot of these remedies work all too well. Herbs like aloe, buckthorn (frangula), cascara sagrada, rhubarb, and senna contain powerful laxatives that will solve your constipation problem in a hurry but may also give you severe cramps and diarrhea. Also, the effects of just one dose could be with you for several days. Take the natural approach to constipation and use bulk-forming herbs such as psyllium or flax

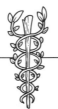

The Healing Arts

Because stomach ulcers are really, really painful, and because for a long time there wasn't much doctors could do for them, there are a lot of herbal ulcer remedies. The best-known and most effective is licorice, in the form of **deglycyrrhizinated licorice** (DGL). You can get this at most health-food stores. Today we know that most ulcers are caused by pepsin. If you think you have an ulcer, don't treat it yourself with herbs—see your doctor at once. Antibiotics and pink bismuth (Pepto-Bismol®) generally get rid of ulcers for good in just a couple of months.

seeds—these give you the fiber you need to stimulate a normal bowel movement. If you must use a laxative, try a traditional one that's safe, effective, and cheap: prune juice. Some people even like the taste.

Skinny Herbs

Wouldn't it be great if there was a magic herb you could take to lose weight? If there was, we'd be selling it, not writing books for a living. You can try one of the many weight-loss teas carried at your health-food store. Sometimes called "yogi" teas, these blends generally contain *diuretic* herbs such as uva-ursi, buchu, and dandelion, often along with the stimulant herb ephedra (more about this one a little further on) and caffeine. Because diuretics make you pass more urine, you lose some water weight right away; the stimulants get you so wired that you lose your appetite. There aren't too many more unhealthy ways to lose weight. Stay away.

Herbs for Heart Health

Many of today's valuable drugs for heart problems, circulatory problems, and high blood pressure have roots in herbal medicine. Digitalis, for example, is a heart drug made from the beautiful foxglove plant.

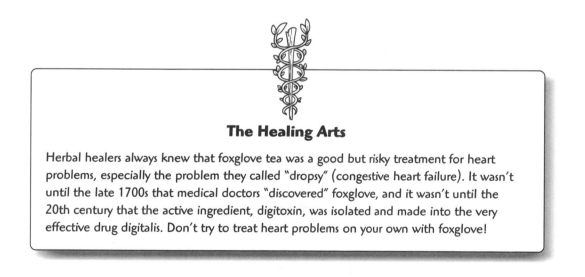

The Healing Arts

Herbal healers always knew that foxglove tea was a good but risky treatment for heart problems, especially the problem they called "dropsy" (congestive heart failure). It wasn't until the late 1700s that medical doctors "discovered" foxglove, and it wasn't until the 20th century that the active ingredient, digitoxin, was isolated and made into the very effective drug digitalis. Don't try to treat heart problems on your own with foxglove!

We're not suggesting that you treat serious medical problems such as angina with herbs, but some herbs could be useful along with your medicine. We've already talked about how garlic, ginger, and ginkgo can help your heart and circulation. There are two other herbs that are definitely useful:

➤ **Hawthorn.** A traditional herbal remedy in Germany, hawthorn has been shown to help congestive heart failure and angina and to help lower blood pressure. It's widely prescribed in Germany as a general heart tonic, but here in the United States, it's strictly a dietary supplement. Hawthorn is powerful stuff, so talk to your doctor before you try it.

➤ **Horse chestnut.** Traditionally, varicose veins have been treated with an extract made from horse chestnut. This is another of those herbs that are safe, effective, and widely prescribed in Europe but available here only at the health-food store. If you want to try it, use only a standardized extract and follow the directions on the label.

Other herbs that are often recommended for heart and circulatory health include angelica (dong quai, in traditional Chinese herbal medicine), blueberry, butcher's broom, purslane, and rosemary. Use them all with caution and only after discussing them with your doctor. Do not use herbs instead of your prescribed medicine!

The Herb that Helps Depression

You've probably been hearing a lot about *St. John's wort* (*Hypericum perforatum*) as a natural treatment for depression and anxiety. St. John's wort is sometimes called *Hypericum*; it's also sometimes called "herbal Prozac®" because it works so well. We don't want to mislead you. St. John's wort can help lift your mood, but only if you're just mildly depressed or anxious or going though a bad period—if you're in a deep depression, you need real medical help.

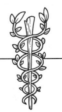

The Healing Arts

St. John's wort gets its name from the folk belief that if you gather the plant (*wort* is an Old English word for "plant") on St. John's Day (June 24) and sleep with it under your pillow, you'll be safe from witchcraft for the coming year.

The National Institutes of Health (NIH) started a three-year study of St. John's wort in October 1997. It'll take a while to get the results, but let's hope they'll be positive. A month's worth of St. John's wort costs about $10; a month's worth of Prozac® costs about $75.

St. John's wort is basically safe and doesn't have the side effects of many drugs used to treat depression. In Germany, doctors write about three million prescriptions for St. John's wort every year—and far fewer for antidepressant drugs such as Prozac®. Your doctor here in America can't prescribe St. John's wort, but you can get it in a lot of standardized forms at your health-food store. Look for a version that's standardized to 0.3 percent hypericin, which is the most active ingredient in St. John's wort. We like the brand HyperiCalm®, but whichever standardized brand you choose, the usual dose is 200 to 300 mg two to three times a day. You'll probably need to take it for three to six weeks before the effects really kick in. If St. John's wort makes you nauseous, tired, restless, or dizzy, or if it gives you a rash, stop taking it.

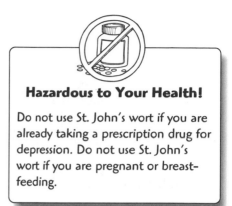

Hazardous to Your Health!

Do not use St. John's wort if you are already taking a prescription drug for depression. Do not use St. John's wort if you are pregnant or breast-feeding.

Herbal Ups: Caffeine and Ephedra

The most commonly used herbal drug in the world is *caffeine*, the stimulating chemical found in coffee, tea, cola, and some one 100 other herbs such as maté (a popular beverage in South America). In general, herbs containing caffeine are a safe and legal way of getting a mild energy lift.

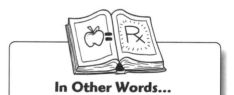

In Other Words...

Caffeine is an alkaloid chemical found in many plants. It was first isolated from coffee in 1820. Caffeine in general is a mild stimulant that improves alertness and concentration.

Ephedra: Is It Safe?

Also known by its Chinese name, *mahuang*, *ephedra* is one of the world's oldest drugs. It's been used for thousands of years to treat asthma and other respiratory problems. It works because Ephedra contains ephedrine, a chemical that relaxes the smooth muscles around the bronchioles and stimulates the central nervous system. In fact, synthetic ephedrine is found in many popular over-the-counter cold, allergy, and asthma remedies. These medicines, when used as directed on the package, are very helpful for relieving stuffiness, congestion, and coughing.

Ephedra is a powerful stimulant. It's so strong that it's banned by the National Collegiate

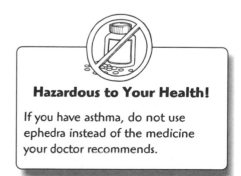

Hazardous to Your Health!

If you have asthma, do not use ephedra instead of the medicine your doctor recommends.

Athletic Association (NCAA) and the U.S. Olympic Committee, even though you can buy drugs containing it at the supermarket. Ephedra, often combined with caffeine, is also sold as a drug for recreational use and is said to be a "natural high" or "herbal ecstasy." Unfortunately, large doses of ephedra can be very dangerous or even fatal—as a number of young people tragically proved in the 1990s. Today ephedra products are regulated in more than 20 states, and there is serious discussion of further regulation at the federal level.

Ephedra has its uses, but recreational highs isn't one of them. Stay away.

Calming Down with Herbs

The most widely prescribed drug in America is diazepam (Valium®), a muscle relaxant that helps relieve tension and anxiety. Why take addictive prescription drugs for tension or to get to sleep when there are so many herbs that do the same thing, safely and without side effects? Here's a rundown of calming herbs:

➤ **Kava.** One of the hottest herbs today, kava comes from the Polynesian islands of the South Pacific. Prepared fresh the traditional way, it's recreationally much like alcohol, without alcohol's unpleasant side effects or chance of addiction—and without alcohol's hangover. More commonly outside Polynesia, Kava is used as a safe, effective natural sleeping pill, muscle relaxant, and treatment for anxiety. It's now available in standardized capsules and as a concentrated tincture; follow the directions on the label. Skip kava tea bags—the active ingredients don't dissolve in water, so you won't get any effect.

➤ **Valerian.** Nature's best-known tranquilizer is valerian root. It really works to help you get to sleep—and it's safe, nonaddictive, and doesn't interact with alcohol or other drugs. Valerian is also a good muscle relaxant. Many women find that it really helps for PMS and menstrual discomfort. You can make a tea from powdered valerian root, but to put it bluntly, the stuff stinks. Old gym socks smell better. We suggest using standardized valerian extract; the usual dose is 150 to 300 mg. Take it about an hour before you're ready for bed.

➤ **Hops.** A traditional European sleep aid, hops can be taken as an infusion. Some people swear by pillows filled with hops—try it for yourself and see.

The herbs skullcap and passionflower are used in a lot of nonprescription sleep aids in Europe. In the United States, the FDA has banned passionflower in nonprescription drugs. If you'd like to try either of these herbs for insomnia, look for them in the health-food store.

Other Healing Herbs

There are so many herbs that are valuable for so many health problems that all we can do here is hit some more highlights:

➤ **Fenugreek.** In the traditional medicine of India, fenugreek is used for treating diabetes. Recent studies have shown that it can help regulate blood-sugar levels and control high cholesterol. If you have diabetes or high cholesterol, talk to your doctor about fenugreek before you try it. Don't use it if you're pregnant.

➤ **Feverfew.** Feverfew leaves have been shown to be an effective treatment for preventing migraine headaches. If you get migraines, discuss feverfew with your doctor before you try it. Buy a standardized extract from a reliable manufacturer.

➤ **Lemon balm (melissa).** For treating cold sores and herpes blisters, try making an infusion of lemon balm, then dabbing it on the sore with a cotton ball. Repeat several times a day.

➤ **Milk thistle (silymarin).** Milk thistle is very helpful for people with liver problems such as hepatitis. Buy it in capsules at the health-food store.

➤ **Red pepper ointment (capsaicin).** For painful skin conditions like shingles or herpes blisters, try a commercial red pepper (cayenne) ointment such as Zostrix®.

➤ **Witch hazel.** An excellent home remedy for hemorrhoids, witch hazel reduces swelling and pain. Look for nondistilled (no alcohol) witch hazel extract at your health-food store.

Time after time, modern research shows that traditional herbal remedies have healing value. Be cautious with the herbs you try, however, and talk to your doctor first if you have a serious medical condition.

Your Herbal First-Aid Kit

Herbs are handy around the house for minor medical emergencies. Here's what we suggest for your herbal first-aid kit:

➤ **Aloe.** This fleshy plant grows easily in a flowerpot on the kitchen windowsill. To relieve the pain of a minor burn or cut, break off a piece from one of the plant's thick leaves and rub the gel inside onto the affected area. Aloe gel is also effective on minor sunburns and dry skin.

➤ **Arnica.** For bruises, bumps, and muscle aches, rub some arnica ointment into the skin where it hurts. Don't use arnica internally or on broken skin.

➤ **Calendula.** Calendula cream is good for minor skin problems, like insect bites, scratches, and scrapes.

➤ **Clove oil.** As an emergency treatment for toothache, clove oil is effective—but it's only temporary. Soak a cotton ball in the oil and rub it directly against the aching tooth and gums. See your dentist as soon as possible.

➤ **Ginger.** As discussed earlier, ginger is a good treatment for indigestion, gas, and nausea. For your first-aid kit, get some ginger capsules or ginger tea bags.

➤ **Peppermint.** This is another good treatment for indigestion, gas, and nausea. Keep some peppermint tea bags in your emergency kit.

➤ **Tea-tree oil.** We talk about this useful antiseptic in detail in Chapter 24, "Aromatherapy: The Nose Knows." Use it on minor cuts, scrapes, and burns.

You should be able to deal with a lot of minor household accidents and illnesses using your herbal first-aid kit. Know the difference between minor problems and a real emergency, though, and get medical help fast if you need it.

Herbs to Avoid

Just because it's natural doesn't mean it's good. Many herbs have healing qualities—and there are some herbs that can kill you. In between, there's a large group of herbs that could do more harm than good. Unfortunately, a few books still recommend herbs such a coltsfoot or lobelia, which are known to have serious side effects even in small doses or to contain cancer-causing compounds. Always be extremely careful about using any herb—when in doubt, skip it.

Check out this table to see the herbs you should definitely avoid. Among the herbs to skip, some are more dangerous than others. We've noted the ones that are especially toxic.

Herbs to Avoid

Herb	Comments
Aconite (*Aconitum napellus*)	Very toxic
American hellebore (*Veratrum viride*)	Very toxic; skin irritant
Angelica (*Angelica archangelica*)	
Arnica (*Arnica montana*)	Safe for external use
Autumn crocus (*Colchicum autumnale*)	
Bayberry (*Myrica cerifera*)	
Black hellebore (*Helleborus niger*)	Very toxic; skin irritant
Bloodroot (*Sanguinaria canadensis*)	
Blue cohosh root (*Caulophyllum thalictroides*)	
Broom (*Cystisus scoparius*)	Very toxic
Coltsfoot (*Tussilago farfara*)	

Herb	Comments
Comfrey (*Symphytum officinale*)	
Deadly nightshade (*Atropa belladonna*)	Very toxic
Ephedra (*Ephedra spp.*)	
European mandrake (*Viscum album*)	Very toxic
Eyebright (*Euphrasia officinalis*)	
Foxglove (*Digitalis purpurea*)	Very toxic
Hemlock (*Conium maculatum*)	Very toxic
Jimsonweed (*Datura stamonium*)	Very toxic
Juniper (*Juniperus communis*)	
Licorice (*Glycyrrhiza glabra*)	Toxic in large doses
Life root (*Senecio aureus*)	
Lobelia (*Lobelia inflata*)	Very toxic
Mayapple (*Podophyllum peltatum*)	Very toxic
Mistletoe (*Phoradendron serotinum* or *Viscum album*)	Very toxic
Pennyroyal (*Hedeoma pulegioides* or *Mentha pulegium*)	Toxic internally
Pokeweed (*Phytolacca americana*)	Very toxic
Rue (*Ruta graveolens*)	Toxic; skin irritant
Sassafras (*Sassafras albidum*)	
Sweet flag (*Acorus calamus*)	
Tansy (*Tanacetum vulgare*)	
Wahoo (*Euonymus atropurpurea*)	
Wormwood (*Artemisia absinthium*)	

Sources: FDA; Varro Tyler, The Honest Herbal *(Pharmaceutical Products Press, 1993).*

Finding a Qualified Herbalist

You're pretty much on your own when it comes to finding a qualified herbalist. No national organization certifies herbalists, and there's no recognized degree in the subject. Naturopathic physicians are well trained in the use of healing herbs, so we suggest consulting one if you want advice on herbal remedies for a medical problem. (For more information on finding a naturopathic physician, see Chapter 4, "Naturopathy: The Healing Power of Nature.") Some health insurance policies cover visits to naturopathic physicians, but none that we know of cover herbalists or herbal remedies.

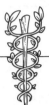

The Healing Arts

In Germany, medicinal herbs are studied for their safety and effectiveness by the doctors and scientists of the E Commission, which advises the German government. Many of today's most popular herbs have been approved as over-the-counter drugs by the E Commission. Here in the United States, the FDA used to keep a list of herbs generally regarded as safe (GRAS). Although the FDA doesn't keep the list anymore, a lot of herbs are still advertised as GRAS.

The complete set of German E Commission reports on specific herbs is available from the American Botanical Council. You can get the 600-page book at your public library or from:

American Botanical Council
P.O. Box 201660
Austin, TX 78720
Phone: (800) 373-7105
Fax: (512) 331-1924
E-mail: ABC@herbalgram.org

The E Commission book is pricey at nearly $200. There are many, many other outstanding books on herbs that are a lot less expensive. They're also in most public libraries. We recommend *The Healing Herbs*, by Michael Castleman (Rodale, 1991), and *The Honest Herbal*, by Varro E. Tyler, Ph.D. (Pharmaceutical Products Press, 1993).

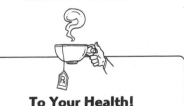

To Your Health!

Don't trust your health to a part-time clerk at the health-food store. Do your research, talk to your doctor, and always use herbs with caution.

Rules, Rules, Rules

When you buy a bottle of herb capsules, there's not much information on the label. Generally there's just some vague wording about "promotes relaxation" or "supports healthy circulation," followed by an asterisk. The asterisk then points out "This statement has not been evaluated by the Food and Drug Administration. This product is not intended to diagnose, treat, cure, or prevent any disease." Supplement makers have to use this roundabout language because the FDA, the federal agency in charge of these things, doesn't allow herb manufacturers to say anything on the label that suggests the herb is a drug or treats a particular disease. We could rant on for a while about how illogical this attitude is, but it won't help you much (although it would make us feel better). The only advice we can offer is to be an informed consumer.

Herbal Help or Herbal Hype?

Most doctors would agree that herbs are useful for minor problems like an upset stomach. They worry, however, that you'll treat a serious problem with herbs instead of coming in for treatment. The delay could make the problem that much worse and harder to treat. They also worry that you'll diagnose yourself incorrectly and treat yourself for the wrong problem, or that you'll use the wrong herbs. Again, that could make your real problem worse. Doctors also point out that in most cases, standard drugs—prescription or nonprescription—are safe, effective, inexpensive, and work better and faster than herbs. In fairness, we should also say that many doctors have become a lot more open-minded about combining standard medicine with herbal approaches to some problems, such as insomnia, migraines, and PMS.

The Least You Need to Know

➤ Traditional herbal remedies are safe and helpful for minor health problems and first–aid emergencies when used cautiously.

➤ Traditional herbal remedies can be helpful for asthma and for heart and circulatory problems.

➤ Women can benefit from herbal remedies for PMS, menstrual discomfort, breast-feeding problems, cystitis, yeast infections, and other problems.

➤ Digestive problems—nausea, indigestion, gas, diarrhea, and constipation—can be helped with herbs.

➤ Herbs can be used to treat depression and insomnia safely and without side effects.

Chapter 16

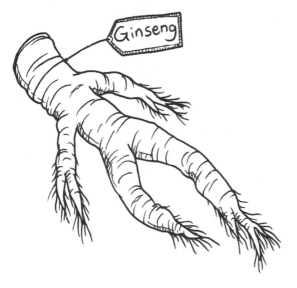

Ginseng and More: Traditional Chinese Herbs

In This Chapter

➤ Herbs in traditional Chinese medicine

➤ Which herbs for what?

➤ The most common Chinese herbs and what they do

➤ Preparing Chinese herbs

➤ Using Chinese patent medicines

➤ Ginseng—the Chinese cure-all

The legendary Chinese emperor Shen Nung is revered for two things. First, he introduced agriculture to China—that's why he's sometimes called the Divine Farmer. Second, he introduced herbal medicine to his people. Legend tells us Shen Nung had a transparent abdomen, which must have been handy for his herbal experiments. Unfortunately, Shen Nung experimented on himself once too often and managed to kill himself accidentally with a poisonous herb—but not before he wrote down more than two hundred herbal remedies.

Five thousand years later, the Chinese tradition of herbal medicine is still going strong—and not just in China. Some Chinese herbs, like ginseng, have become a regular part of herbal treatment here in the West as well. We still have plenty to learn from the mysterious East.

The Herbal Wisdom of China

When it comes to herbs, nobody beats the Chinese. We're not exaggerating when we say that some six *thousand* herbs are part of Chinese herbal lore. In practice, of course, far fewer—only about five hundred—are regularly used, but you can easily see why students in China have to study for years just to learn the basics of herbal medicine.

Not only do they have to learn about each herb individually, they have to learn about how the herbs work in combination. Western herbal medicine generally uses just one or two herbs to treat a problem—peppermint tea to treat indigestion, for example. In traditional Chinese medicine, this approach would be seen as very crude. A Chinese herbalist would decide *why* you're having indigestion and then would prescribe an herbal combination based on the diagnosis. What exactly goes into the combination? That's what you'll spend the rest of this chapter finding out.

Five Energies, Five Tastes

In traditional Chinese medicine, the energies of herbs affect your balance of *Yin* and *Yang*, and the tastes of herbs affect the flow of your *Qi*. (Remember those from Chapter 6, "Traditional Chinese Medicine"?) Let's look more closely at how this works.

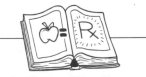

In Other Words...

Yin and **Yang** are the opposing, balancing forces of the universe. Everything and everyone contains both Yin and Yang aspects. **Qi** (sometimes written *chi* or *ch'i* and pronounced *chee*) is the invisible but fundamental energy that flows through everything and everyone in the universe. Qi is the life force of all living things, but it's also the energy found in all nonliving things.

Back in Chapter 6, we talked about the Five Energies. Something that is very Yin is cold, while something that is very Yang is hot. In between are moderately Yin things (cool), moderately Yang things (warm), and balanced Yin-Yang things (neutral). The idea of Five Energies applies to Chinese herbs. An herb that is very Yin is said to be cold. And in *traditional Chinese medicine* (TCM), cold Yin herbs are used to treat Yang conditions, such as heartburn, which are hot. So your *Oriental medical practitioner* (OMP) decides which herbs to prescribe based on your balance of Yin and Yang.

Herbs also have tastes or flavors. We talked about the Five Tastes in foods back in Chapter 6. The same Five Tastes apply to herbs: sour, bitter, sweet, pungent, and salty. Herbs have different effects on you depending on their taste. Here's the rundown:

➤ **Sour.** Herbs that are sour have a tightening effect and concentrate your Qi. Your liver and gallbladder are most affected by sour herbs.

➤ **Bitter.** These herbs reduce excess Qi and dry up excess moisture. Your heart and small intestine are most affected by bitter herbs.

➤ **Sweet.** Sweet herbs strengthen your Qi and invigorate and cleanse your Blood. Your spleen and stomach are most affected by sweet herbs.

➤ **Pungent.** Spicy or pungent herbs get your Qi moving and tonify (generally improve) your Blood (check back to Chapter 6 for more on Blood). Your lungs and large intestine are most affected by pungent herbs.

➤ **Salty.** Herbs that are salty are said to be softening. Your kidneys and bladder are most affected by salty herbs.

The Five Tastes aren't absolutes. A lot of herbs have more than one. Cinnamon, for instance, is said to be both sweet and pungent.

Channeling Herbal Energy

What happens when you take an herb? In TCM, the herb moves through the energy channels (meridians) in your body—the same meridians that your Qi flows through. (Check back to Chapter 6 for more on meridians.) The herb "moves" through your body by:

➤ **Ascending and floating.** These herbs move up and out. They influence the top part of your body and your fingers and toes.

➤ **Descending and sinking.** These herbs move down and in. They influence the lower part of your body and your interior organs.

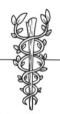

The Healing Arts

In traditional Chinese medicine, your Qi moves through your body along invisible pathways called **meridians.** You have 12 regular meridians, each relating to one of the 12 major organs in traditional Chinese medicine. You also have eight extraordinary meridians that tie in closely to the regular ones. Blockages in the meridians interrupt the smooth flow of Qi and cause health problems. Acupuncture and herbs are the main treatments used to remove the blockages and to get your Qi flowing again.

In addition, herbs can "enter" different channels and affect the Zangfu organs. (Remember them from Chapter 6? The most important are your liver, lungs, spleen, heart, and kidneys.)

Your OMP chooses which herbs to prescribe based on what your Zangfu organs need to get your Qi flowing smoothly again. In general, the effects of the herbs fall into four categories:

➤ **Strengthening.** These herbs strengthen or supplement your Qi.

➤ **Moving.** These herbs redistribute your Qi.

➤ **Dispersing.** These herbs get blocked Qi moving again and relieve stagnation.

➤ **Purging.** These herbs relieve conditions related to blocked or excess Qi and get toxins out of your body.

Some herbs are considered tonics that strengthen your overall Qi and keep you healthy. They're used when you're well to keep you that way, instead of as treatments when you're sick.

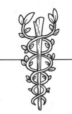

The Healing Arts

The concept of Yin and Yang applies to your organs. You have five solid Yin organs: your lungs, heart, spleen, liver, and kidneys. Collectively, these organs are called the **Zang organs**. You also have six hollow organs that are Yang: your small intestine, large intestine, gallbladder, bladder, stomach, and the Triple Heater. The Triple Heater isn't really an organ; it's more a sort of pathway connecting your organs, but especially your lungs, spleen, and kidneys. Collectively, these organs are called the **Fu organs**. When speaking of organs in general, then, TCM talks about the Zangfu system.

Harmonizing with Herbs

Once your Chinese doctor has decided what your problem is based on the traditional diagnostic ideas we talked about in Chapter 6, the next step is to come up with an herbal formula that will help. Your practitioner starts with a basic, time-tested formula that helps your particular type of imbalance. The basic formula could be pretty complicated, with at least five or six herbs and often 10 or 12 or even more. Each herb is chosen for its particular effect; in combination, the herbs help restore your internal

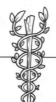

The Healing Arts

In China, herbal prescriptions are filled at herbal pharmacies, just as we go to the drugstore to get our drugs. The highly trained staff at the herbal pharmacy measures out the right quantities of the dried herbs and combines them all together. Rather than getting pills in a bottle, you get a pile of dried herbs. The pharmacist divides a week's worth of herbs into daily doses and puts them into small paper bags.

balance. But because each patient is different, the basic formula is just a starting point. Your herbalist may modify the prescription by adding or changing some of the herbs to fit your case; some changes may also be made because of your age. As you continue to take the formula, additional changes may be made, especially if the formula is giving you digestive upset or doesn't seem to be working as well as it should.

Who's in Charge Here?

To design your personal herbal prescription, your OPM follows some basic principles to make sure the herbs all harmonize with each other. The primary herb in the mixture is known as the *king* or *lord* herb. This herb is targeted at the main symptom or cause of the disease and dominates the formula. The *minister* herb strengthens the effect of the king herb and is also aimed at symptoms. The *assistant* or *servant* herbs help strengthen the king and minister herbs, treat less-important symptoms, and reduce any unpleasant side effects the king and minister herbs cause. Some herbs act as *guides* or *envoys* that lead the other herbs to the right part of the body. Other herbs *harmonize* the mixture and coordinate the action of the various herbs.

Let's look at an example. A common prescription for arthritis is a tea called Du Huo Ji Sheng Tang. The *du huo* part of the name is the Chinese word for the herb angelica root. The *ji sheng* part of the name is the Chinese word for "mistletoe." The *tang* part means this mixture should be taken as a tea. The du huo is the king herb. It expels wind, damp, and cold from the lower part of the body and from the bones and joints. The ji sheng is the minister herb; it also expels cold and damp. The 12 other herbs in the mixture act in varying ways to expel wind, cold, and damp; tonify various organs; invigorate the Blood; and guide and harmonize the mixture.

Healing with Chinese Herbs

In China, herbs are used for minor ailments just the way we in the West pop a couple of aspirins or buy an over-the-counter cough medicine. Westerners usually turn to Chinese herbs for ongoing problems such as PMS, menstrual difficulties, asthma, arthritis, fatigue, headaches, insomnia, depression, poor concentration, and the like. These are problems Western medicine treats with powerful drugs that may have unpleasant side effects like sleepiness or stomach upset—and that don't deal with the underlying causes of the problem.

Your OMP will come up with an herbal mixture designed to treat your particular health problem by correcting your particular imbalance. The process could take a while. You'll probably have to take the herbs for at least a couple of weeks before you notice any improvement. If you don't get better, your OMP may adjust the herbal mixture a bit, which should speed up your healing.

Chinese herbal mixtures have evolved over centuries of experience and are used to treat even serious problems such as high blood pressure and high cholesterol. However—and this is a very big however—they usually don't work as well, as quickly, or as predictably as standard Western drugs, and sometimes they don't work at all.

They can also interact in unknown ways with any drugs you are taking. If you take medicine for a problem such as asthma, heart disease, diabetes, high blood pressure, high cholesterol, or any other condition that you think could be treated with Chinese herbs, *talk to your doctor first. Never stop taking your medicine on your own.*

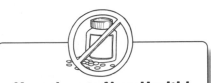

Hazardous to Your Health!

If you take medicine for a problem such as asthma, heart disease, diabetes, high blood pressure, high cholesterol, or any other condition, talk to your doctor before you try Chinese herbs. Dangerous drug interactions could occur. Never stop taking your medicine on your own.

Broadly speaking, it's usually safe to take Chinese herbal remedies along with any medication your Western doctor prescribes, but be sure to discuss your drugs with your herbalist first. Be very cautious with the herbs and stop taking them if you notice any sort of side effect, such as nausea, headache, dizziness, shortness of breath, or diarrhea.

In some cases, the Chinese herbs may work so well that your doctor will lower the dosage on your medicine. *Do not lower the dose or stop taking the drug on your own.*

Ginseng

Ginseng is one of the most commonly used herbs in China. It's become so popular that it's part of Western herbal medicine as well. Between 1687 and 1975, more than a thousand books and papers were published on the value of ginseng. Since 1975, hundreds if not thousands of additional books and papers have been written. Ginseng is one of the best-understood herbs available today.

In the West, ginseng is used mostly as a general tonic and pick-me-up. In China, ginseng is more likely to be used as part of an herbal formula, although it's also used by itself.

In traditional Chinese medicine, ginseng is a very valuable Qi tonic. It has different effects on different people, depending on the state of their Qi. If you're healthy, ginseng improves your stamina, helps you cope with stress, and keeps you alert. It's also said to preserve male virility. If you're sick, ginseng may have a positive effect on your immune system. It also helps you recover faster and lifts your mood. Ginseng is most often used as a tonic for the elderly to improve their overall well-being.

Generally, ginseng isn't used by itself in Chinese medicine. In fact, using it alone is not recommended. Instead, ginseng is an important ingredient in many herbal mixtures. Chinese herbalists also caution against using ginseng too frequently. If you take it over too long a period, you could get insomnia, headaches, high blood pressure, or even heart palpitations.

There are five different kinds of ginseng, but only two are really ginseng in the scientific sense. They're all roots, but each is botanically different, and each has different uses in traditional Chinese herbal medicine.

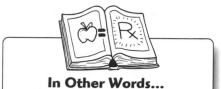

In Other Words...

Ginseng is actually a generic name for several different types of roots used in traditional Chinese medicine. The word comes from the Chinese word *gin* or *jen*, meaning "shape or form of man" and *seng* or *shen*, meaning "spirit of the earth" or "strengthening root." In modern Chinese, ginseng is called **ren shen**.

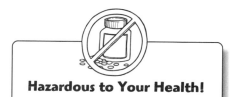

Hazardous to Your Health!

Do not use ginseng if you have high blood pressure.

Chinese Ginseng

Chinese ginseng (*Panax ginseng*) is the traditional ginseng that has been used in China for thousands of years. It's called *ren shen* in Chinese and is also sometimes called *red ginseng* or *Korean ginseng*. It's usually taken as a tea made from sliced or ground roots, although some people prefer capsules or pills. It's used as a general Qi tonic and is said to strengthen the immune system and increase energy. In herbal terms, Chinese ginseng is Yang and has a warming, stimulating effect. Its taste is sweet, and it mostly affects the spleen, heart, and lung channels. Many herbalists recommend taking ginseng for a month in the fall to get your body ready for the cold weather.

American Ginseng

American ginseng (*Panax quinquefolium*), or *xi yang shen* in Chinese, is also sometimes called *white ginseng*. It's been prized by the Chinese since the early 1700s, when Native Americans, who knew all about its medicinal uses, introduced it to European settlers, who then brought it to China by roundabout routes. In China today, American ginseng is taken as a tea. Chinese herbalists feel it is milder than Chinese ginseng and is better for elderly patients. It's also recommended for fever and lung problems. American ginseng is said to prevent wrinkles and to be rejuvenating—and also to cure hangovers. In herbal terms, American ginseng has a cooling, moistening effect that's especially valuable when the weather is hot or dry.

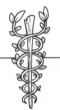

The Healing Arts

A study in the prestigious *Journal of the American Medical Association* back in 1979 claimed that heavy users of ginseng could develop ginseng-abuse syndrome. Symptoms were said to include insomnia, high blood pressure, and diarrhea. In fact, the study was badly flawed, and doctors today agree there's no such thing as ginseng-abuse syndrome. And ginseng is on the FDA's list of herbs that are generally regarded as safe.

American ginseng grows wild in cool, wooded areas of the Northeast and Midwest. Wild ginseng has been so intensively hunted that it's now an endangered species—there's an official wild ginseng season, and you need a permit to harvest it. Almost all the American ginseng sold today is commercially grown in Marathon County, Wisconsin, and exported to China. The roots take at least six years to grow large enough to harvest. Today ginseng is one of the most profitable crops you can grow legally—high-quality roots sell for $50 or more a pound.

Pseudoginseng

As you might guess from the name, pseudoginseng (*Panax notoginseng*) is a close relative of Chinese and American ginseng, but it's not quite the same thing. It's used in the same way, but in China it's also used for heart and circulatory problems. It's said to be very helpful for relieving bruises and stopping bleeding. Pseudoginseng (*tien chi* in Chinese) is usually taken as a powder mixed in water. When the raw root is used, it has a cooling effect; when the root is steamed and then powdered, it has a warming effect. It's often recommended as a spring tonic to get your blood moving. A drink made from pseudoginseng flowers is said to help problems such as nausea, insomnia, and headache.

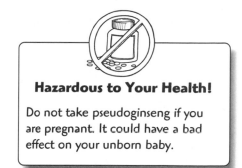

Hazardous to Your Health!

Do not take pseudoginseng if you are pregnant. It could have a bad effect on your unborn baby.

Siberian Ginseng

Siberian ginseng (*Eleutherococcus senticosus*) is in the same botanical family as Chinese and American ginseng, but it's not a true ginseng. To avoid confusion, Western herbalists often call it *eleuthero*; in Chinese, the name is *wu cha seng* or *ci wu jia*. In general, Siberian ginseng has most of the benefits of Chinese or American ginseng without the chance

of insomnia. In fact, Siberian ginseng is usually recommended as a nerve tonic to help you deal with stress. It's usually taken as a liquid extract— a spoonful before bedtime has a soothing effect that helps you sleep. Some bodybuilders take capsules that contain high doses of Siberian ginseng. We advise against this—it could cause dangerous hormonal changes. In herbal terms, Siberian ginseng has a warming effect. Taking Siberian ginseng in the autumn is said to help you adjust better to the upcoming cold weather.

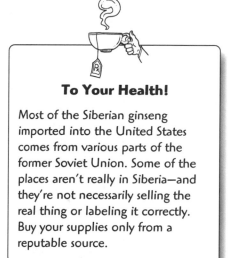

To Your Health!

Most of the Siberian ginseng imported into the United States comes from various parts of the former Soviet Union. Some of the places aren't really in Siberia—and they're not necessarily selling the real thing or labeling it correctly. Buy your supplies only from a reputable source.

Dang Shen

An inexpensive substitute for Chinese ginseng, *dang shen* or *Asian red sage (Salvia multiorrhiza)* has many of the same benefits as a Qi tonic at less cost. It's sometimes called *neutral ginseng*, because it's not as warming as ren shen. In China, dang shen is said to be very helpful for weight loss. It supposedly also keeps your hair from turning gray or falling out. Does it? If you believe that, we've got a Great Wall you might want to buy.

Using Ginseng

In TCM, ginseng alone isn't recommended on a daily basis. If you use it every day as a general tonic, it's best to take it for three weeks running and then take a week off. Because ginseng is generally stimulating, avoid caffeine and other stimulants while you're taking it.

Ginseng can be prepared in a lot of different ways. The root can be used whole (very extravagant), sliced, or powdered. It's also available in tea bags, capsules, and extracts.

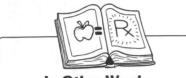

In Other Words...

Standardized herbs have been lightly processed to make sure that each dose has the same basic amount of the major active ingredients.

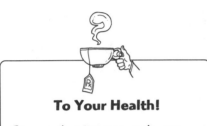

To Your Health!

Ginseng chewing gum, soda pop, and other commercial products sold as "energy boosters" don't really have enough ginseng in them to be of use. One recent study showed that some of these products don't have any ginseng in them at all.

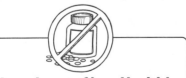

Hazardous to Your Health!

Pregnant women must be very careful about using herbs. If you're pregnant, be sure to stay away from angelica, astragalus, cinnamon bark, ephedra, ginkgo, licorice, mugwort, and rhubarb.

Here in the United States, most people take a more straightforward approach and use commercial ground ginseng root prepared as a tea or take ginseng as an extract or capsule.

To make ginseng tea, put half a teaspoon of ground ginseng root in a cup of water. Bring it to a boil, then simmer for 10 minutes. Don't strain the tea before drinking. It's safe to drink 2 cups daily.

If you go the capsule route, look for a *standardized* brand made from whole, dried roots. These products usually contain about 8 percent ginsenoides, the active ingredients in ginseng. The usual dose is one or two 150 mg capsules daily. If you want to take the extract, choose a brand that contains from 5 to 9 percent ginsenoides. Popular brands include Ginsana® and Ginsun®. You could also try one of the commercial mixtures that combines ginseng with other herbs and/or vitamins.

Siberian ginseng is usually taken in capsules, although you can find it in tea bags. Look for brands that say the product is standardized for eleutherosides, the active ingredients in Siberian ginseng. If the capsules aren't standardized, the usual dose is one to three 500 mg capsules daily. If the capsule is standardized, use a lower dose—one to three 100 or 200 mg capsules daily.

Beyond Ginseng

Even though there are a lot of exotic Chinese herbs, some are used much more often than others. We don't have space here to go into a lot of detail (the classic text on Chinese herbs was written in the late 1500s and runs to 52 volumes), but the following table shows some of the most common Chinese herbs and what they're usually recommended for. We've selected herbs that have become popular in the West and are easily available in any health-food store. Some of these herbs also have uses in Western herbalism, but the Chinese uses are often not quite the same.

As with all herbs, use Chinese herbs only occasionally and be careful. Don't mix them, and stop taking them if they make you feel worse or you notice any sort of reaction.

Popular Chinese Herbs

English/Chinese Name	Uses
Angelica/Dong quai	Treats women's problems, especially menstrual problems; treats liver problems; relieves pain; blood tonic
Astragalus/Huang qi	Qi tonic to boost energy; improves immunity; treats allergies and asthma; treats blood problems
Bupleurum/Chai hu	Treats fever, liver diseases, menstrual problems, headaches, dizziness
Cinnamon bark/Qui zhi	Balances upper and lower body energy; improves circulation, digestion, and respiration; treats fever, menstrual problems; good tonic for kidneys and spleen
Ephedra/Mahuang	Treats asthma, hay fever, colds, coughs; also used as a stimulant and a weight-loss tea
Gentian/Qin jiao	Relieves damp and wind conditions such as arthritis; treats fevers and inflammation
Ginger/Gan jian	Improves digestion, circulation; helps lungs; relieves nausea; treats colds and coughs
Ginkgo	Improves circulation; helps dizziness, headache, depression, senility, lack of concentration
Licorice/Gan cao	Treats coughs, sore throat, ulcer pain, upset stomach, liver problems
Mugwort/Ai ye	Used in moxibustion; treats bleeding problems, menstrual problems, digestive problems
Polygonum/Fo ti	Helps prevent premature aging; treats skin problems, back and knee pain
Rehmannia/Shou di huang	Treats aging problems such as hearing loss; treats fever and night sweats, insomnia, constipation, joint pain
Reishi mushroom	Treats insomnia, anxiety, chronic bronchitis; improves immune system; heart tonic
Rhubarb/Da huang	Laxative; relieves pain and inflammation, improves circulation

continues

Popular Chinese Herbs   (continued)

English/Chinese Name	Uses
Schisandra/Wu wei zi	Treats liver problems, urinary and sexual problems, dizziness, headaches, blurred vision; male tonic
Skullcap root/Huang qin	Relieves fever; treats diarrhea, upper respiratory infections, urinary tract infections, liver problems, headaches, PMS

Note: There are several species of angelica. *Angelica archangelica* is the species generally used in Western herbalism. In Chinese herbal medicine, the species used is *Angelica sinensis*, sometimes known as *Chinese angelica*.

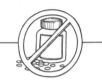

Hazardous to Your Health!

Do not use licorice if you have high blood pressure, kidney disease, congestive heart failure, or glaucoma. Do not use ephedra if you have diabetes, heart disease, glaucoma, or hyperthyroidism.

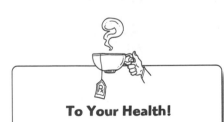

To Your Health!

You can use Tiger Balm, a popular liniment for sore muscles sold in many health-food stores and Oriental groceries, with a clear conscience. It's just a brand name—no tigers are harmed to make it.

Note: Fo ti is used as a general Qi tonic, but many Chinese believe it has near magical rejuvenating powers. They claim that it preserves youthfulness, restores sexual function, and keeps your hair from turning gray. Does it? Doubtful, but give it a try if your health insurance won't cover Viagra® or Grecian Formula®.

Minerals and Other Ingredients

Traditional Chinese herbal medicine also includes minerals, such as calcium from ground oyster shells, and other, more exotic, nonplant ingredients. You might be willing to experiment with Chinese herbs, but are you ready to try dried gecko powder? What about silkworm droppings or deer antler?

Fortunately, these ingredients are rarely used even in China (although the gecko, a type of lizard, is popular as a cough remedy). Instead, herbalists substitute plants that do pretty much the same thing. Even so, if you have any problem with using an animal product, be sure to tell your herbalist. And as we'll discuss later in this chapter, be careful about which Chinese patent remedies you buy.

Everyone should have a really big problem with using any sort of remedy that contains animal parts from endangered species. Sadly, there are still people who will pay handsomely for the supposed aphrodisiac effects of substances like rhino horn or the sexual organs of tigers. We urge you not to encourage or participate in the illegal and immoral trade in endangered animals by even asking about such products.

Choking Down Chinese Herbs

Traditionally, Chinese herbs are made into a "soup" or *decoction* (a very strong tea). The pile of dried herbs—roots, leaves, seeds, flowers, powders, and other weird stuff—you get at the Chinese pharmacy is put into a glass or ceramic pot, 3 to 6 cups of pure water are added, and the mixture is simmered for anywhere from 30 minutes to an hour. Sometimes certain ingredients need special preparation before they're added to the soup; other ingredients might not be added until the last minute. You'll get some careful instructions on how to make the mixture.

When it's ready, drain off the liquid part into a container. Save the herbs; they can be cooked a second time (discard them after that). If you started with 6 cups of water, there should be about 2 cups left.

Cooking your herbal "soup" is the easy part. Drinking it down is hard. Chinese herbal mixtures taste just terrible—there will be no doubt in your mind that you're taking medicine as you try to choke it down. The usual dose is half a cup of the decoction twice a day. If you really can't force it down, try diluting the mixture with hot water, but don't add fruit juice, honey, sugar, or alcohol.

Although "soup" is the preferred way to get the most out of Chinese herbs, powdered herbs in capsules work well and are a lot more convenient. To get the most from them, you may have to take several capsules at a time three times a day. Some herbs are available as tinctures. These generally contain at least 25 percent alcohol, however, and should be avoided if possible. You'll probably have to take a couple of spoonfuls several times a day, which means you'll be taking in a lot of alcohol.

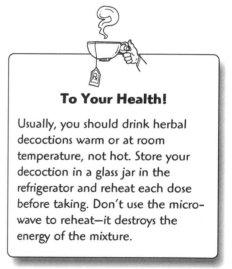

To Your Health!

Usually, you should drink herbal decoctions warm or at room temperature, not hot. Store your decoction in a glass jar in the refrigerator and reheat each dose before taking. Don't use the microwave to reheat—it destroys the energy of the mixture.

No matter how you take them, Chinese herbs take a while to kick in. You may not feel any real change in your condition for a couple of weeks. If you have a chronic condition like arthritis, you may have to continue your herbal treatment for several weeks or even longer.

Sometimes an ingredient in the herbal mixture really disagrees with you. If you're getting nauseous from the mixture or have any other unpleasant side effects such as headaches or diarrhea, stop taking it and discuss the problem with your herbalist. Often a change in the formula solves the problem.

In general, it's best to take your herbs about an hour before eating. If you're taking the herbs to treat a problem above the diaphragm, though, take them an hour after eating. The idea is that the food in your stomach gives the herbs a platform to rise up into the upper part of your body. If you're using a calming formula to treat insomnia, take it two hours before bedtime.

Patent Medicines

It's a lot of work to prepare your Chinese herbs—and let's not even mention what it's like to drink them down. Many of the most common basic formulas are available in pill form. In general, these herbal mixtures are called *patent medicines*, a term that dates back to the late 1800s in America, when various manufacturers patented their own formulas for all sorts of cure-all pills and tonics.

Chinese patent medicines are often imported from China, Taiwan, or Korea. They have names that sound a little odd to American ears, like Six Gentlemen Decoction, Minor Green-Blue Dragon Decoction, or Women's Precious Pills. In general, Chinese patent medicines are based on tried-and-true traditional formulas. They're just a safe, more convenient way of taking your herbs. Be very cautious, however. A lot of the ingredients in a patent medicine may not be familiar to you or might not be translated correctly on the label. Also, some patent medicines also contain drugs such as acetaminophen (Tylenol®) or even diazepam (Valium®) that you might not want to take.

Just as you shouldn't self-treat with Chinese herbs, you shouldn't self-treat with patent medicines. Always get the advice of an experienced herbalist before you try them. And remember, if you're already taking any sort of medicine, prescription or nonprescription, you're at risk for a drug interaction.

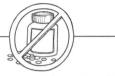

Hazardous to Your Health!

Be very cautious about taking Chinese patent medicines. In a recent study, one popular arthritis remedy known as **Black Pearl, San Kee,** or **black pills for arthritis** was shown to contain not only herbs but also one or more drugs such as diazepam (Valium®), steroids (prednisone), acetaminophen (Tylenol®), and indomethacin (Indocin®). A number of Chinese patent medicines for asthma contain powerful drugs such as theophylline.

Rules, Rules, Rules

For centuries, traditional Chinese herbalists told patients to take *hongqu*, made by fermenting rice with red yeast, for stagnant blood and to strengthen the spleen. Just folklore? No—modern research has shown that red yeast rice contains lovostatin, the same enzyme-blocking substance that's in the prescription drug Mevacor®, which is widely prescribed to lower high cholesterol.

But when a food supplement acts like a drug, the government can get into the act. That's exactly what happened with a very popular red yeast rice product called

Cholestin®. The FDA says it's an unapproved drug; the American importers says it's a dietary supplement because lovostatin occurs naturally in the rice. So far, the importers have been winning in court, but stay tuned—the battle is far from over.

Finding Chinese Herbalists

As you've gathered by now, Chinese herbal medicine is pretty complex. It's not for do-it-yourselfers. If you diagnose yourself incorrectly and choose the wrong herbs or mix up the wrong combination, you could make yourself sicker. And as we'll discuss in just a little bit, some herbs are dangerous and need to be used very cautiously.

In the right hands, though, Chinese herbal medicine can be very helpful. If you're interested in trying it, visit a well-trained OMP and get an herbal prescription designed for your particular health problem.

How can you find someone knowledgeable about Chinese herbs? By looking very hard—there just aren't that many trained Chinese herbalists in the United States. Also, a lot of them trained at universities in Taiwan or China and may not be able to communicate in English very well. In the United States, you'll find them in the Chinese neighborhoods of big cities. If you don't live in a city with a large Chinese population, you'll have an even harder time finding a knowledgeable practitioner. For help in locating one and understanding his or her credentials, check back to the sources listed in Chapter 6 on traditional Chinese medicine.

Your insurance company almost certainly won't pay for your consultation and herbal prescription, even if you go to a licensed acupuncturist. The only way you're likely to be covered is if the consultation is with an herbalist who is also licensed to practice medicine in the United States. Even then, you'll have to pay for the herbs yourself.

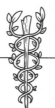

The Healing Arts

Tea (*Camellia sinensis*) is the original Chinese herb. Legend has it that centuries ago, some tea leaves blew into a pot of water being boiled for the great Emperor Shen Nung. He daringly drank the water anyway and thus discovered the world's most popular human-made drink. In TCM, tea (*cha* in Chinese) is used as a stimulant, as Qi tonic, and to help digestive problems. Recent research suggests that Chinese green tea contains catechins, potent antioxidants that could help prevent cancer. Another recent study suggests that drinking tea could lower your risk of stroke or heart attack and bring down your high cholesterol.

Chicanery from China?

As the Cholestin® fight shows, traditional Chinese herbal medicine is controversial. Critics say that the underlying concepts of Yin and Yang, the Five Elements, and all the rest have no relation to what's really wrong with you or how herbs really work. While critics generally agree that some of the herbs in a complex Chinese prescription could be mildly helpful, they're not so sure about the others. There's very little research to show that traditional Chinese herbal formulas actually help. If you have a cold or flu, for instance, you'd probably get better anyway, with or without the herbs.

Critics of Chinese herbal medicine rightly point out that the herbs can easily be mislabeled or adulterated. You also have no way of knowing what pesticides and other dangerous substances were used on them. And they're right to be worried about exactly what's in those patent medicines.

Most important, though, is the question of whether a Chinese herbal remedy could interact badly with any drugs you are taking. The answer is that in most cases, nobody really knows (of course, that's true for Western drugs as well).

Until more research is done, be very careful about using Chinese herbs. Get the best advice you can find, use the smallest possible doses, and stop taking the herbs if you notice any unpleasant side effects.

The Least You Need to Know

➤ The goal of any Chinese herbal remedy is to restore your internal balance and to get your Qi (energy) flowing smoothly again.

➤ Chinese herbs generally are used in combinations that include anywhere from five to a dozen herbs.

➤ To get the right herbal prescription for you, consult a trained herbalist. A do-it-yourself mixture could make your problem worse.

➤ Be very cautious about taking Chinese herbs and patent medicines. The herbs could interact badly with any drugs you take.

➤ Ginseng, one of the most popular Chinese herbs, is a common ingredient in many herbal remedies. By itself, it is a Qi tonic that restores energy.

➤ Chinese herbal remedies can be very helpful for health problems such as arthritis, fatigue, PMS, headaches, insomnia, depression, and poor concentration.

Part 5
You Are What You Eat

Alternative medicine emphasizes diet and nutrition. Why? Because, by some estimates, 80 percent of all serious health problems, like heart disease and cancer, relate to your diet. If everybody in the country would just eat right and take their vitamins, doctors would have a lot of spare time!

In this section, we guide you through the maze of nutritional supplements, explain juice therapy and macrobiotics, and discuss detoxification treatments.

Chapter 17

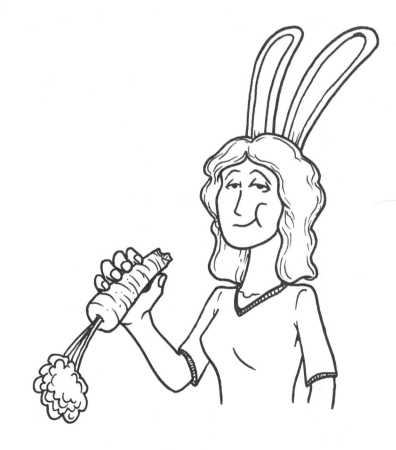

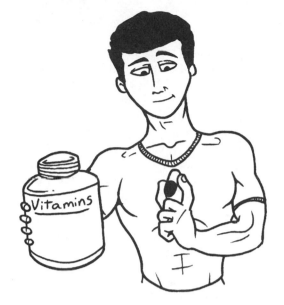

Nutritional Supplements: Extra Help for Health

In This Chapter

➤ Why vitamins and minerals are essential for your health

➤ How large doses of vitamins and minerals may help some ailments

➤ Using amino acids to help your health

➤ The many health benefits of flavonoids

➤ Which fats are good for you

➤ Natural hormones, enzymes, and other supplements that heal

Hang around in the nutritional supplements section of a well-stocked health-food store, and here's what you'll see: utter confusion. We've seen executives who can reorganize an entire corporate division in an afternoon reduced to asking complete strangers whether vitamin E or evening primrose oil is better for PMS. We can understand why everyone's so confused. There are so many supplements out there and so much hype surrounds them, that it's often hard to know what's best for you. Fortunately, it's easy to go from confusion to enlightenment.

What Are Nutritional Supplements?

One reason everyone's so confused about nutritional supplements is that there are an awful lot of them. In fact, there are so many, we've already written a whole book about them—it's called *The Complete Idiot's Guide to Vitamins and Minerals*.

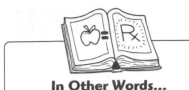

Broadly speaking, a *nutritional supplement* is any substance you take in addition to your normal diet, usually for the purpose of improving your health in some specific way. You may already be taking the most commonly used nutritional supplement, a daily multi-vitamin tablet. Sometimes people with serious health problems, like kidney disease or cancer, need prescription nutritional supplements. In this chapter, we'll focus on supplements anyone can get at the health-food store. If you have special nutritional needs, discuss any supplements with your doctor before you try them.

When you look more closely at all the common nutritional supplements, they fall into some fairly well-defined categories:

➤ **Vitamins.** From vitamin A to vitamin K, you need 14 different vitamins to stay alive.

➤ **Minerals.** You need at least 10 different minerals, including calcium, magnesium, zinc, and potassium, for good health.

➤ **Flavonoids.** This is a general term for a wide range of plant substances, such as the cancer-fighting flavonoid lycopene, found in tomatoes.

➤ **Amino acids.** These are the building blocks of protein.

➤ **Essential fatty acids.** These are good fats, including fish oil and evening primrose oil.

➤ **Hormones.** These include substances such as melatonin and DHEA, which supplement your body's normal hormones. (For more information on DHEA, see "Other Nutritional Supplements" later in this chapter.)

We'll go into each of these categories in more detail in the rest of this chapter. (If you're wondering where the herbs are, we had to give them their own chapter—check back to Chapter 15, "Traditional Herbal Medicine," for more information.) Before we do, though, let's take a look at one of the most exciting areas in all of alternative medicine.

Orthomolecular Medicine: Megadoses

The basic idea of using vitamins, minerals, amino acids, and other supplements to treat health problems has been around for a long time. By the 1920s, for example, doctors knew that large doses of vitamin A can help kids get over the measles faster and with fewer complications. It wasn't until 1968 that the medical practice of using *megadoses* of vitamins, minerals, and amino acids got an official name: *orthomolecular medicine.*

The phrase was coined by Linus Pauling, a brilliant scientist and two-time winner of the Nobel Prize. The basic principle of orthomolecular medicine is that an underlying chemical imbalance in the body causes illness. To correct the problem, the patient takes very large doses of vitamins, minerals, amino acids, and sometimes other nutritional supplements. Because of its emphasis on vitamins, orthomolecular medicine is sometimes called *megavitamin therapy*.

Orthomolecular medicine is very controversial in medical circles, but we don't really understand why. The basic principles make a lot of sense:

➤ Nutrition should be a central part of medical diagnosis and treatment.

➤ Restoring the right nutritional balance helps cure health problems.

➤ The official recommended amounts of vitamins and minerals are far too low and don't take into account individual needs.

➤ A healthy diet that's high in fiber, low in fat, and has plenty of whole grains and fresh fruits and vegetables is crucial for good health. Additives, sugar, junk food, preservatives, and other harmful substances should be avoided.

➤ Drugs should be used only when absolutely necessary and only for as long as necessary.

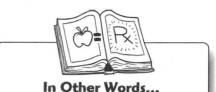

In Other Words...

Megadoses are doses of vitamins, minerals, amino acids, and other nutritional supplements that are much, much larger than normal. **Orthomolecular medicine** uses megadoses to treat health problems that are said to be caused by an imbalance in body chemistry. The word comes from the Latin *ortho-*, meaning "correct," "straight," or "normal," and *molecular*, which refers to the molecules in the body. **Megavitamin therapy** is another way of saying orthomolecular medicine.

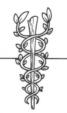

The Healing Arts

Vitamin C and the Nobel Prize seem to go together. The research of Albert Szent-Gÿorgyi (1893–1986) on the role of vitamin C in human health earned him the Nobel Prize in 1937. Linus Pauling is the only person ever to win two unshared Nobel Prizes: for chemistry in 1954 and peace in 1962. Pauling claimed, "We could add an extra 12 to 18 years to our lives by taking from 3,200 to 12,000 milligrams of vitamin C a day." Megadoses of vitamin C seem to have worked for him: Pauling took more than 6 grams a day and lived to 93.

The big objection to orthomolecular medicine is that the megadoses could be toxic. That one really makes us laugh. In 1997, a study in the prestigious *Journal of the American Medical Association* showed that every year, an average of 770,000 patients have bad reactions to the drugs their doctors prescribe and need to be hospitalized. At a conservative estimate, the cost is a whopping $1.56 *billion* a year, to say nothing of the fact that about 140,000 of those patients die. The total number of deaths by vitamin overdose in 1997? Zero.

Mainstream medicine is starting to come around to some orthomolecular ideas, but some remain controversial or unproven. Let's look at some areas where large doses of vitamins and other supplements could help.

Cs for the Common Cold

Do large doses of vitamin C cure the common cold? No—nothing does. Taking 1,000 to 2,000 mg of extra Cs while you have a cold or flu could help you feel a little better while you're sick and get over the illness a little sooner. The older you are, the better this seems to work.

Hazardous to Your Health!

Always talk to your doctor before you start taking large doses of a vitamin or mineral. Never substitute large doses of a nutritional supplement for your regular medicine.

Cs for Cardiac Cases

According to the National Center for Health Statistics, if every adult in the U.S. took an extra 500 mg of vitamin C every day, about 100,000 of them wouldn't die of heart disease every year. Large doses of vitamin C can help lower your cholesterol and your blood pressure. Look at it this way: A year's supply of vitamin C costs about $45. A coronary bypass operation costs about $45,000.

Fabulous Folic Acid

A member of the B vitamin family, folic acid (also called *folate*) is crucial for all women of child-bearing age, because it helps prevent birth defects. The *Daily Reference Intake* (DRI) is 400 mcg, but almost all doctors tell women who could be pregnant to get at least 800 mcg a day. Recent research shows that folic acid could be very important for preventing heart disease. That's because you need folic acid to remove homocysteine, a normal waste product of your metabolism, from your blood. If you're short on folic acid, the homocysteine can build up and cause the kind of artery damage that can lead to a heart attack. Orthomolecular physicians have known for decades that all the B vitamins are crucial to your health, but now other doctors are catching on. If you're an older adult, talk to your doctor about checking your homocysteine level—high homocysteine levels could be as dangerous as high cholesterol for damaging your arteries. Taking 1 to 2 mg a day of folic acid has been shown to lower homocysteine levels and reduce the odds of a heart attack.

Vitamin E: Excellent for Immunity

Vitamin E supplements can really improve immunity in older adults. In a 1997 study that appeared in the *Journal of the American Medical Association*, older adults who took 200 mg a day of extra vitamin E for 33 weeks had more active immune systems. There's no way you can get that much vitamin E from your food—you have to take supplements.

E-luding Heart Disease

Several important recent studies have shown that vitamin E can help prevent heart disease, probably because it helps prevent atherosclerosis. If artery-clogging plaques don't build up inside the arteries that nourish your heart, your chances of a heart attack plummet. And even if you already have heart disease, vitamin E can help keep it from getting worse.

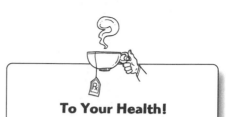

To Your Health!

To make sure that everyone, especially women, gets at least 400 mcg of folic acid every day, the FDA began a fortification program in 1998. Manufacturers now add folic acid to breakfast cereals, baked goods, pasta, rice, and many other grain products.

Calculating Your Calcium

To prevent *osteoporosis* (thin, brittle bones that break easily), all women over the age of 30 should get at least 1,000 mg of calcium a day. That's the amount you'd get by drinking three glasses of milk every day. Do you? If you're like most women, you don't, which means that you almost certainly should be taking extra calcium.

Potassium and Your Blood Pressure

If you have high blood pressure, your doctor has probably told you to cut back on the salt in your diet. An orthomolecular physician would say that's only half the solution—you also need to increase the amount of potassium in your diet. That's easy to do—plenty of fresh fruits and vegetables, like bananas, oranges, and beans, are great sources of potassium.

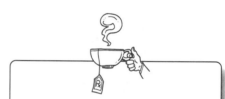

To Your Health!

To be effective, calcium supplements need to dissolve completely in your digestive system. For the best results, choose supplements that are made with calcium citrate or calcium lactate. Two popular brands are Os-Cal® and Caltrate®.

Aid from Amino Acids

Some orthomolecular physicians use large doses of amino acids such as tryptophan to help treat mental and emotional problems such as retardation and depression.

Phenylalanine, for instance, is said to help depression, anxiety, and poor concentration. Using aminos in this way is very controversial, and we can't really advise you on whether or not they work. We'll discuss the basics of amino acids in more detail later on in this chapter.

We could go on—and on and on—about how large amounts of vitamins and minerals may help you avoid serious health problems. We do need to point out, though, that they don't cure anything. There's no evidence, for example, that megadoses of vitamin C or any other substance cures cancer, schizophrenia, or any other disease, although they may help treat the symptoms.

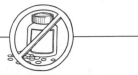

Hazardous to Your Health!

Do not take any amino acids if you have kidney disease. Do not take large doses of lysine if you have diabetes.

Radicals on the Loose!

One reason megadoses work is that they mop up the extra free radicals you make when you're sick. Let's take a closer look to see why that's so important.

What happens when you drive your car? Gasoline is combined with oxygen in the pistons of your engine. The released energy moves the car, but it also gives off exhaust fumes as a byproduct. That's a lot like what happens in the cells of your body. When oxygen combines with glucose in your cells, for example, you make energy—and you also make *free radicals*, your body's version of exhaust fumes. Free radicals are oxygen atoms that are missing one electron from the pair the atom should have. That makes the atom unstable and very reactive. A free radical desperately wants to find another electron to fill in the gap, so it grabs an electron from the next atom it gets near. But when a free radical seizes an electron from another atom, the second atom then becomes a free radical, because now it's the one missing an electron. One free radical starts a cascade of new free radicals in your body. When free radicals start grabbing electrons from your cells, they damage them.

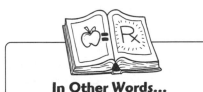

In Other Words...

Free radicals are unstable oxygen atoms created by your body's natural processes and also by the effects of toxins such as cigarette smoke. Free radicals, especially the types called singlet oxygen and hydroxyl, are very reactive and can cause cell damage.

Antioxidant enzymes protect your body by capturing free radicals and removing them before they do any extra damage.

Antioxidants are your body's natural defense against free radicals. Antioxidants are enzymes that patrol your cells looking for free radicals. When they find one, they neutralize it, stop the cascade, and carry the free radical out of your body.

To make those antioxidant enzymes, you need to have plenty of vitamins and minerals in your body. If you're short on the right vitamins and minerals, the free radicals can get the upper hand and do extra damage to your cells before they get neutralized. And as we'll discuss throughout this chapter, lots of other substances, such as flavonoids, are valuable antioxidants on their own.

Free radicals can come from other sources. The ultraviolet light in sunshine can trigger free radicals, leading to skin cancer and cataracts. Toxins of all sorts—tobacco smoke, the natural chemicals found in our food, the poisonous wastes of your own metabolism, and man-made toxins like air pollution and pesticides—trigger free radicals as well.

Every cell in your body comes under attack from a free radical at an average rate of once every 10 seconds. Your best protection is to keep your antioxidant levels high. That's where supplements come in—if you're low on antioxidants or their building blocks, your health could suffer.

Your Daily Dose

Now that we've told you what big doses of vitamins can do, it's time to backtrack a little and talk about why you need vitamins and minerals at all. (If you've already read *The Complete Idiot's Guide to Vitamins and Minerals*, you can skip to the next section.) To maintain basic good health and keep your body running normally, you need 14 *vitamins* and at least 10 *minerals*. Each and every vitamin is equally important to your health—you can't skimp on any of them. Likewise for the minerals. Check out the following table to see which vitamins do what.

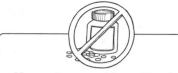

Hazardous to Your Health!

If free radicals damage the DNA in your cells often enough, they can cause the genetic changes that trigger cancer. If free radicals oxidize cholesterol in your blood, they can cause the artery-clogging plaque that leads to heart disease.

In Other Words...

A **vitamin** is an organic chemical compound that is essential in small amounts for normal health. A **mineral** is an inorganic chemical element you need in small amounts for normal health. Your body can't make vitamins and minerals—you have to get them from the foods you eat and from any supplements you decide to take.

The Value of Vitamins

Vitamin	Function
Vitamin A	Prevents infection. Needed for healthy skin, hair, mucous membranes, and strong bones and teeth.
B vitamins	Converts food to energy. Creates neurotransmitters. Needed for healthy skin, hair, blood, immune system, nerves, and cell growth and division.

continues

The Value of Vitamins (continued)

Vitamin	Function
Vitamin C	Provides very powerful antioxidants. Crucial for connective tissue, strong bones, and healing of wounds.
Vitamin D	Enables you to use calcium properly. Needed for normal muscle and nerve function.
Vitamin E	Provides a powerful antioxidant. Needed for immune system and hormone production.
Vitamin K	Provides necessary elements for blood clotting, bone formation, and kidney functions.

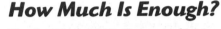

Hazardous to Your Health!

Don't give yourself megadoses of vitamins or minerals. If you want to try megadoses, discuss it with your doctor first.

How Much Is Enough?

The Institute of Medicine, a division of the National Academy of Science, has the job of deciding how much of a vitamin or mineral you need for basic good health. This amount is called the *Recommended Dietary Allowance* (RDA). Starting with some new recommendations in 1997, though, the term *Daily Reference Intake* (DRI) is being phased in. The RDAs or DRIs are the basic amounts that other agencies and organizations, like the FDA and the U.S. Department of Agriculture, use to set their standards. The following tables give the current RDAs/DRIs for vitamins and minerals.

Adult RDAs/DRIs for Vitamins

Vitamin	RDA/DRI for Men	RDA/DRI for Women
Vitamin A	1,000 RE or 5,000 IU*	800 RE or 4,000 IU
B vitamins		
Thiamin (B$_1$)	1.5 mg	1.1 mg
Riboflavin (B$_2$)	1.7 mg	1.3 mg
Niacin	19 mg	15 mg
Pyridoxine (B$_6$)	2 mg	1.6 mg
Folic acid	200 mcg	180 mcg
Cobalamin (B$_{12}$)	2 mcg	2 mcg
Choline	500 mg	500 mg
Vitamin C	60 mg	60 mg

Vitamin	RDA/DRI for Men	RDA/DRI for Women
Vitamin D	5 mcg	5 mcg
Vitamin E	10 mg or 15 IU	8 mg or 12 IU
Vitamin K	80 mcg	65 mcg

*Vitamin A can be measured in Retinol Equivalents (RE) or International Units (IU). One IU equals 0.3 mcg of retinol, the most common form of vitamin A. One RE equals 1 mcg of retinol.

Adult RDAs/DRIs for Major Minerals

Mineral	RDA/DRI for Adults
Calcium	1,000 mg
Chloride	750 mg
Magnesium	350 mg
Phosphorus	800 mg
Potassium	2,000 mg
Sodium	500 mg

A lot of people involved with holistic healthcare have a big objection to the RDAs/DRIs: They're way too low. Nutritionally oriented practitioners believe that the RDAs/DRIs are the bare minimums needed for survival, not the larger amounts that could help you on the way to better health.

On the other hand, you do have to be careful about megadoses of some vitamins and minerals. You need to be especially careful with vitamins A and D and with *trace minerals* such as selenium. So we've drawn up the following conservative table showing the safe dosage ranges for vitamins and minerals.

Foods or Supplements?

There's an easy answer to that question: Both! It's important to eat a good, well-balanced diet that's low in fat and high in whole grains, fresh fruits, and vegetables. A good diet gives you all sorts of great health benefits, like goodly amounts of flavonoids (we'll get to them in a little bit) and fiber (we'll discuss that more in Chapter 20, "Detoxification Treatments: What a Waste"). But even if you faithfully follow the food pyramid and

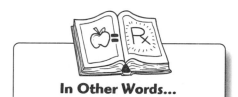

In Other Words...

Trace minerals are minerals you need in very, very, very tiny amounts. The most abundant trace minerals in your body are chromium, copper, iodine, iron, manganese, molybdenum, selenium, and zinc. Your body also contains other trace minerals, like boron, tin, and even gold, but why you have them and what they do is still a mystery.

eat five fresh fruits and vegetables every day, you still may not be getting enough of some vitamins and minerals. The benefits of vitamin E for your heart, for example, don't really kick in unless you take in at least 400 IU to 1,000 IU a day—an amount that's impossible to get from your food alone. And if you want to take extra vitamins and minerals to help a particular health problem, you'll need amounts larger than you can reasonably get from your food.

By taking a daily multivitamin supplement with minerals, you give yourself a health insurance policy—even if you don't eat properly that day, at least you're getting the vitamins and minerals you need. Beyond that, you may want to take additional supplements to help you deal with specific health problems.

Safe Dosage Ranges for Vitamins and Minerals for Healthy Adults

Vitamin	Safe Daily Dosage Range
Vitamin A	5,000–25,000 IU
B vitamins	
Thiamin (B_1)	2–100 mg
Riboflavin (B_2)	50–100 mg
Niacin	20–100 mg
Pyridoxine (B_6)	3–50 mg
Folic acid	800 mcg–2 mg
Cobalamin (B_{12})	500–1,000 mcg
Pantothenic acid	4–7 mg
Biotin	30–100 mcg
Choline	300–3,500 mg
Vitamin C	500–2,000 mg
Vitamin D	400–600 IU
Vitamin E	200–400 IU
Calcium	1,000–1,500 mg
Copper	1.5–3 mg
Chromium	50–200 mcg
Iron	15–30 mg
Magnesium	300–500 mg
Manganese	2.5–5 mg
Molybdenum	75–250 mcg
Potassium	2,000–3,500 mg
Selenium	70–200 mcg
Zinc	15–50 mg

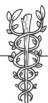

The Healing Arts

According to the Department of Agriculture's *Continuing Survey of Food Intakes by Individuals* (CSFII), most adult women don't meet the DRIs for vitamin B_6 (pyridoxine), vitamin E, calcium, magnesium, iron, and zinc. Only one in five Americans actually eats five fresh fruits and vegetables every day—and one in five doesn't eat any at all. Five servings may sound like a lot to eat, but the servings are small—just half a cup of broccoli, for instance, counts as one serving.

Amino Acids: The Building Blocks of Life

Back in our discussion of orthomolecular medicine, we mentioned other supplements, including *amino acids*. Today there's a lot of interest in supplemental amino acids, for good reason—there's some solid evidence that they really can help. Before we get into the details, though, we'll have to give you some ABCs: amino basic concepts.

Every minute of every day, your body is busy producing 50,000-plus different *proteins*. You use those proteins to make your cells and to keep them running and communicating with each other smoothly. Amazingly, all those proteins are made by various combinations of only 22 amino acids. They're the building blocks of proteins, just as the 26 letters of the alphabet make all the words in the English language.

Amino acids fall into two basic categories: *essential* and *nonessential*. The essential amino acids are the nine you can get only by eating them. The non-essential amino acids are the ones you can make in your body by combining two or more of the essential aminos. Check out the following table to see which aminos are which.

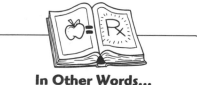

In Other Words...

Proteins are organic substances made up of hydrogen, oxygen, carbon, and nitrogen. Proteins are made from strings of **amino acids**. Each amino acid is a small molecule that has an amino group (a chemical fragment containing nitrogen) and an acid group (a chemical fragment containing carbon, oxygen, and hydrogen).

The Amino Acids

Essential Amino Acids	Nonessential Amino Acids
Histidine	Alanine
Isoleucine	Arginine (essential for babies)
Leucine	Asparagine
Lysine	Aspartic acid
Methionine	Carnitine (essential for babies)
Phenylalanine	Cysteine
Threonine	Glutamic acid
Tryptophan	Glutamine
Valine	Glycine
	Proline
	Serine
	Taurine (essential for babies)
	Tyrosine

How much of each essential amino acid do you need? That depends on how much you weigh. The heavier you are, the more aminos you need. Use this table to work out your personal needs:

Adult RDAs for Essential Amino Acids

Amino Acid	RDA in mg/lb
Histidine	5–7
Isoleucine	6
Leucine	8
Lysine	7
Methionine	8
Phenylalanine	8
Threonine	4
Tryptophan	2
Valine	6

If you're that mythical average woman who stands 5'4" and weighs 120 pounds, you'd need to get 720 mcg of valine every day. To put that in perspective, there's about 650 mcg of valine in a roasted chicken leg.

For basic nutrition, you don't really need all that much in the way of aminos. You can easily get your daily essential amino acids by eating just a few ounces of a complete protein—such as eggs, meat, and milk—that contains all nine essential aminos. Plant foods are incomplete proteins—they're missing one or more of the essential amino acids. You can still easily get your essential aminos without ever eating an animal food just by eating a good variety of plant foods, especially grains and beans.

Aminos for Health

By taking extra amounts of single amino acids, you might be able to help some health problems. Here's a rundown:

➤ **Arginine.** This nonessential amino acid may be helpful for stimulating your immune system, healing wounds, and possibly even slowing the growth of cancer.

➤ **Carnitine.** Your heart contains large amounts of this nonessential amino acid. It's there to help the cells in your heart convert food to energy. Extra carnitine may help people with congestive heart failure by making their hearts work more efficiently. Carnitine also seems to help people with *chronic fatigue syndrome* (CFS), perhaps because it improves energy production in their cells. For CFS, doses of about 3 grams a day seem to help.

➤ **Creatine.** Actually, this is a protein, not an amino acid, but you make it in your body from arginine, glycine, and methionine. Supplemental creatine is very popular today with athletes, especially body builders and weight lifters, because it helps them build strength and muscle size. You need to be very careful with it, though—it's been shown to cause kidney problems for some people.

➤ **Cysteine.** You need cysteine to make glutathione, your body's most abundant natural antioxidant. By itself and as part of glutathione, cysteine helps you corral

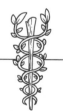

The Healing Arts

You can sell body builders anything if they think it will help them bulk up. Because body builders take protein powders to help them gain weight and build muscle, they're especially gullible when it comes to amino acids, the building blocks of protein. Our current favorite scam is HMB (beta-hydroxy beta-methylbutrate), which is a normal byproduct of amino acid metabolism in your body. On the basis of one questionable study, it's said to stop muscle breakdown during exercise, which in turn makes your muscles grow faster. The claims are no more than the normal byproduct of a large bull.

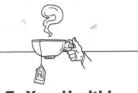

To Your Health!

With plenty of serotonin, you feel calm and confident. If you don't have enough serotonin, you might feel depressed and anxious, and you might also crave carbohydrates and overeat. If you've been having trouble sleeping, try having a high-tryptophan snack about an hour before bedtime. A bowl of bran cereal or a turkey sandwich will help you make more melatonin, which in turn will help you sleep.

In Other Words...

Freeform amino acid supplements contain only those particular amino acids in their pure form. Because the aminos are already in their simplest form, you absorb them into your body right away.

dangerous free radicals and other toxins and remove them safely from your body. (We feel that cysteine and glutathione are extremely important for your health. We don't have the space to discuss it all here, but if you're interested, we modestly recommend our book on the subject, *Glutathione: The Ultimate Antioxidant*.)

➤ **Glutamine.** Glutamine supplements are often extremely helpful for people with intestinal problems such as Crohn's disease. It seems to help because the cells that line your intestines absorb the glutamine directly, which helps to nourish them and get them working properly again. The usual dose is anywhere from 5 to 10 grams a day. If you have a chronic intestinal problem such as irritable bowel or Crohn's disease, discuss glutamine with your doctor before you try it.

➤ **Lysine.** A lot of Dr. Pressman's patients swear that taking 2,000 to 3,000 mg of lysine at the first hint of a herpes blister or cold sore wards it off, or at least keeps it from being as bad. It works even better if you also avoid arginine-containing foods, such as chocolate, nuts, seeds, beer, grains, and soy products.

➤ **Tryptophan.** You need tryptophan to make *serotonin* and *melatonin*, two substances that help control your mood and sleeping patterns (we'll talk more about melatonin in Chapter 25, "Light Therapy: Light Up Your Life"). If you don't have enough tryptophan in your system, you won't be able to make enough of these hormones—which means that you might start to feel depressed and have trouble sleeping. Tryptophan supplements are banned in the United States, so you'll have to get extra tryptophan by eating it. Good choices are turkey, peanuts, oranges, bananas, cottage cheese, whole grains, fish, lean meat, and milk.

Eating Your Aminos

Freeform amino acid supplements are a good way to be sure you're getting enough of the building blocks you need without also getting extra calories. The supplements are available as powders or in capsules. Be sure the label says "freeform" on it; otherwise, you could just be getting ordinary protein powder. Your body will have to break down the protein to release the amino acids. If you prefer the powder, just put a spoonful on your tongue and wash it down with a few swallows of cold liquid. The powders don't dissolve, so you'll have trouble stirring them into drinks.

Help for Arthritis

There's a supplement called glucosamine that can really help people with arthritis. It's not exactly an amino acid, but it's a close relative. We're putting it in here because we think it's wonderful and we don't know where else it can go.

You naturally make glucosamine in your body and use it to make cartilage in your joints. As you get older, you naturally make less glucosamine, which means your cartilage starts to break down. What happens then? Pain and stiffness—arthritis—in the joint.

Glucosamine supplements seem to work by stimulating your body to repair the cartilage, which then helps relieve the arthritis symptoms. It works really, really well for some people, but it can take several weeks to start kicking in. If you're taking medicine for arthritis, keep taking it. As the glucosamine starts to work, you might be able to cut back on your dose.

The only way to get extra glucosamine is to take supplements—it's not found in foods. The tablets are made from chitin, the processed shells of shrimp, crabs, and lobsters. We recommend the version called *glucosamine sulfate*, preferably in a combination formula that also contains some manganese. Choose a good brand from a reliable company such as Solgar or Twin Labs.

Flavonoids for Humanoids

What makes a plum look and taste like a plum? It's the *flavonoids* in it—the brightly colored, complex natural chemicals that give fruits and vegetables their characteristic look and taste. The flavonoids aren't there just for looks, though—a lot of them are powerful antioxidants or offer other important health benefits. We're just beginning to understand how important flavonoids are, and there's still a lot of work to be done in the area. That's why we're always telling you to eat those five fresh fruits and vegetables a day. The more flavonoids you get naturally through your diet, the better—even if we're still not sure just why.

So far, researchers have isolated some flavonoids that are especially helpful.

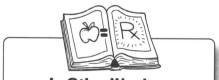

In Other Words...

Carotenes are the orange- or red-colored substances that give veggies like carrots and squash their color. The **flavonoids** are a broad group of natural substances that give color to fruits and vegetables (and also to flowers).

Carotenoids

As you might guess from the name, *carotenoids* are flavonoids found in carrots, sweet potatoes, and other orange- and red-colored fruits and vegetables. They're also found in dark-green leafy vegetables, like collard greens and kale. Carotenoids fall into two categories:

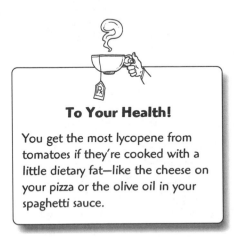

To Your Health!

You get the most lycopene from tomatoes if they're cooked with a little dietary fat—like the cheese on your pizza or the olive oil in your spaghetti sauce.

➤ **Carotenes.** This group includes alpha-carotene, beta-carotene, and lycopene. All the carotenes are great antioxidants, plus the alpha and beta ones are also converted to vitamin A in your body. Lycopene is found in tomatoes—it's what makes them red. Recent studies have shown that lycopene has powerful anti-cancer action. Men who eat lots of tomato-based foods, for instance, are far less likely to get prostate cancer. There's a lot of research now going on about lycopene— stay tuned for more developments and eat plenty of tomatoes in the meantime.

➤ **Xanthophylls.** These are yellow or orange carotenoids that are super antioxidants but don't have any vitamin A activity. Two members of the xanthophyll family—lutein and zeaxanthin—have been shown to be very helpful for protecting your eyes against the free radicals than can cause cataracts and macular degeneration.

Anthocyanins: The Eyes Have It

Anthocyanins are what give fruits and berries like blueberries, raspberries, plums, and red and purple grapes their colors. Like the xanthophylls, the anthocyanins are very helpful for protecting your eyes from free radical damage. To get any real benefit, though, you'll need supplements. Look for capsules made from bilberries (a Scandina-vian berry very similar to our blueberries).

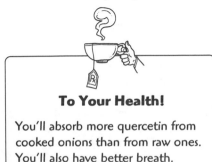

To Your Health!

You'll absorb more quercetin from cooked onions than from raw ones. You'll also have better breath.

Quercetin: How 'Bout Them Onions?

Quercetin is a flavonoid found in lots of plant foods and is most abundant in onions. Quercetin is an excellent natural antioxidant, and it also reduces inflammation and swelling and helps block allergies. Onions are a traditional folk remedy for health problems like bron-chitis and mild asthma, because the quercetin helps relax constricted bronchial tubes. This is another area where some promising research is now going on.

Resveratrol: Why Red Wine Is Good for You

Red wine is crammed with healthful flavonoids, including anthocyanins, but the most healthful of them all is one called *resveratrol*. A 5-ounce glass of red wine has about 800 mcg of resveratrol—an amount that, taken every day, could have a very beneficial effect on your cholesterol level and might even keep cancer from getting started.

If you don't want to drink alcohol to get your resveratrol, you could eat a lot of red and purple grapes or drink purple grape juice. Capsules that contain powdered resveratrol are also now available.

Are OPCs Okay?

Oligomeric proanthocyanidins (OPCs) are flavonoids found in many different plants. OPCs are particularly good at seeking out and destroying free radicals, especially the pesky hydroxyl free radical. Some researchers believe that OPCs can also help circulatory problems such as easy bruising and varicose veins. You can get OPC supplements made from grape seeds or pine bark (the commercial pine bark product is called pycnogenol).

The Good Fats

You'd never know it from the fat phobia we all seem to have, but some fats are actually *good* for you. In fact, you need them to stay alive.

Your body contains about 20 different *fatty acids*, but they're all made from just two: *linoleic acid* and *linolenic acid.* These two fatty acids are essential. Like vitamins, minerals, and essential amino acids, you have to get them from your food—your body can't manufacture them. And have them you must. The fatty acids in your body make your cell membranes, the sheaths that cover your nerves, and are part of the important hormones and other chemical messengers you make to tell your body what to do.

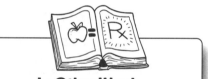

In Other Words...

Fatty acids are molecules made from a chain of carbon atoms bound to hydrogen atoms, with a couple of oxygen atoms near the tail. Fatty acid chains usually have 12 to 24 carbon atoms. **Linoleic acid** is a fatty acid found in fish and many plants. **Linolenic acid** is mostly found in seeds, including corn kernels, and also egg yolks and some fish. Most vegetable oils contain some combination of both fatty acids.

The Alpha and Omega of Fatty Acids

Scientists call the tail end of a fatty acid chain the *omega* end (from the last letter of the Greek alphabet). They then describe the various fatty acids by counting back to find where the oxygen atoms attach. For linolenic acid, that's at the third carbon atom, so another name of linolenic acid is *omega-3*. Likewise, another name for linoleic acid is *omega-6*.

The two essential fatty acids are really groups of fatty acids (in nutrition, nothing is simple). Here's how it breaks down:

➤ **Omega-3 family.** The three members of this family are *alpha-linolenic acid* (LNA), *eicosapentenoic acid* (EPA), and *docasahexanoic acid* (DHA). LNA is found in plant foods, especially nuts, soybeans, canola oil, and flaxseed oil. EPA and DHA are found in fish oil.

➤ **Omega-6 family.** This family also has three members, but the most important is *gamma-linoleic acid* (GLA). It's found in many plants, but evening primrose oil is the best source.

The best way to get more essential fatty acids in your diet is to eat more fish and to use canola or flaxseed oil for cooking and in salad dressings.

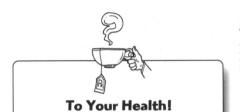

To Your Health!

We've gone into such detail about the essential fatty acids because they're sold under all the different names. Fish oil, for instance, has been shown to help your heart, but the label often says "EPA," not "fish oil." GLA is found in evening primrose oil; sometimes the label says "GLA," and sometimes it says "evening primrose oil" or even "EPO." Be an informed consumer and read the labels carefully.

Nothing Fishy About It

Essential fatty acids, especially the fish oils EPA and DHA, can have important health benefits:

➤ **Heart health.** According to a lot of studies, men who eat fish several times a week are less likely to have a heart attack. Fish oil may also help prevent sudden death from heart rhythm problems and could help prevent artery-blocking blood clots that cause heart attacks.

➤ **Helping cholesterol.** Fish oil supplements (and maybe the GLA in evening primrose oil) can help lower your high cholesterol—but only if you also cut back on saturated fats.

➤ **Crohn's disease.** People with this chronic intestinal problem often are helped by taking fairly large amounts of fish oil. To avoid "fish breath" from the quantities they need to take, they use slow-release capsules.

The GLA in evening primrose oil can be extremely helpful for women with *premenstrual syndrome* (PMS), especially if breast swelling and tenderness are the worst symptoms.

Other Nutritional Supplements

All sorts of other nutritional supplements crowd the shelves of any pharmacy or health-food store. We can't go into all of them here, but here are a few we think are promising:

➤ **Phosphatidyl serine (PS).** This fatty substance is found in your cell membranes. It's possible that it helps improve concentration, memory, and mental focus. It's most often recommended for older adults with memory problems, but today a lot of younger people use it too.

➤ **Coenzyme Q$_{10}$.** Think of this one as the spark plugs in your car engine. Coenzyme Q$_{10}$, also known as *ubiquinone*, works inside your cells to release energy. Not enough CoQ$_{10}$ means not enough energy—especially in your heart muscle. In Japan, Canada, Italy, Sweden, and Denmark, coenzyme Q$_{10}$ is widely prescribed to treat congestive heart failure and to help lower high blood pressure. Here in the U.S., it's a food supplement. You can't really get enough of the foods that contain coenzyme Q$_{10}$—like wheat germ, vegetable oils, and sardines—to be helpful, so you'll have to take supplements. Discuss coenzyme Q$_{10}$ with your doctor before you try it, especially if you have a heart condition.

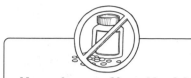

Hazardous to Your Health!

Do not take fish oil if you have diabetes—it can make your blood sugar go up. Do not take fish oil if you are taking any sort of blood-thinning drug, such as Coumadin® or Warfarin®.

➤ **Soy isoflavones.** Complex chemical compounds called *isoflavones* are found in soy foods like bean curd and soy milk. Some of them, like genestein, can act as weak versions of estrogen, the female *hormone* that women stop making when they reach menopause. By eating a lot of soy foods and taking genestein supplements (if needed), menopausal women can help some of the annoying symptoms, like hot flashes, without taking more powerful hormone-replacement drugs. Even better, soy isoflavones may help prevent breast cancer, heart disease, and osteoporosis in older women.

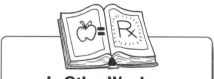

In Other Words...

Hormones are chemical messengers your body makes to tell your organs what to do. Hormones regulate many activities, including your growth, blood pressure, and heart rate. It also determines your glucose levels and sexual characteristics.

➤ **Digestive enzymes.** As you get older, your stomach naturally produces less hydrochloric acid, which can slow down your digestion and cause other digestive discomfort. Digestive enzymes such as papain, bromelain, cellulase, amylase, and lipase can help. There are a lot of different brands that combine several enzymes. You might have to try a few before you find the brand that works best for you. Here's a tip: If you have trouble digesting protein, look for bromelain and papain in the formula. If crunchy vegetables like broccoli, carrots, and kale are the problem, be sure the formula includes cellulase.

There's one popular supplement we'd like to warn you against: DHEA (*dehydro-epiandrosterone*). Your body makes this in your adrenal glands and converts some of it into testosterone, the male sex hormone. You naturally make less DHEA as you get older. Supplements are said to restore your youthful vigor, prevent heart disease, and so on. The catch is that they could also trigger cancer—stay away.

Finding Qualified Practitioners

The importance of nutrition to your health is so obvious that even some mainstream physicians have caught on. The problem is that medical schools haven't. Even today, courses in nutrition aren't always required. If you're looking for a doctor who will take a nutritionally oriented approach to your health, we suggest finding one who's interested enough to belong to one of these professional organizations:

> **American College for Advancement in Medicine (ACAM)**
> 23121 Verdugo Drive, Suite 204
> Laguna Hills, CA 92653
> Phone: (800) 532-3688
> Fax: (949) 455-9679
> E-mail: acam@acam.org

> **American Holistic Medical Association (AHMA)**
> 6728 Old McLean Village Drive
> McLean, VA 22101-3906
> Phone: (703) 556-9728
> Fax: (703) 556-8729
> E-mail: HolistMed@aol.com

> **The Foundation for the Advancement of Innovative Medicine (FAIM)**
> Two Executive Boulevard, Suite 204
> Suffern, NY 10901
> Phone: (914) 368-9797
> E-mail: faim@rockland.net

To find a nutritionally oriented healthcare practitioner in other areas (psychology, for example), contact:

> **Price-Pottenger Nutrition Foundation**
> P.O. Box 2614
> La Mesa, CA 91943
> Phone: (800) FOODS4U
> Fax: (619) 574-1314
> E-mail: info@price-pottenger.org

If you want to use nutrition to help you deal with a chronic health problem such as diabetes or asthma, we recommend the advice of a registered dietitian licensed in your state. To get the details and to find a qualified practitioner near you, contact:

> **American Dietetic Association (ADA)**
> 216 West Jackson Boulevard
> Chicago, IL 60606-6995
> Phone: (312) 899-0040
> Nutrition hot line: (800) 366-1655
> Fax: (312) 899-1979
> E-mail: info@eatright.org

Registered dietitians (R.D.s) have undergraduate and often graduate degrees in nutrition, have done an internship (usually in a hospital), and have passed a stiff exam sponsored by the American Dietetic Association. In addition, R.D.s must usually pass state exams to be licensed to practice in their state. In some states, a nutritionist or other health-care practitioner can take the exam without being an R.D. Those who pass can call themselves *Certified Clinical Nutritionists* (C.C.N.s). Watch out for unlicensed "nutritional advisers," whose degrees come from home-study courses. These people aren't really qualified to give you the advice you need, especially if you have any sort of serious health problem.

Rules, Rules, Rules

Nutritional supplements are regulated by the FDA. The whole regulatory situation is extremely controversial. According to the supplement manufacturers, the FDA would like nothing better than to control them completely and make consumers need a prescription for vitamins, herbs, and all other supplements. According to the FDA, supplement manufacturers make exaggerated and false claims for the health benefits of their products and can't be trusted to regulate themselves.

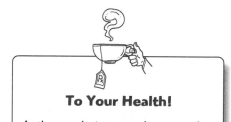

To Your Health!

As the regulations stand now, and as they're likely to become, the only way that you can really know what's right for you is to become an informed consumer.

In 1994 a compromise was reached with the *Dietary Supplement Health and Education Act* (DSHEA). The Act lets manufacturers make structure or function claims on the product labels. In some cases, like "Vitamin E contributes to a healthy heart," the function statement has to be followed by a disclaimer that says "This statement has not been evaluated by the FDA. This product is not intended to diagnose, treat, cure, or prevent any disease." Function claims are a step forward from previous rules that didn't let manufacturers make any claims at all, but they still don't tell consumers very much. In 1998, the FDA proposed new rules that would ban certain types of claims, like "Reduces the pain and stiffness associated

243

with arthritis." Under the proposed rules, manufacturers could only make vague statements on the labels, such as "Helps promote urinary tract health."

With some exceptions, your health insurance generally won't cover the cost of nutritional supplements. Most insurance plans do cover consultations with a dietitian, as long as he or she meets the licensing requirements in your state. Check first, though. Orthomolecular medicine isn't always considered standard medical practice. Your insurance company may or may not cover orthomolecular treatments. Check first.

Flushing Away Your Money

Despite all the evidence of the value of many nutritional supplements, a lot of doctors still scoff and say all you need to do is eat a normal diet (whatever that means). They say the supplements just pass right through without being absorbed, so all you really get is expensive urine. It is true that large doses of some vitamins will mostly pass out of your body, but you can improve your absorption considerably by spreading your dose out over the day.

Doctors also point that for every supplement that helps, there are others that are just hype. They also point out that just taking supplements won't really solve any health problems if you don't also make lifestyle changes and take your prescribed medicine. They're absolutely right there. So lose weight, stop smoking, cut back on alcohol, get more exercise, and take your medicine—and don't forget the vitamins.

The Least You Need to Know

➤ Orthomolecular medicine is based on the belief that large doses of vitamins, minerals, and other nutritional supplements can correct health problems.

➤ You need 14 vitamins and at least 10 minerals for basic good health. If you can't eat a good diet with plenty of fresh fruits and vegetables every day, consider taking supplements.

➤ Extra amounts of some vitamins and minerals can help treat and prevent some health problems, including heart disease, high blood pressure, and osteoporosis.

➤ Amino acids such as glutamine, tryptophan, and lysine can be valuable for treating health problems such as herpes.

➤ Flavonoids are powerful antioxidants that defend your body against damaging free radicals.

➤ Essential fatty acids such as fish oil and evening primrose oil can help protect your heart and relieve PMS symptoms.

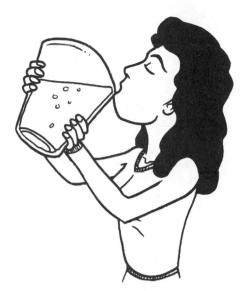

Chapter 18

Juice Therapy: Drink It Down

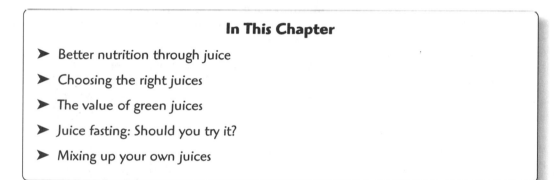

In This Chapter

➤ Better nutrition through juice

➤ Choosing the right juices

➤ The value of green juices

➤ Juice fasting: Should you try it?

➤ Mixing up your own juices

Five a day for better health—you've been hearing that a lot lately. Five what? Fresh fruits and vegetables, of course. And why? Because these foods are crammed with all sorts of things that are good for you: vitamins, minerals, fiber, and lots more. But for all the talk you've been hearing, are you actually eating five a day? If you're a typical American, probably not. Only about one in five of us actually eats five servings of fresh fruits and vegetables every day. We know, we know—you're too busy to keep track of all this. No more excuses. There's an easy, delicious way to get your daily fruits and veggies in one quick dose: Drink them.

A Juicy Idea

Adding a glass or two of fresh juice to your daily diet is a quick and easy way to boost your intake of nutrients. You get all those great vitamins and minerals, of course, but you could get those just by popping some supplements. What juice also gives you are *carotenes* and *flavonoids*, the complex natural substances that give fruits and vegetables

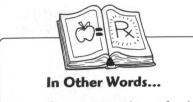

In Other Words...

Dietary **fiber** is a general term for the indigestible parts—mostly cell walls—of plant foods.

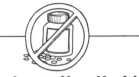

Hazardous to Your Health!

According to the FDA, anywhere between 16,000 and 48,000 cases of food-borne illness each year can be traced back to drinking unpasteurized juice, usually from cider mills and farm markets. If you buy juice, make sure it's pasteurized. The FDA will soon require unpasteurized juice to carry a warning. If you make your own juice, use good kitchen sanitation, wash your hands thoroughly, use only clean equipment, wash fruits and vegetables well, and store leftover juice in the refrigerator immediately.

their vivid colors and distinctive flavors (see Chapter 17, Nutritional Supplements: Extra Help for Health," for more on carotenes and flavonoids). Carotenes and flavonoids aren't just for looks and taste, though—they're also powerful defenses against cancer, heart disease, and more.

When you chomp though a celery stalk or a carrot, you're getting a lot of good nutrition, but a lot of the nutrients stay locked up in the *fiber* of the raw foods. Instead of being absorbed, the nutrients pass out of your body along with the fiber. Don't get us wrong—fiber is crucial for good health, and we're all for plenty of it (in fact, we'll talk a lot more about fiber in Chapter 20, "Detoxification Treatments: What a Waste"). We also want you to get the maximum benefit from the fruits and veggies you eat, though. That's where juicing comes in. Juicing releases the nutrients from the fiber, so you get a concentrated, easy-to-absorb dose of the good stuff in every glass.

If you juice together three celery stalks, two carrots, and one apple, you'll only get about 12 ounces of liquid. In just one tall glass of delicious, refreshing juice, you'll get your five for the day. Total calories? About 120. Total fat and cholesterol? Absolutely none. Taste? Pretty good—try it.

There's one minor problem, though—the juicer takes out a lot, though not all, of the fiber from the plant foods. Since eating plenty of fiber is crucial for good health, you'll still have to make sure you're getting enough. For good health, most nutritionists today suggest at least 25 to 30 grams of fiber every day. You can easily get that amount by eating plenty of whole grains, beans, salads, and fresh fruits and vegetables. If you don't mind the added texture in your juice, you can get more fiber simply by stirring some of the pulp from the juicer back into your drink.

Turning Green with Health

Green vegetables are green because they have a lot of *chlorophyll* in them. Chlorophyll is the complex pigment that makes green plants green. The word comes from the Greek words *khloros*, meaning "greenish yellow," and *phyll*, meaning "leaf."

Some juicing advocates believe that chlorophyll gives you an extra nutrient punch that can stimulate your cells, especially your oxygen-carrying red blood cells and the cells of your immune system. Chlorophyll also has antibacterial action, so it can help you get over an illness or infection. And just a little bit of chlorophyll stops bad breath in a hurry.

Sprouts of leafy plants such as alfalfa, wheat, and barley are naturally very high in chlorophyll—and also vitamins A, C, and E, along with important minerals like calcium, iron, potassium, and zinc. Green drinks can be made by juicing spinach, cabbage, collards, dandelion greens, and other leafy green vegetables, but fresh leafy sprouts are the best way to get the chlorophyll boost. In fact, 1 ounce of wheat-grass juice is the nutritional equal of a big spinach salad.

You can grow, harvest, and juice your own sprouts. If you identify with Eddie Albert on *Green Acres*, that might be the way for you. If you're more the Eva Gabor type, though, you can easily buy your green-drink stuff at the health-food store. You have a choice of liquid or freeze-dried powder with brand names like Green Magma® or Kyo-Green®. It's strong-tasting stuff. You can take it straight, but most people prefer to add an ounce of the liquid or a few spoons of the powder to their daily juice blend.

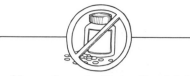

Hazardous to Your Health!

Don't drink grapefruit juice if you take the prescription drugs felodipine (Plendil®) or nifedipine (Adalat® or Procardia®) to treat high blood pressure or angina; lovastatin (Mevacor®) to lower your cholesterol; calcium-channel blockers such as Cardizem® to treat heart disease; carbama-zepine (Tegatrol®) to treat seizures; and terfenadine (Seldane®) to treat allergies. The grapefruit juice increases the amount of these drugs in your blood—in effect, it gives you an overdose.

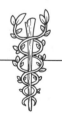

The Healing Arts

Variety is the spice of juicing. It's important to use a variety of fruits and vegetables in your juices. Fruit juices add sweetness to your drinks, but too much sorbitol, the sugar in fruit, can cause diarrhea and digestive upset. Try to drink at least equal amounts of vegetable and fruit juices. As a good rule of thumb, use one vegetable for each fruit. If your juice mixture tastes too bitter or too "green," add some carrot or apple juice.

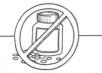

Hazardous to Your Health!

The FDA has recently warned that raw alfalfa sprouts may carry salmonella or E. coli, bacteria that can cause food poisoning or severe gastrointestinal illness. If you get digestive upset after drinking alfalfa juice, see your doctor as soon as possible. And don't give alfalfa juice to kids, the elderly, or anyone in poor health or whose immune system is weak.

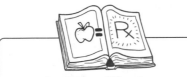

In Other Words...

When you go on a **therapeutic** or **juice fast**, you take in only juice, not solid food. Many naturopaths recommend a juice fast of one to three days twice a year as a way to rejuvenate and cleanse your system.

The Fast Way to Better Health

Therapeutic fasting, also called *juice fasting*, is an important treatment in naturopathic medicine (check back to Chapter 4, "Naturopathy: The Healing Power of Nature," for more on this). This fasting is used to activate your own healing processes and to remove stored toxins from your body. Naturopaths believe that fasting is very helpful for stimulating the liver and treating painful chronic conditions such as arthritis.

During a therapeutic fast, you don't eat for anywhere from one to three or more days. Instead, you drink plenty of fresh juice and may have some raw fruits and vegetables. Why? Because the juice gives you all the nutrients and water you need, but it doesn't take any effort to absorb. Your body can concentrate on healing, not digesting.

If you feel the need for a quick pick-me-up during the day, stop in at your local juice bar for a green drink. You'll get a shot of green juice freshly made from your choice of wheat, barley, or alfalfa.

Juicing Away Food Allergies

According to naturopathic theory, a lot of chronic illnesses, like arthritis and asthma, are caused by food sensitivities. To figure out which foods are causing the problem, a naturopathic physician might suggest a juice fast for several days. If your symptoms get better during that time, you know that food sensitivities are the real culprit. By gradually adding your normal foods back to your diet after the fast, and noting any symptoms that occur when you do, you can figure out which foods make your symptoms kick up.

Recipes for Juicing Up Your Diet

You can juice just about anything that grows—even string beans and beets. To do it, you'll need a high-quality electric juicer. We've found that the most important thing to look for in a juicer is the motor. It should be at least 0.4 horsepower—anything less just doesn't do the job fast enough or well enough. A good juicer costs over $100, but it will easily last for 20 years. It's a very worth-while investment in your health.

Although we're about to give you some juicing recipes, the fun thing about juicing is that you don't really need recipes. Be open-minded (or maybe that should be open-mouthed) and mix up your own combinations. The only things to avoid are OJ and tomato juice—many juicing experts feel they're too acidic.

All-Purpose Vegetable Juice

> 3 carrots
> 2 celery stalks
> 2 beets (with greens if possible)
> $^1/_2$ small green cabbage
> $^1/_4$ onion, peeled
> $^1/_2$ cup fresh parsley

Juice all ingredients together, stir well, and drink at once.

A Glass of Green

> 6 spinach leaves
> 3 collard leaves
> 4 carrots
> 2 celery stalks
> $^1/_2$ cucumber
> 1 apple

Juice all ingredients together. Stir well before drinking.

Fruit Cocktail

> 1 cup fresh strawberries
> $^1/_4$ fresh pineapple, peeled and cut into chunks
> 1 cup red or purple grapes (remove stems)

Juice all ingredients together. To make this into a smoothie, pour juice into a blender and add a cup of plain, nonfat yogurt and add a few ice cubes. Process until smooth.

If your juice mix tastes too bitter, try adding an apple or carrot to the mixture to sweeten it. Half a lemon and/or a piece of fresh ginger about the size of a quarter adds tang.

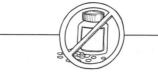

Hazardous to Your Health!

Fasting isn't for everyone and should never be tried on your own. Always discuss fasting with your doctor, naturopathic physician, nutritionist, or other professional before you try it. If you have diabetes or blood-sugar problems, or if you have heart disease or any other serious medical condition, do a juice fast only under your doctor's supervision.

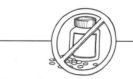

Hazardous to Your Health!

If you have diabetes or blood-sugar problems, watch out for fruit juices and carrot juice. The sugar in them could make your symptoms worse. Drink these juices in small amounts or dilute them with water or vegetable juices.

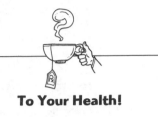

To Your Health!

Always thoroughly rinse all your produce—even the organically grown kind—under running water before you use it.

Juicy Tips

Juicing is basically very easy—just chop up the raw foods, toss them into the juicer, and let 'er rip. To avoid a nice juicy kitchen disaster, though, follow these guidelines:

➤ Remove hard inner pits from peaches, nectarines, cherries, melons, and other fruits.

➤ Core apples before you juice them. The seeds contain tiny amounts of cyanide.

➤ Peel oranges, lemons, and other citrus fruits, but leave on as much of the white pith as you can— it has lots of vitamin C and flavonoids in it.

➤ Leafy carrot and rhubarb tops are toxic—don't juice them.

➤ Peel fruits with tough or hairy skins, like kiwi, pineapple, melons, and mangoes.

➤ Bananas and avocados just can't be juiced—they don't have enough liquid. Mash them and stir them into a juice blend. For a smoother drink, process them with the juice in a blender.

It's always best to drink your juice as soon as you make it. If you have some left over, store it in the refrigerator and use it as soon as possible. Fresh juices tend to settle as they sit, so stir before using.

The Least You Need to Know

➤ Juicing is a quick, easy, and delicious way to get the valuable nutrients in fresh fruits and vegetables.

➤ Green drinks are made from green vegetables like spinach, dandelion greens, and leafy sprouts such as wheat or barley grass. These drinks are high in chlorophyll and also contain vitamins and minerals.

➤ Juice fasts of one to three days can be helpful for removing toxins, stimulating your healing processes, and cleansing your body.

➤ Juice fasts are sometimes helpful for identifying food sensitivities.

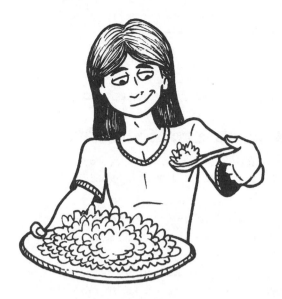

Chapter 19

Macrobiotics: The Brown Rice Way to Health

In This Chapter

➤ The benefits of a balanced whole-food diet

➤ How the macrobiotic diet can help your health

➤ Choosing the right macrobiotic foods for you

➤ Tips for macrobiotic cooking

➤ Learning to live the macrobiotic way

Someday we're going to write a book called *The Encyclopedia of Diets*. It'll be a thick, depressing book, filled with page after page of fads and failures. There will be some bright spots here and there, though—diets that actually work. First among that select group will be the macrobiotic diet.

"Not macrobiotics!" we hear you groan. "Isn't that the diet where all you eat is brown rice and burdock root? How can anyone stick to that?" Read on—there's a lot more than brown rice to this very effective approach to your diet and your health.

Macrobiotics: Change Is Good

Macrobiotics is both a philosophy of life and an approach to nutrition. Philosophically, macrobiotics is a way of seeking order and balance in a changing universe. Nutrition-ally, macrobiotics is a way of eating based on a balanced whole-foods diet.

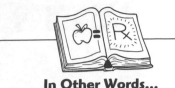

In Other Words...

Macrobiotics comes from the Greek words *macros*, meaning "big," and *bios*, meaning "life." Overall, macrobiotics is a dietary and philosophical approach to life that emphasizes balance and simplicity. The macrobiotic diet emphasizes whole grains and vegetables.

Most people approach macrobiotics from the diet side and get into the fairly sophisticated philosophy as they get further along. We'll take the same approach.

Eating the Macrobiotic Way

The basic macrobiotic diet is heavy on grains and vegetables and very low in fat. Here's how it breaks down:

➤ **Whole grains.** Half of your daily diet comes from whole grains such as rice, millet, barley, buckwheat, whole wheat, and oats. Noodles and yeast-free breads made from whole grains fall into this category.

➤ **Vegetables.** About 20 to 30 percent of your diet comes from fresh vegetables. Vegetables such as potatoes, eggplant, tomatoes, sweet potatoes, peppers, and zucchini should be avoided.

➤ **Beans and sea vegetables.** Anywhere from 5 to 10 percent of your diet comes from legumes such as soy products (tofu, tempeh, soy milk, and the like), adzuki beans, lentils, kidney beans, pinto beans, and bean sprouts. Sea vegetables are various Japanese edible seaweeds, including nori, wakame, Kombu, and hiziki.

➤ **Soups.** Miso (soybean paste) soup, bean soups, and noodle soups should be about 5 to 10 percent of your diet.

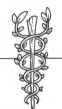

The Healing Arts

Macrobiotics today has its roots in Japan almost a century ago. The basic dietary and philosophical concepts were developed by George Ohsawa (1893–1966). Diagnosed with incurable tuberculosis at the age of 15, Ohsawa sought out alternative approaches to diet and health and overcame his disease. He devoted the rest of his life to the idea of macrobiotics. His work is carried on today by the George Ohsawa Macrobiotic Foundation and by his students, including Michio Kushi and the late Herman Aihara.

➤ **Fish and seafood.** You should eat these only a few times a week.

➤ **Fruits.** Eat these only a few times a week for dessert.

➤ **Snacks.** Eat nuts and seeds as occasional snacks.

➤ **Sweeteners.** Avoid refined sugar; use rice syrup or barley malt instead.

➤ **Salt and condiments.** Use mineral-rich sea salt instead of processed table salt. You can use shoyu (Japanese soy sauce) or tamari (a Japanese condiment similar to soy sauce) to flavor most dishes.

So far, so good. Now comes the hard part: eliminating foods for better health. Here's what the macrobiotic diet *doesn't* have:

➤ Meat, poultry, eggs, and dairy products

➤ Refined sugar, honey, chocolate, and vanilla

➤ Tropical fruits such as mangoes, pineapples, and bananas

➤ Alcoholic beverages, coffee, soda pop, fruit juice, and stimulating herbal teas, such as mint

➤ Refined grains, processed foods, artificial ingredients, food additives, and preservatives

➤ Canned and frozen foods

These foods aren't so easy to give up; it's also hard to give up the convenience of prepared foods. The beauty of macrobiotics is that it's flexible. Change your diet gradually and in a way that works for you.

The Yin and Yang of Yens

There's an underlying logic to the foods that are recommended in the macrobiotic diet. The choices are based on the traditional Oriental idea of balancing Yin and Yang. (We talked a lot about this back in Chapter 6, "Traditional Chinese Medicine.") Yin and Yang are the opposing, balancing forces of the universe—the two sides of the same coin. To put that in Oriental terms, Yin and Yang are the sunny and shady sides of the same mountain—different but inseparable. In general, things that are Yin are inside, descending, contracting, solid, and cold; things that are Yang are outside, ascending, expanding, hollow, and warm.

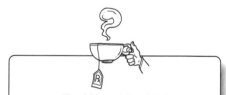

To Your Health!

For a good general introduction to macrobiotics, we suggest *Basic Macrobiotics*, by Herman Aihara (George Ohsawa Macrobiotic Foundation, 1997), and *The Macrobiotic Way*, by Michio Kushi (Avery Publishing, 1985).

According to macrobiotic thinking, different foods have different qualities. Some are very Yin, some are less Yin, some are more Yang, and some are very Yang. Among the vegetables, for instance, mushrooms, okra, and Brussels sprouts are considered very Yin. Chinese cabbage, peas, radishes, broccoli, and beets are more Yin; while kale, acorn squash, and onions are less Yin; and turnips, carrots, and burdock root are less Yang. Remember, though, that Yin and Yang aren't sharp divisions—they're more like points along a continuum. We don't have space to list the Yin and Yang of all the foods—any good book on macrobiotics will give you detailed information.

The goal of macrobiotic eating is to balance the Yin and Yang in your food in a way that matches your environment and your individual health. Extremes should be avoided, but even so, it's okay to eat foods that are very Yin or very Yang, as long as you balance them out with other foods.

The Acid Test

Another important aspect of macrobiotic eating is balancing *acid* and *alkaline* foods. Your body is naturally a bit on the alkaline side. If you get even a little too acidic or too alkalotic, you die. To prevent this, your body has a lot of natural mechanisms to keep you at exactly the right level of alkalinity. If you eat the typical American diet, however, you're making your body work overtime to keep your alkalinity in balance. According to macrobiotic theory, foods such as sugar, dairy products, refined grains, meat, and eggs all create excess acid that has to be neutralized to keep your alkalinity balanced.

Simply put, on the macrobiotic diet, you eat foods that help balance the acid and alkaline content of your body. It's a little more complex in practice, but here, too, any good book on macrobiotics will explain the basics and list acid- and alkaline-forming foods.

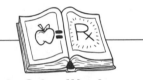

In Other Words...

Acid substances taste sour and sharp; **alkaline** substances taste bitter or slightly salty. The chemical measure of a substance's acidity or alkalinity is called the **pH.** Something with a pH of 7.0 is neutral. If its pH is below 7.0, a substance is acid; if its pH is above 7.0, it's alkaline. Your body's normal pH is between 7.35 and 7.45.

Macrobiotics and Your Health

Many people turn to the macrobiotic diet in search of better health. Do they find it? Yes. The macrobiotic diet emphasizes a low-fat, high-fiber diet with lots of whole grains, beans, and fresh vegetables. If that sounds familiar, it's because that's what every health professional concerned with diet also recommends.

The macrobiotic diet is especially helpful for people with chronic health problems:

➤ **High blood pressure.** If you have high blood pressure, your doctor will tell you to avoid salt because it has a lot of sodium. But even though the macrobiotic diet uses salty condiments such as shoyu (soy sauce), people who go on it often see their blood pressure drop. Why? It's probably two things. First, a few splashes of shoyu have a lot less sodium than a few good shakes of salt. Second, the macrobiotic diet is high in beans and vegetables, which are good natural sources of potassium. For reasons too complex to go into here, getting more potassium and less sodium often makes your blood pressure go down naturally.

➤ **High cholesterol.** The macrobiotic diet is very low in fat, which helps lower your cholesterol levels.

➤ **Diabetes.** Many diabetics find they can control their blood-sugar levels more easily if they follow the macrobiotic diet. That's because there's very little sugar in the diet. Also, beans help slow down the absorption of glucose into your system, so you don't get blood-sugar spikes.

➤ **Chronic pain.** The macrobiotic diet can do wonders for people with chronic pain from arthritis, nerve problems, headaches, and other problems. We don't know why it works, but it's certainly worth trying.

➤ **Chronic fatigue syndrome (CFS).** Some CFS patients get a lot better on macrobiotics. CFS is a mysterious and very individual disease, so this may not work for you, but again, it's worth trying.

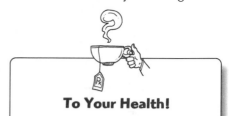

To Your Health!

Studies show that people who follow the macrobiotic diet consistently have much lower blood pressure and cholesterol than the average American.

One side benefit of the macrobiotic diet is that you'll probably lose weight if you're too heavy. The diet is low in sugary foods and calorie-dense fats and meats, and high on satisfying, low-calorie grains, beans, and veggies. Overweight people who go on a macrobiotic diet find that they lose pounds steadily without feeling hungry.

Macrobiotics and Cancer

The macrobiotic diet is sometimes called the anti-cancer diet. One reason is that it's not too different from the cancer-prevention diet recommended by the American Cancer Society. No diet alone has ever been shown to treat or "cure" cancer (or AIDS or any other deadly disease). What the macrobiotic diet might be able to do is prevent cancer. Because it's high in fiber and emphasizes fresh vegetables, the macrobiotic diet gives your body the sort of nutrition we know helps to fend off cancer. And because the diet avoids fat, meat, and processed foods, you're not eating some things that many researchers think help cancer get started. If you're at high risk for cancer or are recovering from it, macrobiotics could help you stay cancer-free—maybe not forever, but maybe for longer.

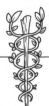

The Healing Arts

Soybean foods such as tofu and miso are an important part of the macrobiotic diet. There's some evidence that natural substances called **soy isoflavones** in these foods protect women against breast and ovarian cancer (see Chapter 17, "Nutritional Supplements: Extra Help for Health," for more on soy isoflavones). They may also help prevent hot flashes during menopause. Studies show that Japanese women who eat a traditional diet that's high in soy foods have less breast cancer. There's also no word for "hot flashes" in Japanese. Other traditional Japanese foods, such as green tea and seaweed, also have anti-cancer properties.

Cooking the Macrobiotic Way

Macrobiotic cooking is very simple once you get the hang of it. Ingredients like seaweed are a little exotic, but you can generally find almost all of them at health-food stores—and today you can buy brown rice in any supermarket.

In general, macrobiotic cooking emphasizes using the freshest possible, organically grown seasonal produce. Again, you can find organic produce at health-food stores and lots of supermarkets. Be sure to check out your local farmers' markets—many small farmers now grow organic produce.

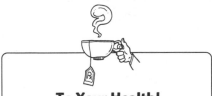

To Your Health!

For help with macrobiotic recipes, we recommend these cookbooks: *Complete Guide to Macrobiotic Cooking,* by Aveline Kushi and Alex Jack (Warner Books, 1985), and *Fresh from a Vegetarian Kitchen,* by Meredith McCarty (St. Martin's Press, 1995).

You don't need lots of fancy equipment to cook the macrobiotic way. A pressure cooker is very helpful for cooking brown rice and other grains quickly. According to macrobiotic principles, pressure cookers are also the most energizing way to prepare food. You'll probably want to buy one if you don't have one already. (Pressure cookers are pretty indestructible—you might be able to find a bargain at a yard sale.) Your other cooking pots should be made of cast iron, stainless steel, ceramic, or glass—avoid cookware made from copper or aluminum or with nonstick coatings. Use serving implements and bowls made of wood, bamboo, or pottery.

Electric cooking devices, like electric ranges, toaster ovens, and microwaves, interfere with the energy in your food. Use a gas or wood stove.

It's surprising how good things like brown rice and burdock root taste when they're cooked the macrobiotic way. The cooking techniques are simple. Grains are generally steamed or boiled; vegetables are steamed or very lightly sautéed. Soups and stews are very easy, especially because they don't involve long cooking times. In macrobiotic thinking, the quality of the water you use has an effect on your food. Use pure well water or spring water free of chemicals such as chlorine. Never use distilled water—its energy has been removed.

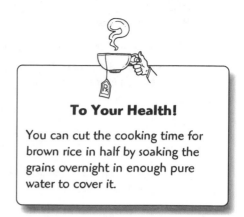

To Your Health!

You can cut the cooking time for brown rice in half by soaking the grains overnight in enough pure water to cover it.

We've also given instructions for making bancha tea, the basic macrobiotic drink. Bancha is made from a mixture of twigs, stems, and leaves of the tea plant; kukicha or twig tea is made just from twigs and stems.

The macrobiotic diet can be very flexible in the hands of a creative cook. We only have space for a few recipes, so we've stuck to the most basic: miso soup and two ways to make brown rice. Use the basic miso soup as your inspiration for other soups and stews. And remember, 1 cup of raw rice turns into anywhere from 3 to 4 cups of cooked rice.

Pressure-Cooker Brown Rice

> 3 cups medium-grain brown rice
> 4$^{1}/_{2}$ cups spring water
> $^{1}/_{2}$ tsp. sea salt

Combine rice, water, and salt in pressure cooker. Fasten lid according to manufacturer's instructions.

Cook over high heat until pressure comes up. Reduce heat to low and cook for 45 to 50 minutes.

Remove pressure cooker from heat and let pressure drop to 0 before removing lid.

Boiled Brown Rice

> 3 cups medium-grain brown rice
> 6 cups spring water
> $^{1}/_{2}$ tsp. sea salt

Combine rice, water, and salt in heavy pot with tight-fitting lid. Bring to boil over high heat. Reduce heat to medium-low and cook 50 to 60 minutes.

Remove pot from heat and let stand five minutes before serving.

Basic Miso Soup

> 1 oz. wakame (sea vegetable)
> 4 cups spring water
> 2 cups assorted vegetables, cut into small pieces
> 4 tsp. miso

Cover wakame in water and soak five minutes or until softened. Cut wakame into small pieces.

Combine wakame with water in medium pot. Bring to boil, then add vegetables. Cook until vegetables are tender, about four minutes.

Reduce heat as low as possible, stir in miso, and simmer gently for three minutes. Don't let the miso boil—it destroys the valuable enzymes in it.

Bancha Tea (Kukicha)

> 2 tsp. roasted twigs
> 6 cups spring water

Combine twigs and water in medium pot. Bring to boil, then reduce heat and simmer for five to eight minutes.

To serve, pour tea through bamboo strainer.

How you eat your food is important in macrobiotics. Try to eat in a calm and relaxed environment and take a moment to be grateful for your food before you begin. Chew your food very thoroughly—some macrobiotic counselors suggest 50 times per mouthful! There's no limit on how much or how often you eat, as long as you're hungry when you do.

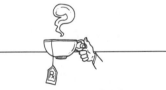

To Your Health!

If you buy your grains and beans in bulk, check them carefully for pebbles, chaff, damaged bits, and other waste before cooking. Put the grains or beans in a large bowl and sort through them. Then add enough cold water to cover to a depth of about an inch. Stir gently with your fingertips and drain into a strainer. Rinse quickly with cold water.

Nutrition and Macrobiotics

The macrobiotic diet is low—some experts say dangerously low—in vitamins and minerals. Rice has no vitamin A or vitamin C. Brown rice is often touted as a good source of B vitamins, but that's only relative to white rice. Brown rice still has its outer husk, or bran, on it (that's what makes it brown), and the bran has most of the Bs. Of the most important B vitamins, brown rice is especially low in folic acid and doesn't have any cobalamin (vitamin B_{12}) at all. Cobalamin is found naturally only in animal foods such as meat, fish, and eggs—foods that aren't eaten much, if at all, on the macrobiotic diet. Soy foods such as miso, tempeh, and soy milk do have some cobalamin, but you'd have to eat a lot of them—more than most people can manage—to get enough cobalamin from your diet alone. And although plant foods such as sea vegetables and shiitake mushrooms contain cobalamin, it's not in a form your body can use. As you can see in the following table, there just aren't that many Bs in brown rice. And if you check back to Chapter 17, you'll see that even eating 6 cups of brown rice a day doesn't give you all the Bs you need.

Rice Nutrition

Nutrient	Brown Rice	White Rice
Protein	5 g	5.5 g
Carbohydrates	45 g	57 g
Fiber	3.3 g	0
B vitamins		
Thiamin (B$_1$)	.20 mg	.33 mg enriched; .04 mg unenriched
Riboflavin (B$_2$)	.02 mg	.03 mg
Niacin	2.6 mg	3.0 mg enriched; .8 mg unenriched
Pyridoxine (B$_6$)	.29 mg	.19 mg
Folic acid	8 mcg	7 mcg
Cobalamin (B$_{12}$)	0	0
Calcium	20 mg	23 mg
Iron	1 mg	2.25 mg enriched; .41 mg unenriched
Magnesium	86 mg	26 mg
Phosphorus	151 mg	95 mg
Potassium	153 mg	80 mg
Sodium	2 mg	4 mg
Zinc	1.2 mg	.94 mg
Total Calories	**218**	**264**

Amounts are for 1 cup. Federal law requires packaged long-grain white rice to be enriched with B vitamins.

Source: Bowes and Church, Food Values of Portions Commonly Used *(1997).*

You don't eat just brown rice on the macrobiotic diet, although it may seem that way. You also eat plenty of other grains, along with vegetables, beans, and other nutritious plant foods that provide vitamins and minerals. Beans and grains have little or no vitamin C, however, and in general, grains aren't a good source of minerals. The diet avoids dairy products and animal foods, which are the best food sources of calcium and iron. Another problem is that most of the vegetables are served lightly cooked, which lowers their vitamin content. Cooking reduces the amount of vitamin C in food by about half or more, for example. The best natural sources of vitamin C are fruits, which are also not a big part of the macrobiotic diet.

All this means that if you follow the macrobiotic diet carefully, you have a good chance of ending up short on some important vitamins and minerals, no matter how much you eat. We strongly suggest that you take vitamin and mineral supplements to make sure your needs are being met. That goes double for women, especially pregnant women, and children.

Brown rice is an excellent source of dietary fiber (we'll talk more about fiber in Chapter 20, "Detoxification Treatments: What a Waste"). There's over 3 grams of fiber in 1 cup of brown rice (there's none in a cup of white rice). That's about as much fiber as you'll find in an apple, a cup of Brussels sprouts, or half a cup of corn kernels.

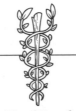

The Healing Arts

Starting in the early 1800s, rice mills in Asia began removing the brown outer covering—the bran—from rice grains. **Polishing**, as it was called, produced white rice that cooked quickly and tasted good. People who ate a lot of white rice and little else, however, developed a disease called **beriberi**. They became weak, had leg pain or paralysis, and became mentally confused. It wasn't until the late 1890s that researchers realized people who ate brown rice and not much else didn't get beriberi. That's because rice bran contains the B vitamin thiamin—polishing the rice removes the bran and the vitamin, causing a serious deficiency. The symptoms of beriberi can start after only 10 days without enough thiamin.

Learning to Live with Macrobiotics

Macrobiotics isn't just a diet—it's a lifestyle. Like any other lifestyle change, switching to macrobiotics can be difficult at first.

Many people find that the change in diet causes digestive problems. As they start eating more fiber and beans, they start having gas and sometimes diarrhea. To a degree, this is normal. Your system has to adapt to handling a lot more fiber. The best approach is to change over gradually to the new foods, giving your digestion a few days after each change to get used to it.

A bigger problem for some people is being the only macrobiotic person in the family. In our experience, that can cause family friction in a major way. If you're not the main family cook, you may have to persuade whoever is to learn how to cook some macrobiotic dishes, or learn how to make them yourself. And if you are the main family cook, good luck convincing your family to trade their French fries for brown rice.

If you're interested in macrobiotics, the best way to get started or to learn more is to take a course. Macrobiotic classes and weekend programs are fairly easy to find—check with your local health-food store or alternative health practitioners. You can also contact these organizations, which sponsor courses, camps, conferences, and other programs around the country:

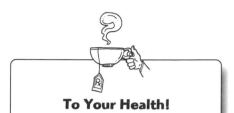

To Your Health!

Eating out the macrobiotic way can be a problem, but cheer up—it used to be a lot worse. Thirty years ago, only weirdos and hippies were vegetarians, and menus didn't have meatless dishes. Today it's a lot easier to get a vegetarian meal along macrobiotic lines.

George Ohsawa Macrobiotic Foundation
P.O. Box 426
Oroville, CA 95965
Phone: (800) 232-2372
Fax: (916) 533-7908

Kushi Institute
P.O. Box 7
Beckett, MA 01223
Phone: (413) 623-5741
Fax: (413) 623-8827
E-mail: info@macrobiotics.org

Macrobiotic programs are fun—you learn a lot, the people are interesting, and the setting is somewhere peaceful. Costs for programs vary, but they're usually quite reasonable—and of course, your macrobiotic meals are part of the fee.

Macrobiotics for Micro Benefits?

A lot of nutritionally oriented healthcare professionals feel that the macrobiotic diet is too bland and restrictive to stick to easily. It does take some getting used to, but once you get the hang of it, macrobiotics is pretty easy to follow. Nutritionists are also rightly concerned about the low vitamin and mineral content of the macrobiotic diet. They have a good point, but supplements can easily provide the missing nutrients.

Exaggerated claims that macrobiotics "cures" cancer, AIDS, and other deadly diseases have given it a bad reputation in medical circles. As we've already explained, macrobiotics doesn't cure cancer or anything else, but it may prevent some diseases or keep them from getting worse. It's hard to prove a negative, though, and there have only been a few useful studies that show the value of the macrobiotic diet from a medical perspective.

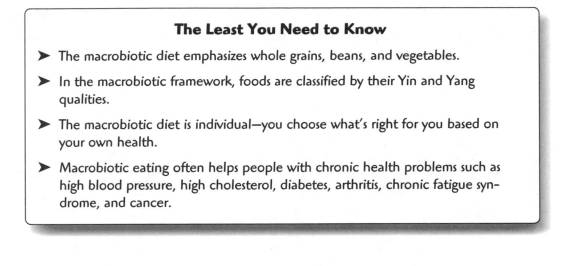

The Least You Need to Know

➤ The macrobiotic diet emphasizes whole grains, beans, and vegetables.

➤ In the macrobiotic framework, foods are classified by their Yin and Yang qualities.

➤ The macrobiotic diet is individual—you choose what's right for you based on your own health.

➤ Macrobiotic eating often helps people with chronic health problems such as high blood pressure, high cholesterol, diabetes, arthritis, chronic fatigue syndrome, and cancer.

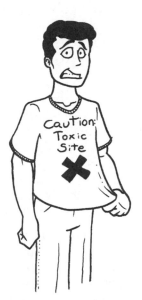

Chapter 20

Detoxification Treatments: What a Waste

In This Chapter

➤ How health–damaging toxins can accumulate in your body

➤ Detoxifying yourself through diet

➤ Heavy metals and your health

➤ The crucial role of fiber

➤ Balancing your bowel bacteria

➤ Colon hydrotherapy for better health

You take good care of your health. You don't smoke and you drink in moderation, and you're careful about your diet. You buy free-range eggs and meat and organically grown fruits and vegetables. You even have water filters on the taps in your house. On the whole, you think you're doing a pretty good job of avoiding environmental toxins.

Think again.

Where were you today? Maybe you worked all day in an office, breathing in fumes from the copying machines and printers as well as formaldehyde from the carpeting. On the way home, you breathed in gas fumes when you filled your car's tank and then got more toxins, including dioxin and carbon monoxide, while you were held up in a traffic jam. Then you stopped at the dry cleaner and breathed in benzene fumes as you picked up your cleaning. In today's world, toxins are all around you, all the time.

Your Body as Toxic Dump

Most of us, most of the time, manage to deal with *environmental toxins* pretty well—they're eliminated through our normal metabolic processes. But sometimes, for reasons we'll discuss more in the rest of this chapter, toxins can build up in your system and cause health problems. If they build up enough, the health problem could be serious.

Take that whiff of benzene you got at the dry cleaner. It probably won't hurt you, but years of exposure to benzene—from working in a dry cleaning shop, for instance—increases your risk of getting leukemia.

What about all the other thousands of chemicals all around you every day? A typical fabric softener you can buy in any supermarket contains nine different chemicals that the Environmental Protection Agency says can cause central nervous system damage or cancer. What happens when those chemicals are combined? The answer to that is really scary: Nobody knows. Most of the chemicals in use today have never been studied for their effects on humans, much less for their effects in combination.

Then there are the heavy metals—lead, aluminum, cadmium, and others. We're surrounded by them, but our bodies are terrible at getting rid of them. If you take any sort of drug—alcohol, prescription drugs, even nonprescription painkillers like acetaminophen (Tylenol®), your body has to deal with the toxic breakdown products. And then there are toxins your own body sometimes makes—you might be making yourself sick.

We think it's important for everyone to be aware of how their environment—outside and in—affects their health. The picture isn't really that dark, though. There's plenty you can do to help your body get rid of toxins.

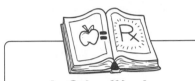

In Other Words...

Environmental toxins are harmful poisons found all around us. Examples include dioxin, carbon monoxide, formaldehyde, lead, pesticides, and other dangerous substances. Many environmental toxins are the result of modern industrial processes, but some, such as cadmium, come from harmful activities such as cigarette smoking.

Living with Your Liver

Your liver is the largest internal organ in your body, weighing in at around three pounds. It's an amazing chemical factory that performs literally thousands of functions every second of every day. One of your liver's biggest jobs is to remove waste products and toxins from your body. To do that, your body pumps just under a quart of blood through your liver every minute.

The processes your liver uses to capture and remove wastes and toxins are called *detoxification pathways*. They're very complex, but simply put, detoxification is

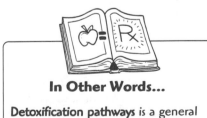

In Other Words...

Detoxification pathways is a general term for all the various ways your body removes wastes and toxins from your system.

done in your liver by a whole bunch of enzymes and antioxidants, all working together. One of the best ways to keep your liver functioning well, then, is to make sure you have enough vitamins and minerals so you can make all those enzymes and keep your antioxidant level high (see Chapter 17, "Nutritional Supplements: Extra Help for Health," for more information). Drinking plenty of fluids—at least 64 ounces a day—also helps keep your liver working well.

If you're exposed to a lot of toxins—and who isn't these days?—some holistic health practitioners recommend a metabolic cleansing program. The idea is that for about a week every few months, you follow a diet that gives your liver a chance to clean out accumulated toxins. While you're on the cleansing program, you eat very lightly—mostly fresh fruits and vegetables—and also take special supplements that support the liver by providing the amino acids, vitamins, minerals, and other nutrients it needs.

Metabolic cleansing isn't for everyone—you shouldn't do it if you're pregnant, diabetic, or have a chronic health problem like heart disease, for example. You also shouldn't do it on your own. The advice and supplements you need are available only through nutritionally oriented health practitioners.

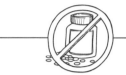

Hazardous to Your Health!

Follow a metabolic cleansing program only with the help of a nutritionally oriented healthcare practitioner. Do not go on a metabolic cleansing diet if you are pregnant; diabetic; or have hypoglycemia, kidney disease, liver disease, heart disease, or any other serious medical problem. Always discuss metabolic cleansing with your doctor before you try it.

It's Heavy, Man

Part of the environmental pollution that surrounds us all is made of tiny bits of *heavy metals* such as aluminum, arsenic, cadmium, lead, mercury, and nickel. If these toxins accumulate in your body, they can cause serious problems. Even low exposure to lead, for example, can cause permanent nerve and brain damage, especially to children. That's because for most of human history, there was no way to get exposed to these metals, so our bodies never evolved in ways to get rid of them—we didn't have to.

As you can see from the following table, it's easy to be exposed to heavy metals—they're all around you. One problem with heavy metal exposure is that by the time it shows up on conventional blood tests, a lot of damage may have been done. For that reason, some alternative health practitioners recommend testing hair samples to check for heavy metal

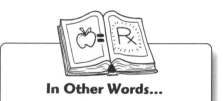

In Other Words...

Technically speaking, **heavy metals** are metals that have high atomic weights. The term has come to include any metal that's dangerous to your health even in moderate amounts, including aluminum, arsenic, cadmium, lead, mercury, and nickel.

exposure. Hair testing is more than a little controversial. That's because your hair naturally contains some heavy metals, so the test results will always show some heavy metals as well. Today better lab techniques have made hair-testing results more meaningful, but you still need to be cautious. Unscrupulous practitioners have used perfectly normal hair-analysis results to convince people they have to go through an expensive detoxification process.

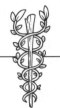

The Healing Arts

According to the federal *Centers for Disease Control and Prevention* (CDC), about 9 percent of American children between the ages of one and five have dangerously high levels of lead in their bodies. Most of these children live in poor neighborhoods where lead paint is still found in the housing. Not surprisingly, these kids often have learning and behavioral problems and score low on intelligence tests. Kids aren't the only ones at risk. In 1997, the CDC said that over 4,000 adults had dangerously high lead levels from lead exposure on the job.

Common Sources of Heavy Metal Poisoning*

Metal	Source
Aluminum	Foil, cans, deodorants, buffered aspirin, some antacids, aluminum utensils and cookware, baking powder
Arsenic	Insecticides, herbicides, paints, some ceramics
Cadmium	Paints, metal plating, colored plastics, gasoline, fertilizers, fungicides, cigarette smoke, batteries, solder
Lead	Chips or dust from lead-based paint, leaded gasoline, solder, inks and dyes, pottery glazes, batteries
Mercury	Paints, fungicides, fabric softeners, floor waxes and polishes, photo film, some plastics, latex house paints before 1990, batteries
Nickel	Metal alloys in costume jewelry, cigarette smoke

All these metals have many industrial uses and are often found in the soil, air, and water of industrialized areas.

If you have severe heavy metal poisoning, you'll need medical treatment with a *chelating* drug—a drug that attaches to the metal and removes it from your body (see Chapter 8, "Chelation: Grabbing for Good Health," for more information). For less severe cases, treatment with a high-fiber diet, along with large doses of vitamin C, antioxidants, and other supplements, can be very helpful.

Don't decide that you have heavy metal poisoning on your own—and don't try to treat it on your own. Follow the advice of a nutritionally oriented healthcare provider.

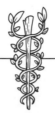

The Healing Arts

The old expression "mad as a hatter" dates back to the days when mercury was used to make the felt used in hats. The hatters got mercury poisoning from the fumes, which made them very irritable and anxious, gave them memory problems, and caused tremors and convulsions. Today very little mercury is used to make hats and very few people are likely to be exposed to such high levels. Low-level mercury poisoning still happens, though.

I'm Sick of This: Environmental Illness

For some people, environmental toxins are a serious problem. That's because their systems, for any one of several possible reasons, just can't get rid of the toxins efficiently. In a less toxic world two hundred years ago, that wouldn't matter. In today's world, they get sick with what some doctors call *environmental illness* (EI).

It's not easy to diagnose environmental illness. As you can see from the following table, the symptoms cover a broad range and aren't very specific. Also, people with EI find that their symptoms change from day to day as their exposure to environmental chemicals changes.

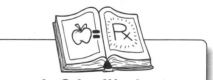

In Other Words...

Environmental illness (EI) is caused by an overload of toxins in the body. The symptoms are often mysterious and variable, and include depression, forgetfulness, headaches, fatigue, rashes, and loss of appetite.

Common Symptoms of Environmental Illness

Nervous System/Brain

depression

fatigue

poor memory

inability to concentrate

headaches

dizziness

"spaciness," "fogginess," or feelings of unreality

insomnia

excessive sleepiness

irritability

restlessness

lethargy

panic attacks

behavior or personality changes

lack of coordination

claustrophobia

Muscles and Bones

fatigue

joint pain

swollen joints

arthritis

aching muscles

muscle twitches and spasms

muscle weakness

lack of coordination

Digestive System

loss of appetite

food cravings, especially for sugar

nausea

vomiting

abdominal pain or cramps

constipation

diarrhea

weight loss

Heart and Lungs

heart arrhythmias

chest pain or tightness

wheezing

shortness of breath

Nose, Mouth, Sinuses, Throat

inability to taste foods well

inability to smell well

sore throat

persistent hoarseness

laryngitis

nasal or sinus burning

Skin and Nails

acne

skin rashes

dry skin

flushing

sensitivity to sun

increased sweating

discolored or deformed nails

slow healing of cuts

Menstrual

severe PMS

severe menstrual symptoms

Immune System

swollen glands in neck and armpits

chronic fatigue syndrome

mononucleosis or Epstein-Barr infection

yeast infections

worsening food or inhalant allergies

Source: Sherry A. Rogers, M.D., Tired or Toxic.

Some people are more at risk than others for EI because their environments contain more toxins. You might be at risk if:

➤ You work in one of those "sealed" office buildings where you can't even open a window.

➤ You're exposed to chemical fumes a lot—you work in a factory, a garage, a copy shop, a dry cleaning shop, for example—or you're a painter, a welder, or in a similar profession.

➤ You work with agricultural chemicals such as fertilizers and pesticides.

You might also be at risk if you work at a construction site or do maintenance work that involves a lot of cleaning chemicals.

Environmental illness is usually treated first by getting you away from the chemicals that are causing the problem and then using nutrition, supplements, and sometimes a detoxification program to flush the toxins from your system.

Diagnosing EI isn't easy—a lot of conventional doctors don't even believe the illness exists. If you think your health problems are caused by your surroundings, you need the help of a doctor who specializes in environmental medicine. To find one near you, contact:

> **American Academy of Environmental Medicine (AAEM)**
> P.O. Box CN 1001-8001
> New Hope, PA 18938
> Phone: (800) LET HEAL

Send a self-addressed stamped envelope with 55¢ postage along with your request.

Plugging Up Leaky Gut Syndrome

Sometimes the toxins that are making you sick come from your own body. To understand how that can happen, bear with us as we take you on a little tour of your small intestine.

Understanding Your Interior

Your small intestine isn't really small—it's actually anywhere from 15 to 20 feet long. It's called *small* because it's only about $1^1/_2$ inches wide, or about as wide as an average garden hose. (Now that you understand how misleading names for parts of your body can be, you understand how your boss can call the thing he sits on his brain.) Your small intestine's job is to take partially digested food from your stomach, break it down even more, and absorb the nutrients into your body. To do that with maximum efficiency, your small intestine is lined with millions of tiny, fingerlike projections called *villi*. The villi make the total surface area of your small intestine much larger—so large, in fact, that your small intestine has about the same surface area as a tennis court. A dense network of blood vessels surrounds the villi and carries the nutrients to your liver for further processing. The cells lining your small intestine are continually being replaced by new cells; the old lining is shed and eliminated along with other waste products.

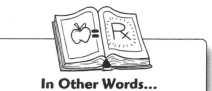

In Other Words...

The **villi** (singular **villus**) lining your small intestine are tiny, fingerlike projections designed to increase the total area available to absorb nutrients. The word comes from the Latin word for "hair" or "fleece"—you have so many villi, the lining of your small intestine looks hairy.

Leaks in the System

What the villi keep out is as important as what they let in. Your intestinal lining is supposed to let in only small molecules of digested food; it's supposed to keep out bacteria, toxins, and large molecules of undigested food.

If your small intestine has been damaged by a lousy diet, an illness, high stress levels, certain drugs, or food allergies, the villi may not be working too well. Large molecules of undigested food can "leak" through the villi and end up in your bloodstream. They're not supposed to be there, though, and your body reacts to them as if they are toxins or invading germs. The result is what's called *leaky gut syndrome*. The symptoms of leaky gut syndrome vary a lot from person to person, ranging from minor skin rashes up to asthma attacks and arthritis. Leaky gut syndrome also puts extra stress on your liver, since the food particles end up there and have to be removed.

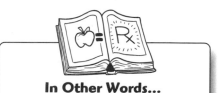

In Other Words...

If the villi of your small intestine are damaged, you develop **leaky gut syndrome**. Instead of keeping out large molecules of undigested food, the villi "leak" and let the particles enter your bloodstream. Your body reacts as if the molecules are invaders, causing symptoms such as skin rashes, digestive upsets, joint pain, and fatigue.

Many holistic health practitioners believe that leaky gut syndrome is at the root of a lot of chronic poor health. Take a look at the following table and see if you've had more than two of the symptoms in the past few weeks.

Leaky Gut Syndrome Symptoms

Physical Symptoms	Mental/Emotional Symptoms
bloating	depression
gas	mood swings
cramps	poor memory
diarrhea	anxiety or nervousness
constipation	fatigue
fatigue	confused or "fuzzy" thinking
food allergies	
skin rashes	
headaches	
joint pain	
frequent colds and minor illnesses	

Source: Dr. Alan Pressman.

If you're having the symptoms of leaky gut syndrome, you may need to take a test called a *comprehensive digestive stool analysis* (CDSA) to make sure. (We'll talk more about doing a CDSA a little further on in this chapter.)

Once it's diagnosed, leaky gut syndrome is fairly easy to deal with. The first step is to decide what's causing it—food allergies, for example, or overuse of drugs such as ibuprofen (Advil®) or aspirin. Next is to switch to a diet that's low in fat and high in fiber from plenty of whole grains and fresh fruits and vegetables. You might also want to take glutamine supplements. This amino acid nourishes and strengthens the walls of your small intestine. Supplements containing rice-bran oil (also called *gamma oryzanol*) also help strengthen the villi.

Moving Things Along with Fiber

Fiber, fiber, fiber. Why are we so obsessed with fiber? To understand why, let's take another little detour into your body. This time we'll visit your large intestine, also known as the *bowel*.

Your large intestine is only about five feet long—it's called *large* because it's about two inches wide. Actually, your large intestine has two main sections. The first is the colon. This part joins up with your small intestine on the lower right side of your abdomen. From there, the colon goes upward for a bit, then across your abdomen under your rib cage, and then down again on the left side of your abdomen. From there, the contents of your colon empty into the other section of your large intestine, the rectum, and are eliminated from your body through the anus. Your rectum is about five inches long.

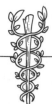

The Healing Arts

Study after study shows that people who eat a high-fiber diet are just plain healthier. They have lower cholesterol, less heart disease, and fewer bowel problems like diverticulitis and constipation. They also have a lot less colon cancer—and today colon cancer is one of the three leading causes of cancer death in the United States. You can sharply reduce your odds of being one of the 50,000 people who will die this year from colon cancer by adding fiber to your diet. The American Heart Association, the American Cancer Association, and just about everybody else says you should aim for 20 to 30 grams of dietary fiber every day.

Everything that doesn't get absorbed by your small intestine passes into your large intestine. That includes your own wastes, along with cholesterol-containing bile acids, pesticides, food additives and preservatives, heavy metals, and pollutants of all sorts. Obviously, the faster these toxic wastes leave your body, the better off you are.

Dietary fiber is what makes it all move along quickly through your bowel. There are basically two kinds of fiber:

➤ **Soluble fiber.** Most of the fiber found in plant foods is soluble—that is, it dissolves in water to form a soft gel.

➤ **Insoluble fiber.** This fiber is mostly cellulose, the indigestible fiber found in the cell walls of plant foods. Insoluble fiber absorbs water and swells up, but it doesn't dissolve. Bran of any sort is a good source of insoluble fiber.

Both kinds of fiber help keep your *stool* soft, bulky, and easy to pass. The fiber also binds up the waste products and toxins in your stool and keeps them away from contact with your colon and rectum.

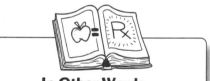

In Other Words...

Dietary fiber is a general term for the indigestible parts of plant foods. There are two kinds of fiber: soluble, which forms a soft gel in water, and insoluble, which absorbs water and swells. **Stool** is a polite word for your body's solid waste.

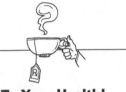

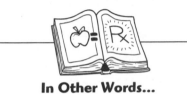

Bacteria Battles

Your small intestine contains literally billions of bacteria; your large intestine has *trillions* of them. Don't panic—you need all those little guys to digest your food and even to make some vitamins, like vitamin K. The bacteria come in hundreds of different kinds. Most are beneficial, but there are some bad guys lurking around. If for some reason the balance of good bacteria and bad bacteria in your intestines gets out of whack, the bad guys can start to multiply and crowd out the good guys. When that happens, you have *dysbiosis*, also known as *bacterial overgrowth*. When the overgrowth is in your large intestine, it's sometimes called *toxic bowel.*

The bad bacteria not only crowd out the good ones, they give off toxins and waste products that can seriously upset your digestion and even cause cancer. The most common symptoms of dysbiosis are digestive problems such as cramps, bloating, and gas that happen about an hour after you eat. After several days, you might start having alternating bouts of diarrhea and constipation. Other, less obvious symptoms like skin rashes, weight loss, and fatigue might also start turning up. As with leaky gut syndrome, the toxins can enter your bloodstream and cause a range of symptoms, including joint pain and mood swings. Also, clearing the toxins out of your system puts a strain on your liver.

The Fungus Among Us

A yeast-like organism known as *Candida albicans* also lives in your intestines. When conditions are right for bacterial overgrowth, they're also right for *Candida*. A yeast overgrowth can get out of hand very quickly and cause many of the same symptoms as bacterial overgrowth. If the yeast spreads to your mouth, you can get a painful condition called *thrush*; women can also get annoying vaginal yeast infections.

Discovering Dysbiosis

What can make the balance tip in favor of the bad guys? Sometimes drugs such as antibiotics, hormones, or steroids can throw the balance off; so can illnesses and intestinal parasites. The most common culprit, though, is a bad diet that's too high in fat and sugar and way too low in—you guessed it—fiber.

To be sure dysbiosis is the problem, a holistic healthcare practitioner will arrange for you to have a *comprehensive digestive stool analysis* (CDSA). A stool sample is sent to a lab, where a variety of tests help determine, among other things, how well you're digesting your food and what your balance of good and bad bacteria is.

Dissing Dysbiosis

If dysbiosis is the problem, you can take steps to treat it. First, you'll need to improve your diet by getting rid of the junk food and sugar and adding more fiber, especially soluble fiber from fruits such as bananas, pears, and apples. The fiber helps eliminate the bad bacteria and their toxins quickly and gives the good bacteria a chance to recover. Fiber also nourishes the good bacteria in your colon and helps them get back in charge.

To help the good guys along, you might want to try beneficial bacteria supplements containing acidophilus, bulgaricus, bifidobacteria, or lactobacillus. A type of yeast called boulardii is also helpful. Here's what to look for when you buy these supplements at the health-food store:

➤ Products that contain just one kind of bacteria, preferably the DDS-1 acidophilus strain or the Malyoth bifidobacteria strain

➤ Products that have been cultured in a milk-based medium and then ultrafiltered

➤ Products certified to contain one billion (yes, billion) active bacteria per gram

➤ Products that have been kept refrigerated at all times

The usual daily dose for treating mild dysbiosis is 1 gram of acidophilus (about $1/2$ teaspoon) and 250 mg of bifidobacteria ($1/8$ of a teaspoon) mixed into 3 ounces of pure, chlorine-free water. Swallow it down on an empty stomach before each meal, along with one or two 300-mg capsules of boulardii. You may need larger doses if your overgrowth is severe or if it's affecting your liver.

To help the bacteria get established in their new home, you might also want to take *fructooligosaccharides* (FOS for short—you can see why) supplements. FOS are simple sugars that the bacteria love but your body doesn't really absorb. Take 1 gram a day for as long as you're taking the beneficial bacteria supplements.

Soon after you start taking the beneficial bacteria, you may feel worse for a couple of days, with unpleasant gas and diarrhea. That's because the bad guys are being killed off by the new good guys and are releasing toxins as they die. Stick with it—in a few more days, you'll probably feel a lot better.

Colon Hydrotherapy

Sometimes bowel problems can be helped by *colon hydrotherapy*, also sometimes called a *high colonic* or *colonic irrigation*. This is a safe, effective way to remove wastes from the large intestine without the use of drugs. During a colon hydrotherapy session, pure water is gently introduced into the last few inches of the lower colon. The water softens and loosens accumulated wastes, which then are eliminated naturally. The process is repeated several times during a session.

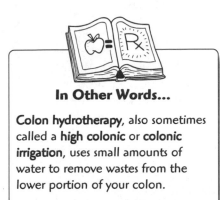

In Other Words...

Colon hydrotherapy, also sometimes called a **high colonic** or **colonic irrigation**, uses small amounts of water to remove wastes from the lower portion of your colon.

Colon hydrotherapy sounds like it could be an unpleasant experience, but it's not if it's done by a properly trained professional. Although you will have to remove some clothing, you don't have to strip, and you're always modestly covered with a drape or robe. You lie on a comfortable padded table and insert the nozzle yourself. There are no unpleasant odors and, because the nozzle is sterile and used only once, there's little chance of infection.

Many people who've tried colon hydrotherapy say it helps them improve their bowel function—they have more regular movements and less constipation and gas. In general, they often say they feel more energetic and healthier.

You do need to be cautious about colon hydrotherapy. Doing it once in a while may be beneficial, but too often—more than once every couple of weeks—can make your body fluids get out of balance. It can also make problems such as hemorrhoids or ulcerative colitis worse. In general, if you have any sort of chronic bowel problem, skip the colon hydrotherapy.

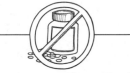

Hazardous to Your Health!

Some alternative medicine practitioners claim they can "cure" cancer through intensive colon hydrotherapy using mysterious herbs or even coffee. There is no evidence at all that these "therapies" work, but there's plenty of evidence that they're harmful. Stay away.

Do not use colon hydrotherapy if you have any sort of bowel problem such as severe hemorrhoids, Crohn's disease, or colitis.

Most colon hydrotherapists today are also trained and licensed in other fields, such as massage therapy. Right now only the state of Florida requires colon hydrotherapists to be registered, so you need to be careful about finding a qualified practitioner. Your best approach is to find someone who is licensed by your state in some other area—as a chiropractor, for instance—and who also has met the certification requirements of the *International Association for Colon Hydrotherapy* (I-ACT). For more information, contact:

> **International Association for Colon Hydrotherapy (I-ACT)**
> P.O. Box 461285
> San Antonio, TX 78246-1285
> Phone: (210) 366-2888
> Fax: (210) 366-2999
> E-mail: iact@healthy.net

I-ACT can provide a list of certified colon hydrotherapists near you.

Rules, Rules, Rules

When it comes to detoxification, you may be financially on your own. Insurance companies don't always recognize environmental illness or dysbiosis as valid conditions and may refuse to pay for your treatment, even if it's coming from a medical doctor. You'll almost certainly have to pay for metabolic cleansing programs, hair analysis, and the like out of your own pocket. And don't even think of asking your insurer to cover colon hydrotherapy.

Detox for Big Bucks

According to many doctors, detoxification is just a way for unscrupulous practitioners to make money. Take environmental illness, for instance. The symptoms are so vague and contradictory, and cover such a broad range, that a lot of conventional doctors say EI doesn't even exist. The same goes for leaky gut syndrome, dysbiosis, and yeast overgrowth—conventional doctors say these problems are actually relatively rare and don't happen anywhere near as often as alternative practitioners claim. The medical profession objects to metabolic cleansing programs and detoxification diets for two reasons. First, they're not convinced the programs are really needed or really help anything. Second, they claim that naturopaths, chiropractors, and others push the programs just as a way to make money by selling you the supplements. We leave it to you to decide if you really need the programs and the supplements that go with them. If you're in doubt, don't do it.

Colon hydrotherapy really bothers a lot of doctors. They say there is rarely, if ever, any need for a normally healthy person to do it and that it can be harmful. They do have a point—colon hydrotherapy washes out both good and bad bacteria, and it can be irritating to the bowel. It's also possible that poor sanitation or carelessness with the hydrotherapy equipment could spread illness from client to client.

The Least You Need to Know

➤ Detoxification programs use diet and supplements to help remove built-up toxins, wastes, and heavy metals such as lead from your body.

➤ Frequent exposure to toxins can lead to environmental illness.

➤ A high-fiber diet helps move toxins and waste products out of your body quickly.

➤ Intestinal problems such as leaky gut syndrome or bacterial overgrowth can produce internal toxins that cause serious health problems.

➤ Colon hydrotherapy can be used to remove wastes from the lower portion of the colon.

Part 6
Getting in Touch

High-tech medicine, with all its fancy machines, has its uses, but there's nothing quite like the human touch to make you feel better. And as you'll learn in this section, touching is what chiropractors do best—especially when they're touching your aching back. When it comes to lower-back pain, chiropractic is the treatment of choice. Don't just listen to us, though—in a major 1994 study, the federal Agency for Health Care Policy and Research *(AHCPR) said so as well.*

Massage and bodywork programs, such as Rolfing or the Alexander Technique, are hands-on techniques for straightening out the kinks in your sore muscles and bones and teaching you ways to keep them out.

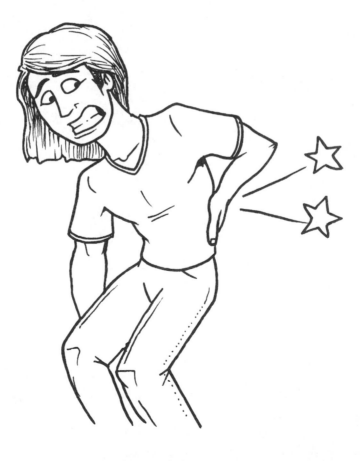

Chapter 21

Chiropractic: Working Out the Kinks

In This Chapter

➤ Why chiropractic is so popular today

➤ The theory behind chiropractic

➤ Why chiropractic is recommended for back pain

➤ How chiropractic can help headaches, neck pain, and other problems

➤ Finding the chiropractor who's right for you

Before we get into this chapter, we have to confess something: Dr. Pressman is a chiropractor. We'll try to be completely objective here as we explain why chiropractors are the best healthcare practitioners for treating lower-back pain, the best for treating athletic injuries, the best for helping chronic pain, the best for treating most health problems without drugs or surgery, the best for giving you good nutritional advice, and the best for helping you achieve better overall health the natural way. All that, and they're modest, too.

A Touching Story

As a profession, *chiropractic* is just over a century old. It all began back in the 1890s, when a physician named Daniel David Palmer got fed up with some of the worthless medical practices, like purging and magnetic healing, that many doctors of his time used. Dr. Palmer felt that doctors should encourage the body's natural healing processes and not just use drugs and other methods to treat symptoms. Then in 1895,

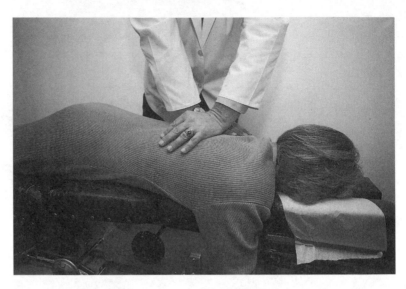

Chiropractic treatment is comfortable, safe, and easy. It's the preferred treatment for most cases of lower-back pain. Photo © American Chiropractic Association, by Jack McGuire.

Dr. Palmer examined a janitor who had lost his hearing years before, right after he hurt his back. Dr. Palmer saw that one of the vertebrae in the man's upper spine was out of position. He gently pushed it back into place—and a few days later, the janitor got some of his hearing back.

Dr. Palmer realized he was on to something and began studying the effects of spinal manipulation, now a basic principle of chiropractic. He felt that many health problems can be traced back to spine problems. In particular, he felt that *subluxations*—misalignments in the spinal column—press on the nerves of the spine and not only cause back pain but also affect other parts of the body. In effect, the subluxation pinches off the nerve and blood supply to your body's organs and systems, which in turn limits your body's ability to maintain good health and heal itself. Adjustments to the vertebrae of the spine relieve the pressure on the nerves and help restore the patient to health. The terms *chiropractic manipulation* and *chiropractic adjustment* are interchangeable.

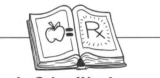

In Other Words...

Chiropractic is a branch of the healing arts that gives special attention to the role of the skeleton and muscles in health. Chiropractic care works with your body's natural strengths to restore and maintain your health—without drugs or surgery. The word comes from the Greek words *cheiro*, meaning "hand," and *praktikos*, meaning "doing." Literally, chiropractic means "done by hand."

Chiropractic Today

Dr. Palmer's idea of one cause, one cure, turned out to be a little too simplistic. Manipulation is still an important part of chiropractic, but today's practitioners are also well trained in other aspects of holistic healthcare, including nutrition and physical therapy. Today, as in Dr. Palmer's time, chiropractors treat the whole person without drugs or surgery.

There are more than 50,000 chiropractors in the United States—every state licenses them to practice. After medicine and dentistry, chiropractic is the third-largest doctoral-level health profession. In terms of alternative medicine, chiropractic is on top. Over 20 million people a year visit a chiropractor, making it the most popular alternative therapy. People go to chiropractors because they get results, as a recent Gallup poll shows:

➤ 90 percent of chiropractic users felt their treatment was effective.

➤ 80 percent said they were satisfied with the services they received.

➤ 68 percent said they would probably go back to a chiropractor again for treatment of a similar condition.

➤ 50 percent said they'd be willing to see a chiropractor for some other problem that chiropractors treat.

And a recent survey by the respected Harris polling service found that 70 percent of patients who went to a chiropractor for back pain were satisfied with their treatment.

Oh, My Aching Back

Chances are pretty good that you've hurt your back at some point in your life. You're hardly alone. Careful studies have shown that at any given time, some 31 million American adults are having lower-back pain, and a third of all Americans over age 18 have had back pain bad enough to seek professional help. In fact, back problems are the leading cause of disability for Americans under the age of 45. And if you've never had back pain, just wait. As many as 80 percent of all Americans will suffer back pain at some point in their lives. What's it all costing? With medical treatment, disability payments, sick days, lost productivity, and all the other related expenses, a staggering $50 billion a year!

Even with today's modern medical technology, we still don't know what causes most cases of *lower-back pain*. Poor muscle tone in the back gets blamed for some of it; so do muscle spasms and tears. Sometimes it's caused by *disc* problems—if that's the case, the pain might actually be in your buttock or leg, and you might also have numbness, tingling, and weakness in the legs. Anyone can get back pain, but it does seem to happen more often to people who are in poor physical condition or who spend a lot of time sitting or standing. If you do a lot of heavy physical work, you're also more likely to hurt your back. Emotional stress or long periods of inactivity often make back symptoms seem worse.

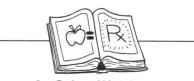

In Other Words...

Lower-back pain (LBP) is a general term for any sort of pain in the lower portion of the back, roughly in the area below your waist. Sometimes the pain is caused by pressure on one of the **discs**—the pads of tough tissue that separate and cushion the vertebrae in your spine. Chiropractic adjustment can fix the misalignment that causes the disc to "slip."

No More Back Pain

If—or more likely when—you hurt your back, your best treatment option is probably to visit a chiropractor as soon as possible. That's not just Dr. Pressman speaking—it's the federal *Agency for Health Care Policy and Research* (AHCPR), the branch of the Public Health Service (a division of the Department of Health and Human Services) that sets guidelines for these things. In a major 1994 study, a panel of 23 experts studied back-pain treatment. Here's what they concluded:

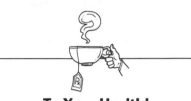

To Your Health!

If you hurt your back, here's a tip from Dr. Pressman: Put an ice pack (use a bag of frozen veggies in an emergency) on the painful area for 20 minutes, then take it off for a couple of hours. Repeat several times a day over the next day or two. If you're still having pain, see your chiropractor.

➤ Spinal manipulation is a recommended treatment for acute lower-back problems in adults.

➤ In most cases, conservative treatment such as manipulation should be pursued before surgery is considered.

➤ Prescription drugs such as steroids, painkillers, and antidepressants are not recommended for treating acute lower-back pain; however, many times muscle relaxers are recommended.

Spinal manipulation to treat back pain varies from patient to patient, of course, but it usually involves gently stretching or moving the spine, neck, and pelvis. Sometimes you hear a popping or crackling noise, just like the sound of cracking knuckles, during the treatment.

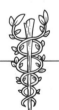

The Healing Arts

Should you have surgery for a lower-back problem? Only if it's absolutely your last resort—and maybe not even then. Careful studies have shown that there just isn't any good scientific evidence on the effectiveness of surgery for treating lower-back pain. And back surgery fails to help anywhere from 15 to 40 percent of the time. Despite all the evidence that surgery doesn't help, the number of back surgeries in the United States continues to climb. In 1998, it was well over 300,000—more than double the number performed in 1980.

Your first treatment may well give you almost instant relief from the worst of your back pain, although the muscles in the area may feel sore for a few days. You might need a few more treatments over the next couple of weeks to get complete relief.

No More Headaches

Chronic tension headaches are a very common health problem, one that medical doctors generally treat with powerful drugs. Chiropractors take a different approach—and it's been proven to work better.

In a 1997 study, 126 patients who got severe tension headaches were divided into two groups. For six weeks, one group got standard chiropractic treatment that included spinal manipulation; the other group got standard drug treatment with the anti-depressant.

During the treatment, both groups said their headaches were better. The chiropractic group had no side effects, but 82 percent of the drug group had side effects such as drowsiness, dry mouth, and weight gain.

Four weeks after the treatment ended, there was a dramatic difference between the two groups. The people who took the drug were right back where they were before the study—their headaches were just as bad. The chiropractic group, however, was doing much better. Even though they weren't getting chiropractic treatments anymore, they still had fewer headaches, the ones they did have weren't as bad, and they didn't need to take nonprescription painkillers as often.

No More...

Chiropractic is often amazingly helpful for all sorts of health problems, especially those that cause chronic pain or are related to your muscles or joints. Neck problems, such as whiplash injuries (caused when the head and neck are suddenly jerked back and forth), are often helped quite a bit by spinal manipulation. So are problems such as ringing in the ears (tinnitus), dizziness, and migraine headaches. Chiropractic can also help joint problems such as a frozen shoulder, carpal tunnel syndrome, and knee and ankle sprains.

Ongoing health problems such as asthma, chronic fatigue syndrome, and chronic digestive problems such as irritable bowel syndrome are helped, sometimes dramatically, by chiropractic. *In these cases, chiropractic treatment is in addition to, not*

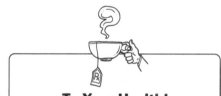

To Your Health!

More and more athletes are using chiropractors to treat sports injuries. That's because chiropractic treatment gets them back on the field faster—and without the use of drugs that might disqualify them from competition. The first chiropractor joined the U.S. Olympic medical team for the 1988 summer games, and today most professional sports teams have chiropractors on staff.

285

instead of, standard medical treatment. Keep taking your medicine! Your chiropractor will help by doing spinal manipulation and giving you dietary advice and sometimes nutritional supplements. Many patients find that chiropractic treatment helps them feel better and need less pain medication.

Chiropractic Approaches

As a profession, chiropractic has evolved quite a bit. Earlier chiropractors took a one-cause, one-cure approach. They believed that almost all health problems were caused by subluxations, which meant that almost all health problems could be helped by spinal manipulation.

This approach still has some validity, and there are some chiropractors who still follow it. As a group, they're called *straight* chiropractors, and they're in the minority. Most chiropractors today are called *mixers*. They use spinal manipulation and most of the usual techniques for chiropractic adjustments. These usually involve gently stretching or moving a joint slightly beyond its range of motion, or applying a very precise, short, sharp thrust to the joint to move it back into position. Mixers also use a variety of other chiropractic techniques as needed, including massage therapy, acupuncture, nutritional supplements, and so on. As a rule, mixers are flexible and tailor their treatments to your individual needs.

Directional Nonforce Technique

Directional nonforce technique (DNFT) is a method used to help cases that don't respond well to more traditional chiropractic approaches. DNFT uses low-force, highly specific adjustments to correct subluxations without the cracking and popping of traditional techniques.

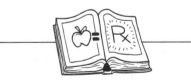

In Other Words...

Applied kinesiology (abbreviated AK and pronounced *kin-EASY-ology*) is a system that uses muscle testing along with other standard methods of diagnosis to find imbalances that harm your health.

Applied Kinesiology

Some chiropractors have also been trained in the techniques of *applied kinesiology* (AK). The basic concept behind AK is that imbalances in your muscles cause blockages in the energy circuits of your body—an idea that's not too different from the concept of subluxations. Applied kinesiologists believe that imbalances such as illness, injury, or toxins from things you're allergic to make the muscle's energy circuits switch off. Because muscles work in pairs (one to contract and the other to extend), if one muscle is weak, the other muscle gets overworked when it tries to compensate.

AK uses *muscle testing* to find the imbalances and what's causing them. The testing is done by having you resist pressure on an arm or leg while the practitioner feels one of your muscles. If the muscle feels "spongy" or "sags," an imbalance could be the problem. Usually imbalances are caused by your muscles, but sometimes food allergies or environmental toxins are the suspects. In those cases, a challenge test may be used: A small glass bottle containing the suspected substance is placed on your abdomen and your arm muscle is tested. Some AK practitioners use medical devices to measure the strength of the muscles. Once the problem has been identified, AK practitioners use manipulation, nutrition, exercise, and sometimes acupressure to help restore balance.

Using AK to find muscle weaknesses has some scientific support, but there's no real evidence for using it to find food allergies or other problems. In the hands of a chiropractor, osteopath, or medical doctor, AK has its uses, but be wary of homeopaths and other healthcare practitioners who use it or teach it as a home self-care technique.

Finding a Qualified Chiropractor

To become a chiropractor, students follow the pre-med curriculum in college for at least two years. After that, they spend five years at an accredited chiropractic college. The curriculum is a lot like what a medical student follows—except chiropractic students get even more training in anatomy, nutrition, physiology, and rehabilitation. Chiropractic colleges are highly selective, and the program is very rigorous. You can feel confident that any graduate of an accredited U.S. chiropractic college has solid medical knowledge and thorough training.

To find a chiropractor near you, contact:

> **American Chiropractic Association**
> 1701 Clarendon Boulevard
> Arlington, VA 22209
> Phone: (800) 986-INFO
> Fax: (703) 243-2593
> E-mail: info@amerchiro.org

To find a "straight" chiropractor near you, contact:

> **International Chiropractors Association**
> 1110 North Glebe Road, Suite 1000
> Arlington, VA 22201
> Phone: (800) 423-4690
> Fax: (703) 528-5023
> E-mail: chiro@erols.com

To find a chiropractor trained in applied kinesiology, contact:

> **International College of Applied Kinesiology**
> 6405 Metcalf Avenue, Suite 503
> Shawnee Mission, KS 66202-3929
> Phone: (913) 384-5336
> Fax: (913) 384-5112
> E-mail: info@icakusa.com

Chiropractors are usually called just that, but sometimes they're known as *doctors of chiropractic* (D.C.s) or *chiropractic physicians*.

M.D. versus D.C.

Daniel David Palmer, the founder of chiropractic, went to jail in 1912 for practicing medicine without a license. For decades after that, medical doctors and chiropractors were at war. According to the chiropractors, the M.D.s were trying to drive them out of business because chiropractic worked so well. The medical types said the chiropractors were quacks who claimed to cure cancer by spinal manipulation. Medical students were taught that chiropractic was worthless at best and could do harm. The American Medical Association banned medical doctors from cooperating with chiropractors.

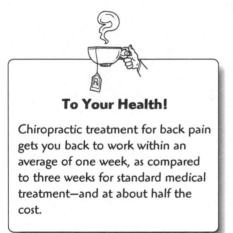

To Your Health!

Chiropractic treatment for back pain gets you back to work within an average of one week, as compared to three weeks for standard medical treatment—and at about half the cost.

The ban was the last straw. The chiropractors fought back on antitrust grounds. The case went all the way to the Supreme Court, and in 1990, the chiropractors won. The cooperation ban was lifted, and the AMA paid a substantial penalty. Most of that money is now being used to fund chiropractic research.

The Insurance Controversy

In almost all cases in almost all states, your health insurance will cover chiropractic treatment, especially if it's for a back injury. In fact, if you can't get to work because of back pain, your employer and insurance company may well encourage you to see a chiropractor.

In many but not all states, your health insurance will cover direct chiropractic treatment—in other words, you don't have to be referred to a chiropractor by your primary physician. Not all HMO plans in all states let you do that, though, so call first to make sure. In almost all cases, Medicaid and Medicare cover visits to the chiropractor.

Your insurance company may be less cooperative about chiropractic treatment for other problems, especially if frequent visits are needed. Unfortunately, sometimes dishonest patients and chiropractors alike have stretched the truth when it comes to disability cases and treatment for people who have been in car accidents. Insurance companies are always on the lookout for fraud. You may have to argue your case with your insurer.

A typical chiropractic treatment lasts about 20 minutes and costs anywhere from $50 to $150.

Rules, Rules, Rules

Chiropractors are licensed to practice in all 50 states and the District of Columbia. To be licensed in their state, they must be graduates of an accredited chiropractic college and then pass a stiff exam—in most states, it's the same exam medical doctors have to take. To maintain their licenses, chiropractors usually have to take continuing education courses to keep their knowledge up to date. If you have any questions about a chiropractor, contact your state medical licensing board.

Yes, But...

A lot of medical doctors have a lingering prejudice against chiropractors. Given all the evidence, most doctors reluctantly agree that chiropractors can often help lower-back pain better than they can. They don't agree with the concept of subluxations as the cause of disease, though, and most don't feel a chiropractor should treat you for anything other than back pain and perhaps minor muscle and joint pain. That's mostly because medical doctors don't think chiropractors have the training to diagnose or treat anything else. They worry that a chiropractor might misdiagnose a serious health problem or try to treat it with chiropractic methods. Either way, the doctors say, that could cause a dangerous delay in getting the right medical treatment. In fact, this happens very rarely—if your medical problem is outside the scope of a chiropractor's expertise, you'll be referred to a medical doctor.

The Least You Need to Know

➤ Chiropractic uses spinal manipulation along with nutritional advice, exercise, and sometimes supplements to treat health problems naturally, without drugs or surgery.

➤ Chiropractic is the most popular alternative therapy. More than 20 million people visit a chiropractor every year—and 90 percent of them are satisfied with their treatment.

➤ Numerous studies prove that chiropractic treatment for lower-back pain is the best choice in almost all cases.

➤ Other health problems, such as chronic tension headaches, sports injuries, whiplash, and ankle and knee sprains are usually helped by chiropractic treatment.

➤ Health problems involving chronic pain are often helped by chiropractic treatment.

➤ Chiropractors are licensed to practice in all 50 states and the District of Columbia. Health insurance almost always covers their services.

Chapter 22

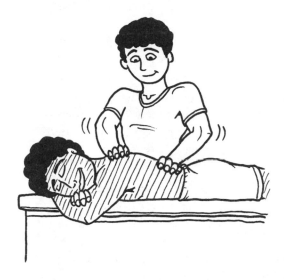

Massage: There's the Rub

> **In This Chapter**
>
> ➤ Relaxing with massage
>
> ➤ How massage can help some health conditions
>
> ➤ Basic massage techniques
>
> ➤ Finding professional help

At the end of a long day, your back aches, your shoulders and neck are tense, you feel all knotted up. Wouldn't a nice back rub feel good? And wouldn't a nice full-body massage feel even better? Actually, it would feel better than good, and not just for your tight muscles. As your body relaxes, so does your mind—massage reduces stress and helps you think more clearly and creatively. It works so well that today some major corporations now provide massage therapists to their workers. You can get a quick back rub right at your desk. And even if your company doesn't provide massage as a perk, today trained massage therapists are easy to find.

The Massage Marvel

Massage—the art of stroking, pressing, kneading, and otherwise manipulating the muscles under your skin—might be the oldest healing therapy of all. It's part of traditional medicine in just about every culture—in fact, there are probably about a hundred different types of massage therapy worldwide. The different approaches fall into five broad categories:

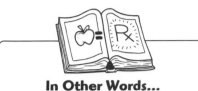

In Other Words...

Massage is the manipulation of your soft tissues (skin and muscles) in order to improve your circulation, help you relax, and relieve pain and soreness. Professional massage is done by a trained massage therapist, also known as a **masseuse**.

➤ **Traditional European massage.** The focus here is on relaxation and improved blood circulation through muscle massage.

➤ **Modern Western massage.** This is a general term for what is also known as deep-muscle or deep-tissue massage. The most common use is for sports massage (we'll discuss that a little further on in this chapter).

➤ **Structural massage and movement integration.** Also known as *bodywork*, these methods use deep-muscle massage and other approaches to correct movement imbalances and posture problems. We'll talk about these methods, such as Rolfing, in the next chapter.

➤ **Oriental methods.** We've already discussed these massage techniques in Chapter 11, "Acupressure and Shiatsu: Press On!"

➤ **Energetic methods.** These are approaches that are said to release blocked energy. We've already discussed reflexology, or foot massage, in Chapter 12, "Reflexology: Rubbing It In." We'll talk about other energy techniques, such as reiki and healing touch, in the next chapter.

In this chapter we'll talk about the traditional European approach and today's Western approach to massage. These are the techniques that focus on improved circulation and overall relaxation through muscle massage. The techniques are also used as therapy for specific health problems, especially those that involve joints and muscles or chronic pain.

Touch for Health

Medical researchers have been looking into massage therapy pretty carefully in recent years. They've discovered that massage doesn't just feel good. It can actually lower your heart rate, lower your blood pressure, improve your circulation, and even increase your production of natural painkillers.

Although therapeutic massage doesn't cure any health problems, it's often very useful for relieving symptoms, especially those related to stress. Massage helps insomnia, depression, and anxiety. It's also great for relieving chronic pain, especially from arthritis, old injuries, headaches, and a painful muscle condition called fibromyalgia. For some people, massage also helps digestive problems such as irritable bowel syndrome; people with asthma, respiratory allergies, and sinus problems also often get relief from massage. Some hospital-based cancer treatment centers have begun offering massage—it reduces the anxiety and stress that go along with a life-threatening illness and helps the patients cope better.

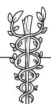

The Healing Arts

A major study in 1986 at the *Touch Research Institute* (TRI) at the University of Miami School of Medicine showed that premature babies who were regularly massaged gained more weight, were more active, and went home from the hospital an average of six days sooner than those who weren't massaged. Another TRI study showed that kids with asthma had fewer attacks if their parents gave them regular massages. And other TRI studies have shown that massage can help lower your blood pressure and relieve migraines.

By itself, massage doesn't increase your muscle strength, but it is helpful for stimulating weak or inactive muscles, especially if you can't move around much because you're sick or injured. If you've been in a cast for a broken arm, for example, massage can help you regain motion more quickly once the cast comes off. Massage can also help improve the range of motion in your joints, so it's helpful for elbow, shoulder, hip, and knee problems.

Massage is generally very safe for everyone, but you do sometimes need to be cautious. If you have some kinds of heart disease or cancer, or if you have an infectious disease, a skin problem such as severe psoriasis, or a circulatory system problem such as blood clots or phlebitis, talk to your doctor before you decide to have a massage.

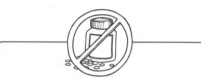

Hazardous to Your Health!

Do not have a massage if you have heart disease, circulatory problems, some kinds of cancer, an infectious illness, or some skin conditions. Do not use massage to treat serious injuries to joints, bones, or muscles—see your doctor or go to an emergency room as soon as possible.

Swedish Massage

Although the art of massage has been around for thousands of years in every culture, *Swedish massage* is the type you're most likely to find today—it's the basic method used in traditional European massage. An active massage system that uses long strokes, kneading, and a variety of rubbing, vibrating, and pressure techniques, Swedish massage works on the surface layers of your muscles.

The basic techniques of Swedish massage were first developed in the 1830s by a Swedish gymnast named Per Henrik Ling. He found that combining five kinds of movements in the massage gave the most effective results. The different basic

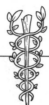

The Healing Arts

Massage is the third most popular alternative therapy in America. Consumers spend between $2 and $4 billion annually on some 75 million visits to massage therapists. The number of massage therapists has been growing rapidly to meet the demand. By some estimates, there are more than 150,000 trained massage therapists in the United States today. Many work in spas and health resorts, but massage isn't just an indulgence—a lot of massage therapists now work in medical offices alongside doctors, chiropractors, and physical therapists.

movements are often referred to by the French words Ling used to describe them or by their English equivalents (we have no idea why a Swede used French for his techniques). Here's a rundown of the basic strokes, in both languages:

➤ **Stroking (effleurage).** Long, firm, gliding strokes usually done with the whole hand or thumbs. The strokes trace the outer contours of your body.

➤ **Kneading (petrissage).** A wide variety of techniques comes under this category. In general, kneading means working on specific muscle groups by rhythmically lifting, rolling, kneading, or squeezing them.

➤ **Friction.** These circular strokes are used for the deeper muscles and for connective tissue such as tendons. Friction techniques often move against the grain of the muscles. Friction has to be used cautiously; it shouldn't be used on an area that's been recently injured.

➤ **Percussion (tapotement).** Also sometimes called *hacking*, percussion is the use of gentle, rhythmic, drumming motions. It's usually done on the back.

➤ **Vibration.** To do vibration, the massage therapist rapidly relaxes and contracts his or her own arm muscles, which transmits the vibrations to whatever part of your body is being touched. Vibration is a lot of work, which is why mechanical vibrators are often used instead. A gentler technique called *jostling* is often used on your arms and legs. The therapist gently shakes your muscles back and forth to relax them.

A trained massage therapist will usually start your massage with stroking, then move on to use kneading and friction on any areas that seem especially tense or sore. Percussion is used to relax the large back muscles. Vibration and jostling are used

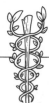

The Healing Arts

Swedish massage techniques date back to the 1830s, but they didn't get to America until the 1850s, when two doctor brothers, Charles and George Taylor, introduced them. By the 1870s, massage was common in the United States—you could even get a massage at your local YMCA. Massage faded in the early 20th century as drug-based medicine replaced older ideas. By the 1960s, sleazy "massage parlors" gave all massage a bad reputation. More recently, however, both doctors and patients have realized that massage and other touch therapies can be very helpful for both general relaxation and as part of medical treatment.

throughout the massage, especially on your arms and legs, whenever the therapist needs to relax your muscles.

As a general rule, massage strokes move inward toward the heart. So, if your arm is being massaged, the strokes will generally start at your hand and move toward your shoulder. Back strokes usually start at the shoulder and move downward. The therapist will use a small amount of oil, lotion, cream, or powder—only about a teaspoonful—to help his or her hands move smoothly on your skin.

Contemporary Western Massage

Sounds like you get a massage while watching a new Clint Eastwood movie, doesn't it? Actually, contemporary Western massage is the American twist to traditional European massage. It uses the same basic techniques as Swedish massage but adds a stronger relaxation element. *Trigger-point massage*, which uses deep massage to relax very specific muscles, was developed as part of this approach. Another important area of contemporary massage is for sports.

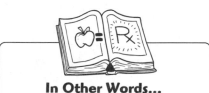

In Other Words...

Trigger-point massage uses strong finger pressure and deep massage to work on trigger points—muscle knots caused by stress, tension, or injury. The trigger points send pain to other parts of the body, so the goal of the massage is to break the pain cycle.

Sports Massage

A lot of athletes find that massage gives them a competitive edge. Sports massage falls into three categories:

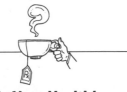

To Your Health!

Any light, nonallergenic oil or cream (jojoba oil, sweet almond oil, unscented cold cream) makes a good massage oil. To make your own, add 10 to 15 drops of your favorite aromatic oil to an ounce or so of unscented oil. If you prefer a lotion or cream, choose an unscented one and blend in just two or three drops of the aromatic oil per tablespoon.

➤ **Maintenance.** Many athletes claim that regular massages help them perform better and more consistently—and avoid injuries. It also helps them recover from heavy workouts faster, so they can train harder.

➤ **Event.** Massage before, during, and after an athletic event can help you warm up faster, perform better, and recover faster.

➤ **Rehabilitation.** Athletic injuries feel better and may heal faster if massage is part of the treatment.

Professional sports teams have had massage therapists on staff for years. Ordinary weekend warriors can get the benefits of sports massage as well—a lot of health clubs now have massage therapists on staff.

Massage for Everyone

Pretty much everyone can benefit from a massage. Mothers know this instinctively—that's why they cuddle, stroke, and rub their babies. When they do, the baby stops fussing or crying, but the importance of touch goes far beyond that—babies who aren't cuddled and touched don't grow and develop normally.

Pregnant women really benefit from massage, especially when it comes from a loving partner. Many of the minor discomforts of pregnancy, like fatigue, anxiety, and backaches, are soothed by massage. Massage is also helpful for general relaxation, especially during the difficult last few months of pregnancy and during and after the birth. It's so helpful, in fact, that massage techniques are taught in natural childbirth classes.

The elderly benefit from massage as well. Having a massage improves blood flow throughout the body, which makes you feel more energetic and positive and also improves your immunity. Massage can often help older adults with painful arthritis regain mobility and get around better.

Enjoying Your Massage

Having a massage should be a relaxing, enjoyable experience. Your massage therapist will work with you to help make sure it is. Here's what to expect:

➤ **Getting started.** If this is your first session, the massage therapist will ask you some questions about your general health, why you want a massage, and if there's any particular body areas that you want massaged—or that you want the therapist to avoid.

➤ **Clothing.** The massage therapist will leave the room as you take off as much of your clothing as you're comfortable with. You'll have a sheet or towel to drape yourself with during the massage. The massage therapist will uncover only the part of your body being massaged, so your modesty is protected.

➤ **The massage table.** You'll usually lie on a comfortable, padded massage table. For a seated massage, you'll sit in a specially designed massage chair that supports the front of your body.

➤ **Music.** Some people like to listen to relaxing music during a massage; some don't. Likewise, some people like to talk with the therapist and others don't. Tell your massage therapist which you prefer.

➤ **Massage oil.** If you're allergic to oil or lotion or have a preference about scented oils, tell your massage therapist. Powder can be used instead of oil.

➤ **Relax.** Breathe steadily and relax your muscles as much as possible. After a massage, you may feel so relaxed that you're a little dizzy or weak in the knees. Get off the massage table slowly and plan to take it easy for a bit.

Any massage is relaxing and enjoyable. The more regularly you get massaged, the more beneficial and long-lasting the relaxation effect is.

Finding a Qualified Practitioner

Finding a massage therapist you're comfortable with is pretty easy—there are anywhere between 120,00 and 160,000 massage therapists in the United States. Many massage therapists operate by word of mouth from satisfied customers. They also advertise in local papers and the Yellow Pages and put up signs in health-food stores and alternative medicine centers.

As we'll discuss a little further on, some states regulate massage therapists and some don't. If your state does regulate the practice, your massage therapist should meet all the requirements. Even if your state doesn't have any regs, at a minimum, your therapist should be a graduate of a training program accredited or approved by the Commission on Massage Therapy Accreditation. The national credential for massage therapists is the designation *Nationally Certified in Therapeutic Massage and Body* (NCTMB). These initials after a massage therapist's name mean that he or she has met a high standard of training and experience and regularly participates in continuing education programs in the field.

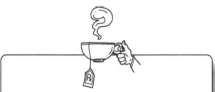

To Your Health!

There's no excuse for not finding a qualified practitioner to give you a massage. While many massage therapists are in private practice, others work at spas, health clubs, sports medicine clinics, or in chiropractors' offices. Some work in hospitals and nursing homes, and a lucky few work on cruise ships.

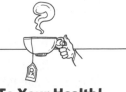

To Your Health!

Before you visit a new massage therapist, ask about his or her qualifications. Also ask for references by past clients—and check them out. Every therapist is different—you may have to try several before you find one you're comfortable with.

To check on whether a massage therapy training program is certified, or for a referral to a qualified massage therapist near you, contact:

> **American Massage Therapy Association (AMTA)**
> 820 David Street, Suite 100
> Evanston, IL 60201-4444
> Phone: (847) 864-0123
> Fax: (847) 864-1178
> E-mail: info@inet.amtamassage.org

Nearly 30,000 massage therapists belong to the American Massage Therapy Association. Members agree to follow a strict code of ethics.

Another good way to find a qualified massage therapist near you is through:

> **Associated Bodywork and Massage Professionals (ABMP)**
> 28677 Buffalo Park Road
> Evergreen, CO 80439-7347
> Phone: (800) 458-2267
> Fax: (303) 674-0859
> E-mail: expectmore@abmp.com

A typical massage session is an hour long. Costs vary, depending on your location, the type of massage, and the experience of your therapist. In general, fees start at around $45 an hour and go up to $100 or more. At-home massage usually costs a little more because of the therapist's travel time.

Becoming a Massage Therapist

As massage becomes more popular, people are turning to it as a profession. If you're interested in becoming a massage therapist, you can probably find a good training program near you—there are some 900 massage therapy schools in the United States. Check out the program carefully before you sign up. For the most thorough training, you want to attend a program that's been accredited or approved by the American Massage Therapy Association or Associated Bodywork and Massage Professionals. To get a current listing of programs, contact AMTA or ABMP.

Rules, Rules, Rules

As of 1998, 26 states and the District of Columbia regulate massage therapists in some way. The requirements vary from state to state, so what's called a *licensed massage therapist* in one state might be a *certified massage therapist* in another. Some local governments also regulate massage therapy—that's usually to keep sleazy sex-for-sale types from calling themselves "massage therapists."

States that regulate massage therapy usually require at least 500 hours of education. Therapists usually also have to pass a standardized entry-level test called the *National Certification Exam* (NCE). To find out if your state regulates massage therapists, call your state medical licensing board or contact the American Massage Therapy Association.

More and more health insurers and HMOs recognize the value of therapeutic massage and cover at least some of the cost, but only if it's provided by a qualified professional. Coverage still varies quite a bit, though, so check with your insurer to get the details. You're more likely to be covered if you live in a state that regulates massage therapists.

There's the Rub

The positive evidence for massage as an effective treatment to aid relaxation and healing is very strong, and there's not much evidence that's negative. As far as we can tell, the reason American doctors don't recommend massage a lot more often seems to be that they just don't think of it.

The Least You Need to Know

➤ Massage therapy helps improve blood circulation and relax tense or sore muscles. Today massage is the third most popular form of alternative therapy in the United States.

➤ The most common form of massage is the traditional European method known as Swedish massage.

➤ Massage helps overall relaxation and is also useful for treating sports injuries, muscle and joint problems, headaches, and chronic pain. It may also be helpful for other chronic ailments, such as digestive and sinus problems.

➤ Everyone—from babies to the elderly—can benefit from massage. Pregnant women find massage very helpful for relieving discomfort before, during, and after childbirth.

➤ Well-trained professional massage therapists are in private practice and also work in health clubs, medical offices, and many other settings.

Chapter 23

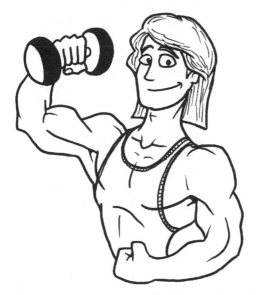

Bodywork: Straightening Yourself Out

In This Chapter

➤ The many types of bodywork—and which is right for you

➤ How bodywork can help with movement and posture problems

➤ Restoring your body's natural structure with bodywork

➤ Using bodywork to reduce stress and restore energy flow

Remember the way your mother was always telling you to stop slouching and stand up straight when you were a kid? Now that you're a grownup, you can admit it: You should have listened to her. Lucky for you, it's not too late to improve your posture; get rid of back, neck, and joint problems; and restore a youthful spring to your step. What you need is some bodywork—any one of the many techniques that help you get yourself moving smoothly again.

The Body of Knowledge

All forms of *bodywork* have one basic goal: to help your body move easily and naturally, the way it's meant to go. Different types of bodywork take different approaches to getting you there. We'll get into specifics a little further on in this chapter, but in general, bodywork falls into two main categories:

➤ **Movement methods.** Bodywork based on movement methods is designed to help you unlearn bad movement habits and learn good new ones. The techniques vary, but most involve some sort of hands-on manipulation of your muscles by an instructor.

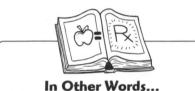

In Other Words...

Bodywork is a general term for any system of movement, touch, and sometimes deep massage designed to help you improve your body's structure and function.

➤ **Energetic methods.** These methods are designed to release blocked energy and restore its natural flow in your body. Some techniques are hands-on; others don't involve any touching.

A basic idea behind all bodywork is that your body's functions and your body's structure—your bones and muscles—can't be separated. Functional problems, such as stress, injury, or illness, affect your structure—and vice versa. Bodywork aims to restore healthy structure *and* function.

Does it? You bet. Bodywork can help you get a wider range of movement with greater ease, increase your flexibility, improve your coordination, and relieve stress-related physical problems. The question isn't really does bodywork help; it's which form of bodywork is best for you. Let's start by looking at the most popular forms.

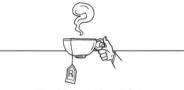

To Your Health!

Insurance coverage for bodywork varies quite a bit. If your health insurance covers massage, it will probably cover at least some forms of bodywork. You're more likely to be covered if the treatment is prescribed by your doctor or chiropractor. It also helps if the bodywork practitioner is licensed in some way in your state—as a massage therapist or physical therapist, for instance.

Rolfing: Meet Dr. Elbow

One of the oldest and best-known forms of bodywork is called *Rolfing® structural integration*, a form of deep-tissue massage that realigns and balances your body. The idea is to bring your head, shoulders, chest, pelvis, and legs into better vertical alignment. Rolfing is named for its developer, biophysicist Dr. Ida P. Rolf. From her studies of the human body, Dr. Rolf knew that your large muscles are actually made up of bundles of smaller muscles. A tough, thin layer of flexible connective tissue called *fascia* wraps around your muscles and forms the tendons that attach the ends of your muscles to your bones. The fascia is supposed to move easily and let your muscles slide past each other. Dr. Rolf realized that injuries, poor movement habits, and chronic muscle tension from stress make the fasciae get stuck—and stuck fasciae keep you from moving freely or even standing up straight. In the 1940s and 1950s, Dr. Rolf developed a system of deep massage that helps the fasciae get unstuck, restores free movement to the muscles, and breaks old patterns of muscle strain and misuse. The result is better body alignment and improved posture.

Rolfing, as the technique came to be called, can be an intense experience. The Rolfer uses his or her thumbs, knuckles, hands, and even elbows and knees as part of the deep massage—grateful patients called Ida Rolf "Dr. Elbow." There can be some discomfort as the fasciae are massaged and released. Rolfing usually involves 10 sessions—lasting

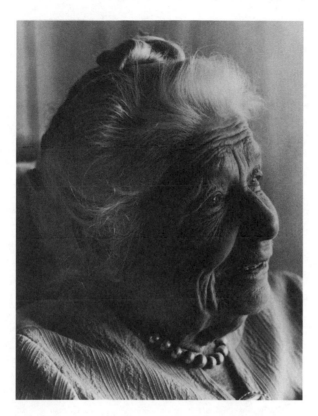

Ida Rolf, the great Dr. Elbow. Photo courtesy of The Rolf Institute.

one hour each—of massage and movement education spaced a week apart; the cost is about $75 to $90 a session.

The results of Rolfing can be amazing. It's particularly helpful for repetitive strain injuries, sports injuries, poor posture, and neck and shoulder pain. Rolfing also helps people with respiratory problems learn to relax their chest and back muscles, which helps them breathe more easily. Many athletes and performers have also found that Rolfing improves their breathing and flexibility.

Finding a Rolfer

The Rolf Institute was founded by Dr. Rolf in 1971 to train people as Rolfing practitioners. Today there are more than 900 certified Rolfers nationwide. For more information, or to find a certified Rolfer near you, contact:

Hazardous to Your Health!

Bodywork usually involves a combination of massage and movement. It's almost always safe and beneficial, but if you have heart disease, circulatory problems, some kinds of cancer, rheumatoid arthritis, an infectious illness, or some skin conditions, certain kinds of bodywork might not be right for you. If you'd like to try a bodywork technique, discuss it with your doctor and an instructor before you start.

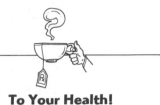

The Rolf Institute
205 Canyon Boulevard
Boulder, CO 80302
Phone: (800) 530-8875
Fax: (303) 449-8788
E-mail: RolfInst@rolf.org

Open-minded doctors see Rolfing as a helpful form of physical therapy or massage that's especially useful for cases of chronic neck, shoulder, and back pain. Rolfing is sometimes covered, at least in part, by health insurance. It's also now being offered by some employers as a way to prevent repetitive strain injuries.

Healing with Hellerwork

A former Rolfer named Joseph Heller (not the novelist by the same name) developed his own system of bodywork in the late 1970s. *Hellerwork*, as it's known, uses deep massage along with retraining in basic movements to help you learn stress-free ways to stand, walk, sit, bend, reach, and so on. Part of Hellerwork treatment is exploring the emotional issues that lead to physical symptoms. Hellerwork teaches you to move more fluidly and gracefully, which relieves discomfort from poor posture, back and neck problems, and the like. The movement retraining also helps you learn how to prevent problems and injuries in the future.

Hellerwork usually involves 11 sessions; each session spends about an hour on bodywork and half an hour on movement education. There aren't that many certified Hellerwork practitioners yet. To find one near you, contact:

> **Hellerwork International**
> 406 Berry Street
> Mount Shasta, CA 96067
> Phone: (800) 392-3900
> Fax: (530) 926-6839
> E-mail: hellerwork@hellerwork.com

Hellerwork sessions usually cost about $100 or more apiece. There hasn't been any real research on its effectiveness, and your insurance company probably won't pay for it.

The Trager® Approach

The Trager® Approach is a mind/body therapy that uses gentle touch and movements to help release deep-seated physical and mental patterns caused by injuries, poor posture, poor movement habits, stress, and emotional traumas. Dr. Milton Trager developed his healing techniques for decades, but it wasn't until 1977 that he brought his ideas to a wider audience and began training students.

Trager Approach sessions have two parts. In the first part, called *table work*, you strip down to your underwear and lie on a comfortable, padded table. The practitioner uses gentle, nonintrusive touching to move your body and limbs. By rocking, swinging, stretching, and pressing, the practitioner helps you realize that it's possible to move freely and gracefully. The practitioner works in a relaxed, meditative state known as *hookup*. Trager practitioners believe this helps them connect deeply with their patients and be sensitive to even slight changes.

The second part of a Trager Approach session teaches you a series of physical movements called *Mentastics® exercises*. The exercises help you re-create the feelings you had on the table and teach you to be aware of your movements.

For more information, and to find a certified Trager practitioner near you, contact:

> **The Trager Institute**
> 21 Locust Avenue
> Mill Valley, CA 94941-2806
> Phone: (415) 388-2688
> Fax: (415) 388-2710
> E-mail: Trageradmin@trager.com

A typical Trager session lasts about 90 minutes. There's no set number of treatments. The effects are cumulative, so the more sessions you have, the more you're helped. Your insurance plan may cover Trager if it's recommended by a doctor to treat a neuromuscular condition.

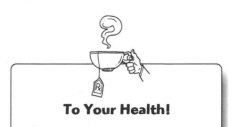

To Your Health!

The Trager® Approach is designed to help sports injuries, back and neck pain, and stress-related problems (tension headaches, chronic digestive upsets). A 1986 study showed that Trager can help patients with chronic lung disease breathe more easily. Although there aren't any good studies to back them up, many patients with neuromuscular disorders (multiple sclerosis, Parkinson's disease) have been greatly helped by the Trager Approach.

Acting Out with the Alexander Technique

Of all the bodywork methods, the Alexander Technique is the one that's most popular with performing artists of all kinds. The famed Juilliard School in New York City teaches this technique to its music and acting students, and actors such as Kevin Kline, Robin Williams, and Jeremy Irons have studied it. Why? Because the Alexander Technique helps actors, dancers, singers, and musicians relax and be more effective on stage. It reduces performance anxiety—the fancy way to say stage fright.

The Alexander Technique was developed more than a hundred years ago by an Australian actor named F. M. Alexander. Today it's a technique for people of all ages and

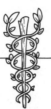

The Healing Arts

As a young man, Frederick Mathias Alexander (1869–1955) was a Shakespearian actor touring in Australia. He was a hit until he started having problems such as chronic hoarseness and losing his voice on stage. When no medical treatment helped, Alexander realized that his voice problems came from his own movements. By studying himself in a three-way mirror, he saw that he was tensing his chest, back, neck, and head muscles so much that his voice box was compressed. It took years, but when Alexander finally taught himself to relax and restored his body's natural posture, his full, rich voice came back.

abilities, because it teaches you how to reduce tension and strain on your muscles and joints; improves your range of motions; and improves your posture, balance, and coordination. It's especially helpful for people with arthritis and other joint problems and for stress-related ailments such as migraines, headaches, and back trouble.

The basic goal of the Alexander Technique is to correct the patterns of muscle misuse you've developed over your lifetime. Years of muscle tension from stress and from sitting and standing incorrectly make you overuse some muscles and underuse others—this throws your natural balance way off.

Patterns of misuse tend to start and show up in the way you hold your head and neck over your body. Tension in the neck and shoulders compresses your spine, which in turn affects how you stand, walk, sit, and even breathe.

To reduce the tension and restore your natural balance, follow the advice of F. M. Alexander: "Free the neck; let the neck go forward and upward; let the back lengthen and widen." Alexander Technique teachers help you become aware of your movements and your patterns of misuse. Through gentle touch and verbal guidance, they show you new ways to move without strain.

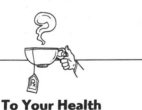

To Your Health

When you keep the Alexander Technique principles in mind as you move, they gradually become part of your normal activities. Your posture improves, you have fewer aches and pains, and you feel more relaxed and energetic.

Finding an Alexander Technique Teacher

The Alexander Technique is easy to learn, but it's hard to teach. Instructors need to have a very thorough understanding of human anatomy. They also need to be very perceptive so they can see the subtle imbalances in your movements and help you learn to correct them. To become a certified Alexander Technique teacher takes 1,600 hours of classroom training over a three-year period. To learn more, or to find a certified teacher, contact:

> **North American Society of Teachers of**
> **the Alexander Technique (NASTAT)**
> 3010 Hennepin Avenue South, Suite 10
> Minneapolis, MN 55408
> Phone: (800) 473-0620
> Fax: (612) 822-7224
> E-mail: NASTAT@ix.netcom.com

NASTAT was founded in 1987. Since then, more than 700 teachers have earned certification.

Certified teachers often offer introductory workshops and group classes through health clubs and continuing education programs. The best way to learn the Alexander Technique, though, is through a series of one-on-one lessons with a trained teacher. For the best results, you'll probably want to take 30 sessions. Each session is about 30 to 45 minutes long and costs anywhere from $40 to $80.

Because the Alexander Technique is so helpful for arthritis, chronic pain, neck, back, and hip problems, as well as repetitive strain injuries, your insurance company may cover some of the cost. You're more likely to be covered if your doctor or chiropractor refers you to a trained Alexander Technique teacher.

The Feldenkrais Method®

The amazing Dr. Moshe Feldenkrais (1904–84) had a fascinating career. Born in Russia, he was trained as a physicist and was also one of the first Europeans to earn a black belt in judo. After World War II, Dr. Feldenkrais settled in Israel, where he cured himself of crippling knee injuries by changing the way he moved. Dr. Feldenkrais became interested in applying his scientific and personal knowledge to the area of human movement. His approach combines gentle touch and movement training to help you increase your range and ease of motion and improve your flexibility and coordination.

The Feldenkrais Method is taught in two ways. In group classes, known as Awareness Through Movement®, a teacher verbally leads students through a sequence of movements, such as standing and sitting, that help you learn easier, more efficient ways to

307

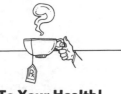

do these basic positions. In private lessons, called Functional Integration®, the teacher tailors the lesson to your individual needs. The lesson may include some gentle touching and manipulation.

To learn more about the Feldenkrais Method and to find a class or teacher near you, contact:

> **Feldenkrais Guild® of North America**
> P.O. Box 489
> Albany, OR 97321
> Phone: (800) 775-2118
> Fax: (541) 926-0572
> E-mail: feldngld@peak.org

Guild-certified practitioners have completed 800 to 1,000 hours of training over three to four years. Insurance companies usually don't pay for Feldenkrais Method classes.

Breaking Bad Patterns

Developed by Judith Aston, a former patient of Dr. Ida Rolf, Aston-Patterning combines movement training, massage, and exercises to help poor posture; back, neck, and shoulder pain; and chronic headaches. It's also helpful for finding the work habits that are causing the discomfort. For more information, contact:

> **The Aston Training Center**
> P.O. Box 3568
> Incline Village, NV 89450
> Phone: (702) 831-8228
> Fax: (702) 831-8955
> E-mail: astonpat@aol.com

Myotherapy: Muscling In

Also known as pain erasure, *myotherapy* focuses on relaxing muscles so tense they've gone into painful spasms. The therapist uses touch to find knots of tension—*trigger points*—in your muscles. Knotted muscles don't just hurt. They send pain throughout your body and distort your posture and movements, which in turn can affect your circulation, your nervous system, and your organs. Pressure on the trigger points relieves the pain and lets the muscles go back to their normal position.

The most popular form of bodywork myotherapy is Bonnie Prudden Myotherapy℠, which combines trigger-point therapy with individualized exercises to help you avoid a return of the pain. Bonnie Prudden, the developer of the technique, has been a fitness advocate for more than 40 years. She began developing her techniques of myotherapy in the 1970s and has been training practitioners since 1979. For more information, and to find a myotherapist near you, contact:

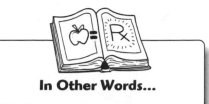

In Other Words...

Myotherapy is any treatment that affects your muscles—the prefix *myo-* is from the Greek word meaning "muscle." There are many types of myotherapy, including physical therapy, massage, and many kinds of bodywork.

> **Bonnie Prudden Myotherapy**
> 7800 East Speedway
> Tucson, AZ 85710
> Phone: (800) 221-4634
> E-mail: info@bonnieprudden.com

Bonnie Prudden myotherapists study for 1,400 hours over a one-year period to become certified. Your insurance probably won't cover this sort of myotherapy.

The Rosen Method

This method sees tension in your body as caused by stress or unexpressed emotions—and as founder Marion Rosen says, "Relaxation is the gateway to awareness." Instructors use gentle touch and discussion to help you become aware of body tension and learn how to release it. Movement exercises help the process along.

To find a trained Rosen Method practitioner near you, contact the Rosen Method Professional Association at (800) 893-2622.

Moving On

The various therapies we've just discussed all involve some sort of movement on your part; most also involve some sort of touch or manipulation from an instructor. There's another way to approach bodywork, though: through energy. In energetic approaches, you may do some moving, but the main goal is to find energy blockages in your system and release them to get your energy flowing smoothly again. The idea of energy flows and blockages is basic to many nonWestern treatments (check back to Chapter 6, "Traditional Chinese Medicine," Chapter 10, "Acupuncture: Getting Right to the Point," and Chapter 11, "Acupressure and Shiatsu: Press On!" for more on this). There are some Western techniques that use the same concept.

Therapeutic Touch

Therapeutic touch (TT) is a healing approach used mostly by many nurses in hospitals. TT practitioners are trained to sense the personal energy fields that are said to surround everyone. By holding their hands just above the body of a patient, they find and "sweep away" blockages in the energy field. In addition, the TT practitioner transfers energy to the patient. The aim of TT is to help the patient heal faster.

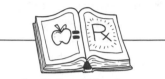

In Other Words...

Therapeutic touch (TT) seems to work by lowering the patient's anxiety level, which lets his or her natural healing process work better. TT is said to be particularly helpful for pain control and healing surgical wounds and burns.

TT was developed in the early 1970s by Dolores Krieger, Ph.D., R.N., a professor at New York University's nursing school. Some 100,000 people worldwide have been trained in the technique. A similar technique, called *healing touch* (HT) is also widely used, especially by nurses.

Therapeutic touch got a lot of attention in 1998, when a nine-year-old girl named Emily Rosa came up with an experiment that proved it didn't work. Her work was published in the prestigious *Journal of the American Medical Association.* Twenty-one trained TT practitioners were asked to place their hands, palms up, through a screen that kept them from seeing young Emily. She then held her hand over either their left or right hand and asked them to say which hand she was holding her hand over. The idea was that they would be able to sense the energy from Emily's hand. In fact, in over 280 tests, most couldn't—their results were actually no better than just guessing.

A 1998 study, however, showed TT helped relieve the pain of arthritic knee. Considering how contradictory the studies are, and how much some of Dr. Pressman's patients have been helped, we'd say give it a chance.

If you'd like to learn more about TT, contact:

Nurse Healers Professional Association
1211 Locust Street
Philadelphia, PA 19107
Phone: (215) 545-8079
Fax: (215) 545-8107

For more information about healing touch, contact:

American Holistic Nurses' Association (AHNA)
P.O. Box 2130
Flagstaff, AZ 86003-2130
Phone: (800) 278-AHNA
Fax: (520) 526-2752
E-mail: AHNA-Flag@flaglink.com

The Pluses and Minuses of Polarity Therapy

According to Dr. Randolph Stone (1890–1981), the founder of *polarity therapy*, "Energy is the vital force in the body." Dr. Stone believed that energy fields and currents exist everywhere in nature. Good health comes from good balance and flow of energy in your body; blocked energy leads to poor health. The idea behind polarity therapy is that your body has a human energy field with electromagnetic patterns. Your energy field has polarity—qualities of both attraction and repulsion—much like the Yin and Yang of traditional Chinese medicine. By stimulating and balancing your energy field, polarity therapy helps restore your health.

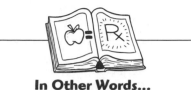

In Other Words...

Because the human energy field is affected by many things, including touch, diet, exercise, mental attitudes, and emotions, **polarity therapy** combines bodywork, diet, exercise, and counseling. You work with a polarity therapy practitioner to discover and deal with physical, mental, and emotional energy blocks.

Polarity therapy bodywork focuses on the craniosacral system—your skull, spine, and sacrum (the bottom part of your spine, found between your hip bones). Polarity practitioners detect the energy imbalances and use gentle touch to correct them. They also teach you simple self-help techniques for relaxing and balancing the flow of energy. You'll also learn easy polarity therapy exercises that help you relax and calm yourself. Polarity therapy also takes an energetic approach to diet, emphasizing fresh fruits and vegetables. Polarity practitioners recommend occasional internal cleansing using herbal drinks, including two special mixtures known as *liver flush* and *polarity tea*. The liver flush combines fruit juices, olive oil, garlic, and other ingredients to cleanse the liver, kidneys, and bowel. It's followed by an herbal tea made with a variety of ingredients, including anise, fennel seed, licorice, and mint.

For more information, and to find a *registered polarity practitioner* (RPP) near you, contact:

> **American Polarity Therapy Association (APTA)**
> 2888 Bluff Street, Suite 149
> Boulder, CO 80301
> Phone: (800) 359-5620
> Fax: (303) 545-2161
> E-mail: SATVAHQ@aol.com

To become an RPP, students have to complete at least 615 hours of training in an APTA-approved program. Many RPPs use polarity therapy as part of their practice as chiropractors or psychotherapists, and in other healthcare areas.

Reach Out to Reiki

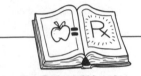

In Other Words...

Reiki (pronounced *ray-key*) is a Japanese word meaning "universal life energy." The *ki* part of reiki is the Japanese word for "energy"—it's very similar to the Chinese concept of Qi. Reiki is found in all things, living and nonliving.

Reiki is a form of energy therapy that has become extremely popular in the last few years. That's because it's easy for anybody to learn just by taking a short course. Once you've learned the basics, you can do reiki healing on yourself and on your family and friends. Even pets and ailing houseplants can benefit!

Reiki is a form of natural healing that uses patterns of touch to channel the energy of life through the hands of the healer to the person being treated. The healer senses where your energy is depleted and sends more energy to those areas of your body.

The basic concepts of reiki were first developed in the late 1800s by Dr. Mikao Usui, a Christian educator in Japan. In search of a way to heal both the body and the soul, Dr. Usui went on a 14-year quest through the world of Eastern philosophy and Tibetan Buddhism. He rediscovered lost Tibetan energy healing methods and brought them back to Japan.

Reiki is said to restore depleted energy and remove energy blockages. It's helpful for relieving stress, including headaches, insomnia, and digestive upsets, and for helping chronic pain. Reiki is not a religion, but it does have a spiritual side. People who have been trained in it say they have a heightened awareness and more emotional peace.

The Usui System of Reiki Healing, as it's formally known, is simple and relaxing. During the treatment, you lie, fully clothed, on a table or on the floor. The practitioner places his or her hands on or over different parts of your body and holds them there

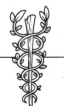

The Healing Arts

Reiki was carried on by a student of Dr. Mikao Usui. Dr. Chujiro Hayashi passed the concept on to a young Japanese-American woman named Hawayo Takata in the 1930s. Hawayo Takata lived and taught in Hawaii for many years. In the 1970s, she began teaching reiki to students across the country and around the world. She died in 1980, but reiki is carried on today by her granddaughter, Phyllis Lei Furumoto, and by the more than 200,000 people who have been initiated into it.

while channeling reiki into you. There are 12 positions altogether: four on your head, four on the front of your body, and four on your back. Channeling energy to all 12 points restores your energy balance.

During the first level of reiki training, you're taught the reiki hand positions for healing. You're also "attuned" or initiated by your teacher. Attuning isn't a healing ceremony—rather, it creates a healer by opening your energy channels and clearing away obstructions. Once you've been attuned, you've become a Reiki I practitioner. You can now access your energy channels to treat yourself. The next level, or Reiki II, involves further attuning and learning three reiki symbols that have powerful healing effects. Once you've become a Reiki II, you can do distance healing and help people who aren't even in the same room. To become a reiki master or teacher, you'll need further study to attain Reiki III attuning.

To learn more about reiki, and to find a practitioner or classes in your area, contact:

> **The Reiki Alliance**
> P.O. Box 41
> Cataldo, ID 83810
> Phone: (208) 682-3535
> Fax: (208) 682-4848
> E-mail: 74051.3471@compuserve.com

Inexpensive weekend courses to learn Reiki I are often given at alternative health centers and in continuing-education programs. Attaining the higher levels takes longer.

Bodywork versus Physical Therapy

Most medical doctors agree that some kinds of bodywork, like the Alexander Technique or Rolfing, can be helpful for people with chronic movement problems. In fact, they will sometimes recommend this sort of bodywork, especially if you have back, neck, or joint problems or painful arthritis. In most cases, though, doctors prefer to recommend standard physical therapy, which is effective, is given by trained therapists, and is almost always covered by your insurance. Doctors are a lot more skeptical about energy therapies such as Therapeutic Touch and reiki. That's not surprising, because there's very little objective evidence to show these treatments work.

The Least You Need to Know

➤ Bodywork uses touch and movement to help your body move more easily and naturally. There are many bodywork techniques.

➤ Bodywork is often very helpful for increasing your range of movement, relieving joint and back problems, and helping chronic pain.

➤ By teaching you better ways to move, bodywork techniques help you stay healthy and avoid injury.

➤ Some bodywork techniques are well-accepted by the medical world as useful therapies. Your health insurance may cover part of the costs for some treatments.

➤ Energy approaches to bodywork remove blockages in your energy flow and restore your natural energy balance.

Part 7
Making Sense of It All

Come to your senses with the information in this section! In the chapter on aroma-therapy, we explain how your nose knows—the scent of essential oils can be very relaxing and soothing to jangled emotions. In the chapter on light therapy, we discuss a very specific medical use: It helps people with seasonal affective disorder (SAD) get over winter depression. We also sing the praises of music therapy in this section.

You may be a little surprised to find a chapter on hydrotherapy in this section. Actually, we are too. We put hydrotherapy, or water treatment, here mostly because it involves your sense of touch—but also because we didn't know where else this important therapy should go.

Chapter 24

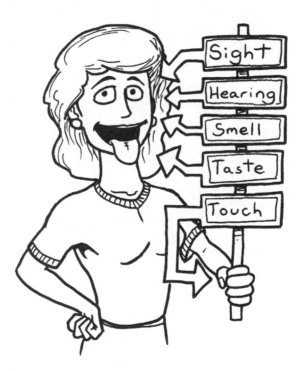

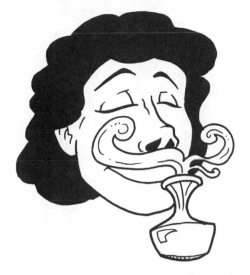

Aromatherapy:
The Nose Knows

In This Chapter

➤ Basic principles of aromatherapy

➤ Essential information about essential oils

➤ Enjoying aromatherapy safely

➤ How aromatherapy helps relieve pain, helps skin problems, and helps you relax

When patients come to Dr. Pressman's office, they often ask, "What smells so good?" It's the gentle, flowery smell of lavender. Dr. Pressman doesn't make his office smell of lavender just to be nice (although he's a very nice guy). He has an ulterior motive: The smell of lavender makes people calm down and relax. And as a very experienced health practitioner, he knows that relaxed patients benefit more from their treatments.

Making Scents of Aromatherapy

Aromatherapy uses *essential oils* made from plants to help treat or relieve the symptoms of many different physical and mental problems. The basic concepts of aromatherapy can be traced back to the ancient Egyptians thousands of years ago. In the centuries since then, various aromatic oils were often used for medicines, perfumes, and cosmetics. By the early 1900s, though, their medicinal use had really dropped off as synthetic drugs took over. In the 1930s, however, aromatherapy returned, this time as a serious science. What happened to bring aromatherapy back? In 1910, a French chemist named Réné-Maurice Gattefossé burned his hand badly. He put lavender oil on the burn and was surprised at how quickly it healed and how little scarring it left. Gattefossé went on to study the medicinal uses of other plant oils. He published his work in 1936 and laid the foundation of modern aromatherapy—he even invented the word. In the 1960s, a French doctor named Jean Valnet began using essential oils to treat medical problems such as burns and diabetes. His work was so successful that today many French doctors and hospitals regularly use essential oils as part of their treatments.

Aromas and Emotions

At the most basic level, aromatherapy seems to work by affecting your sense of smell. You've probably had this experience: A faint whiff of an aroma awakens an incredibly vivid memory or brings out a strong emotion. It might be the scent of lilacs in bloom, for instance, that reminds you of childhood days at your grandmother's house. Or maybe it's the smell of chamomile tea—that's the one, along with the taste of madeleine cookies, that got Marcel Proust started on his monumental seven-volume novel, *Remembrance of Things Past*, back in 1913.

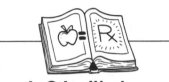

In Other Words...

Aromatherapy is the use of pleasant-smelling **essential oils** to treat physical and emotional problems. Essential oils are natural chemicals extracted from plants by distillation. The term is a little misleading, because essential oils aren't greasy or oily. In fact, they feel very much like water and evaporate very quickly.

Whatever the smell, the reason you get such a powerful response is that the smell receptors in your nose are connected directly to your *limbic system*—the part of your brain that controls your emotions. And the limbic system is directly connected to the parts of your brain that control, among other things, your memory. There's some scientific evidence that pleasant smells have a direct effect on your brain activity.

Some aromatherapy practitioners believe that the molecules of the essential oils, which are extremely small, are quickly absorbed into your system through your skin. When the essential oils are used for massage, applied directly to an irritated area of your skin, or inhaled, the active ingredients enter your bloodstream and can have useful effects, such as stimulating your immune system. Aromatherapists often claim that a particular essential oil is a "nerve tonic" or helps "detoxify" the body. We're not too sure about that sort of thinking—there's no real evidence for those claims. On the other hand, some essential oils, including tea-tree oil and eucalyptus, are indeed antiseptics that can prevent or reduce infection.

Aromatherapy can be very helpful for a number of different conditions, including these:

➤ Stress-related problems such as insomnia, depression, anxiety, or tension headaches

➤ Skin problems such as acne, psoriasis, eczema, and insect stings

318

➤ Mild digestive upsets

➤ Chest and nasal congestion from a cough, cold, or bronchitis

➤ Cystitis and yeast infections

Some aromatherapy fans say the essential oils can influence your mental state. Peppermint and rosemary, for example, are said to be stimulating, while lavender is said to have a sedative effect.

Your Essential Home-Remedy Kit

All told, about three hundred different essential oils are in common use today. You'll find them in cosmetics, perfumes, foods, drinks, and even standard medicines. For practical purposes, though, you need only these 10 for a useful home-remedy kit:

➤ **Chamomile.** Used for tension headaches, digestive upsets, skin problems, and sore joints and muscles. It's very mild, so it's especially good for children.

➤ **Clove.** A whiff of clove oil may send your memory back to the dentist's office. If you've just had a root canal, that might not be a memory you want to keep, but don't hold that against clove oil—it's a valuable antiseptic and can be a good emergency treatment for a toothache.

➤ **Eucalyptus.** This one goes back to the 1780s, when two doctors in Australia distilled it from leaves of the eucalyptus tree. It's used mostly for coughs and colds. It also makes a good natural insect repellent.

➤ **Geranium.** The pleasant, lemony smell of geranium oil makes it a pleasant treatment for skin problems. It also makes a nice addition to massage oils.

➤ **Lavender.** Used for stress-related problems, headaches, burns, insect stings, skin conditions, and more. The most useful and important home remedy of all the essential oils.

➤ **Lemon.** The lovely aroma of lemon is soothing in itself and blends very nicely with almost any other oil. It's also good as an appetite stimulant. Lemon oil helps skin problems.

➤ **Peppermint.** Used for digestive upsets and respiratory problems.

➤ **Rosemary.** Used for digestive upsets, chest and nasal congestion, sore joints and muscles, and headaches.

➤ **Tea tree.** Antiseptic and antifungal, it's useful for skin problems, athlete's foot, burns, insect stings, cold sores, cystitis, yeast infections, and respiratory problems.

➤ **Thyme.** Thyme is helpful for minor skin infections, cuts, and the like. Use it cautiously in very small amounts.

Lavender and tea tree are so useful that we need to look at them more closely.

Lavender

Lavender is the one essential oil that's really essential for the home first-aid kit. It's made from the flowering tops of the lavender plant (*Lavandula angustifolia* or *L. officinalis*) using steam distillation. The oil has a light-yellow color and a sweet, flowery scent. The aroma of lavender is great for relieving stress—something about its delicate floral smell really calms you down. Try putting a few drops on a hanky and breathing in the smell for a few minutes the next time you have one of those annoying tension head-aches.

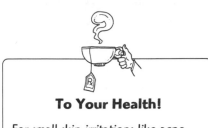

To Your Health!

For small skin irritations like acne, eczema, insect stings, and burns, dab on lavender oil with a cotton swab. It's also excellent for mosquito bites.

For skin irritations that cover bigger areas, like sunburn, use a massage oil with lavender added. Use a lavender massage oil for sore joints and aching muscles, or make a hot compress from a washcloth soaked in warm water with a few drops of lavender. Steam inhalations using lavender are helpful for colds, bronchitis, flu, laryngitis, and sore throats.

Tea Tree

Tea-tree oil is steam distilled from the leaves and twigs of an Australian plant called, not surprisingly, the tea tree (*Melaleuca alternifolia*). Aborigines in Australia used tea-tree leaves and sap as a medicine. Modern research shows that the oil has strong antiseptic and antifungal properties. Tea-tree oil is a light yellow-green color with a spicy, slightly pungent smell that takes a little getting used to. It's very helpful for skin irritations like acne blemishes and insect bites; it's also good for clearing up fungus infections like ringworm and athlete's foot. Some people find that tea-tree oil helps relieve the pain and itching of cold sores and herpes blisters; it also helps them heal faster. In massage oils or compresses, tea tree is good for soothing aching joints and muscles. It also

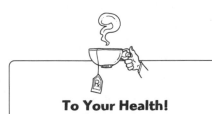

To Your Health!

Many women find that a sitz bath using warm water with a dozen or so drops of tea-tree oil added helps relieve the uncomfortable symptoms of cystitis and yeast infections. Re-peat several times a day.

makes a good inhalation for colds, flu, bronchitis, and sore throats. Tea-tree oil also is helpful for relieving the symptoms of cystitis and yeast infections.

Using Essential Oils

It's easy to enjoy the pleasant aroma of an essential oil. To scent a room, put a few drops on a *scent ring*—a plastic or metal ring designed to sit on top of a light bulb. The heat from the bulb releases the scent. For a longer-lasting effect, use an electric diffuser. For a relaxing scented soak, just add a few drops to your bath water. Try adding a few drops of an essential oil to the water in a room vaporizer or humidifier—some designs have little "medicine cups" that are perfect for holding the oil.

To use essential oils in massage, you'll need to mix them into a *carrier oil*. Carrier oils are light, bland vegetable oils such as sweet almond oil, apricot kernel oil, fractionated coconut oil, jojoba oil, or grapeseed oil. They're used as a base for the volatile and aromatic essential oils, especially for massage oils and skin preparations.

The usual dilution is 10 to 15 drops of essential oil to an ounce of carrier oil. (Check back to Chapter 22, "Massage: There's the Rub," for more information.) You can make an ointment by adding two or three drops of an essential oil to a tablespoon of any nonallergenic cream base, like cold cream. (We like calendula cream, which you can get in any health-food store.)

For skin problems or to soothe aching muscles, essential oils can be used *topically* (directly on the skin), either *neat* (undiluted) or mixed with a carrier oil. The essential oil should almost always be diluted in a carrier oil. The exceptions are tea-tree oil, which is often most helpful when applied neat, and lavender oil when used to treat burns. Play it safe when you use an essential oil on your skin. Do a patch test first to make sure you're not allergic.

To do a patch test, use a cotton swab to rub a drop or two of the essential oil on the inside of your forearm. Cover it with a band-aid and leave it on for 24 hours. If the area gets red, irritated, or itchy, you're allergic to that essential oil—don't use it. The oils most likely to cause skin irritation are chamomile, cinnamon, and clove. Some people are sensitive to oregano, but anyone could be sensitive to any oil. Be cautious and use common sense.

For respiratory problems, essential oils such as eucalyptus work well in inhalations. Add a few drops of the oil to a bowl of steaming hot water. Close your eyes, lean over the bowl, and drape a towel over your head. Breathe deeply for about 10 minutes.

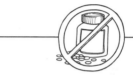

Hazardous to Your Health!

Never put essential oils directly onto a hot light bulb—the bulb might explode! We suggest that you avoid aroma lamps. These devices, while attractive, use a candle flame to heat the oils and consequently are a potential fire hazard.

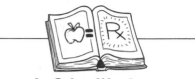

In Other Words...

In aromatherapy, **topical** doesn't mean current events—it means applied directly to the skin. And **neat** doesn't mean tidy—it means undiluted.

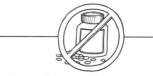

Hazardous to Your Health!

Never swallow any essential oil or use it internally! Keep essential oils away from your eyes. Stop using an essential oil immediately if you develop any sort of reaction to it. And remember, essential oils are volatile, which means they burn easily. Keep them away from open flames, such as candles.

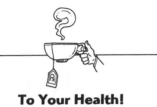

To Your Health!

During the cold and flu season, you may be able to fend off illness by gargling every day with tea-tree oil. Put a couple of drops into a glass of warm water and gargle; stir well after each mouthful. Don't swallow it!

Steam inhalations are helpful and very relaxing when you have a cold or stuffy nose, but they aren't always convenient. Try putting a few drops of an essential oil on a tissue or handkerchief. Hold it to your nose and breathe deeply. Don't sniff directly from the oil container—you'll get a big snootful of scent that could irritate the delicate mucous membranes of your nose.

Peppermint, chamomile, or rosemary often helps digestive problems such as nausea, gas, or heartburn. But because you really shouldn't swallow essential oils, put just one drop of the oil into a cup of hot water and sip it slowly. Alternatively, make an herbal tea, as explained in Chapter 15, "Traditional Herbal Medicine."

Essential oils are really valuable for people who have trouble sleeping. There's nothing like a warm bath scented with a few drops of chamomile, lavender, or lemon to get you ready for a good night's sleep.

In 1998 researchers discovered that, at least in the test tube, several different essential oils destroy the nasty *Streptococcus pneumoniae* germ that causes pneumonia, peritonitis, meningitis, and other serious illnesses. The most effective oils were oregano, thyme, and rosewood; cinnamon and clove also worked, but not as well.

Uses for Essential Oils

Problem	Suggested Essential Oil
Acne	tea tree
Anxiety	chamomile, lavender
Bronchitis	eucalyptus, lavender, rosemary
Burns	lavender, tea tree
Colds	eucalyptus, lavender, peppermint, rosemary
Coughs	eucalyptus, rosemary
Fungal infections	tea tree
Headache	chamomile, eucalyptus, lavender, peppermint, rosemary
Insect bites	tea tree, lavender
Insomnia	chamomile, lavender, lemon
Menstrual discomfort	chamomile
Muscle and joint pain	chamomile, rosemary
Nausea, indigestion	chamomile, peppermint, rosemary
Skin irritation	chamomile, geranium, lavender, lemon, thyme
Toothache	clove

The Scentual Woman

We're grownups, so let's be honest—scent is sexy. If you've bought a popular perfume recently, you know that's why the manufacturers can charge such a high price for just one measly ounce of the stuff. You don't have to spend a lot of money to smell nice, though. You can easily use a few tiny drops of essential oil on your wrists or behind your ears instead. Popular choices are jasmine, lavender, neroli, patchouli, rose, sandalwood, or ylang ylang. You can also mix oils to create your own perfume. For best results, combine only three or at most four essential oils. Perfumers often describe a good mix in terms of sound, saying that a perfume should have top, middle, and base notes. The top note should come from a light, fresh scent, such as lemon or bergamot. The middle note should come from a floral scent, such as rose or geranium. The base note should be a deeper, more complex scent, such as patchouli or sandalwood.

To make your own blends, add a few drops of each scent, starting with the base note, to an odorless carrier oil such as jojoba or fractionated coconut oil. Experiment until you find a mixture you like.

Tip to you guys: Ignore everything you just read. Give the woman in your life expensive perfume.

Tip to you gals: According to Gattefossé and other French researchers, these essential oils are aphrodisiacs—cinnamon, clove, myrtle, rose, sage, and ylang ylang. How do they know? They don't say.

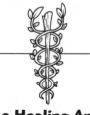

The Healing Arts

The complicated formulas for commercial perfumes are deep, dark secrets, literally locked away in vaults and known only to a select few. "Noses" (as expert perfumers are called) guess that the popular perfume Opium contains bay, benzoin, carnation, cinnamon, frankincense, jasmine, orange, orris root, patchouli, pimento berry, rose, and ylang ylang, along with some other mysterious ingredients. The proportions of these is the deepest, darkest secret of all.

Buying Essential Oils

It might seem outrageous to shell out anywhere from $5 to $15 for a tiny little bottle of an essential oil, but remember, the stuff is very concentrated. You only need a drop of lavender oil to relieve the pain and itching from a bee sting, for example, so a 5 milliliter (about an ounce) bottle could last for months.

Essential oils vary in quality and purity. Unfortunately, price isn't really a guide here. Read the label carefully—it should say the product is an essential oil. If the label says anything else, like "pure botanical oil," skip it.

Some manufacturers of essential oils are on the slippery side. It's easy to substitute lower-quality ingredients in essential oils. The high-priced essential oil German chamomile, for example, is a beautiful deep-blue color—one that's easy to fake with inferior ingredients. To be sure you get what you pay for, buy your essential oils from a well-stocked store that carries reputable brands.

Your oils will come in small, dark-tinted bottles to keep light from affecting them. Store the oils in a cool, dark place and be sure to keep them tightly sealed. If you want to mix your own massage oils or creams, combine the essential oil and the carrier oil or cream base just before you're ready to use them.

Sniffing Out Help

You're on your own when it comes to aromatherapy. Even though American consumers in 1995 spent some $59 million on aromatherapy products sold through health-food stores, it's not recognized as a treatment in the United States, and there's no licensing or certification requirement for aromatherapists. There are some associations, like the American Aromatherapy Association, that offer short courses and a certification program, but they're not exactly rigorous. Anyone can hang out a shingle, with or without taking any courses at all, and take your money for aromatherapy advice. Fortunately, aromatherapy for minor ailments is simple and safe, as long as you use common sense. If you want to use aromatherapy for a serious health problem, discuss it with your doctor before you try it.

Do I Smell a Rat?

Even though aromatherapy is widely used in France by doctors and in hospitals, a lot of American doctors think it stinks, at least as a medical treatment. They point out that there's almost no scientific research to prove that aromatherapy really works on serious illnesses, and they worry about the safety of using essential oils internally. Most doctors wouldn't object to using essential oils in the ways we've discussed here—as inhalations or for minor skin irritations, say—but they would point out that there are plenty of over-the-counter preparations that work just as well and cost less.

The Least You Need to Know

➤ Aromatherapy is based on the use of fragrant essential oils made from plants.

➤ The aromas of the essential oils are said to affect your mental state; some aromas are soothing, calming, or relaxing, while others are stimulating or refreshing.

➤ Aromatherapy is helpful for relieving stress-related problems such as anxiety, insomnia, and tension headaches.

➤ Essential oils are helpful for treating minor health problems such as digestive upsets, skin irritations, insect stings, muscle aches, sore joints, and respiratory problems.

Chapter 25

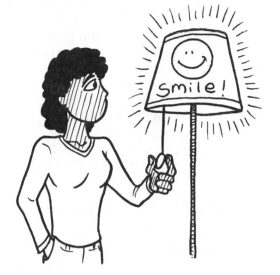

Light Therapy: Light Up Your Life

In This Chapter

➤ How light affects your body rhythms

➤ Treating winter depression with light

➤ How light can reset your body's internal clock

➤ Helping jet lag and sleeping problems with light

➤ Skin problems that light can help

Those short, dark, winter days can really get to you. After weeks of getting up in the dark, working indoors all day, and coming home in the dark, you find yourself eating more, sleeping more, and feeling depressed. You know that a little sunshine, preferably the kind you find on a gorgeous beach in Hawaii, always makes you feel better in the winter, so you arrange a vacation. But what happens when you get to Waikiki after a long flight? Jet lag. Crossing all those time zones has scrambled your sleep patterns. You *need* that sunshine, but you're in no shape to enjoy it. What's going on here?

Your Internal Clock

What's happening is that your internal clock is out of sync with your surroundings. Most living things—even fruit flies—have an internal clock that keeps them on a 24-hour cycle of waking and sleeping. Your *circadian rhythm*, as these cyclic ups and downs are called, is controlled by a complex set of biological timers. The timers are synchronized to the pattern of light and dark—when it gets light, you start to wake up; when it gets dark, you start to get sleepy.

But what if you start doing the night shift and have to sleep during the day? Or quickly pass through a number of different time zones and end up with *jet lag*? That can knock your internal clock completely out of sync. You don't sleep well, your digestion gets out of whack, and you tend to be really cranky. That's bad enough, but if you're a shift worker, it could be downright dangerous. Most industrial accidents happen on the night shift, when workers are fighting their natural instinct to sleep.

More Than Meets the Eye

How does your body know what time it is? From clues in the environment around you, especially light. You see light with your eyes, so it makes sense to think that you have something in your eyes that connects to your brain's sense of time. In fact, researchers have found a couple different light-sensitive substances in your eyes that probably have a lot to do with keeping your circadian rhythms running smoothly.

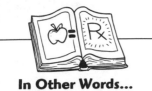

In Other Words...

Your **circadian rhythm** is your natural cycle of sleeping and wakefulness. Your body naturally wants to be awake and active during the daylight hours and asleep during the night-time hours. The word comes from the Latin word *circa*, meaning "about," and *dies*, meaning "a day." **Jet lag** is the fatigue and insomnia you get from traveling rapidly through several time zones.

The eyes don't have it all, though. In 1998, researchers found that shining a light on the back of your knees, where you can't see it, could have an effect on your internal clock. The researchers still aren't sure why, but they think it's because you also have something in your blood that responds to light and carries a message to your brain. And as you'll see a little further on in this chapter, that raises some interesting possibilities.

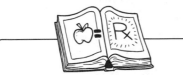

In Other Words...

SAD, or **seasonal affective disorder**, is a type of depression that affects people in the winter when the days are short and dark. SAD people sleep a lot, tend to overeat (especially sugary and starchy foods), have trouble concentrating, and can be very irritable. The symptoms of SAD generally go away when the longer, sunnier days of spring begin.

Making SAD People Happy

In the winter, when the days are short, cold, and often cloudy, you don't get much sunshine. Most of us just grumble a little about how crummy it is outside, but for some people, the sunshine shortage is a real problem. When they don't get enough rays, they start to sleep more, eat more, feel really down and irritable, and have trouble concentrating on their work. What they have is *SAD—seasonal affective disorder*. SAD affects about 6 percent of the American population, or about 11 million people every year. The symptoms usually start showing up in November, as the days get shorter, and peak in the short, dark days of December and January. Most SAD people are between the ages of 20 and 40; for some reason, women are four times as likely to get SAD as men. Another 25 million people (about 14 percent of the population) get a milder form of SAD known as *winter blues*. The big difference between SAD or winter blues and clinical depression is the regular seasonal pattern. If you get depressed in the winter and feel better the rest of the year, SAD could be the problem.

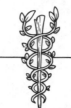

The Healing Arts

Over one million kids may have SAD. In fact, a recent study suggests that at least 3 percent of all American school kids get depressed and tired when the days are short. That makes their schoolwork uneven, to the point that some are diagnosed as having learning disabilities. They also get other symptoms of SAD, including irritability, headaches, appetite loss, carbohydrate cravings, and sleep changes. These kids get better fast when they start getting light therapy.

Scientists aren't really sure why some people get SAD in the winter. Some think SAD happens because your internal clock goes a little haywire when you have to force yourself to get up and get going in the morning while it's still dark. Your body clock tells you that if it's dark, you should be asleep, but your alarm clock tells you that if you don't get up, you're going to be late to work. If your body clock wins out over your alarm clock, you have SAD.

Whatever the reason for SAD, there's a pretty good way to help the problem: *light therapy*. When people with SAD spend at least 30 minutes a day or longer in front of special bright lights that imitate sunlight, they usually start to feel a lot better. The treatment seems to work best if they do it first thing in the morning.

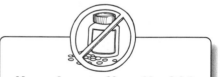

Hazardous to Your Health!

Do not use light therapy if you have eye disease. Talk to your doctor before you buy and use a light therapy lamp.

The secret is in the light. The bulbs or fluorescent tubes inside give off light that's about 20 times as bright as the light in an ordinary room, or about as bright as the sky half an hour after sunrise. What's missing from the light are the *ultraviolet* (UV) rays that could cause skin cancer or cataracts. You can read, work, sew, even watch TV while sitting in front of the light. Most people use a large, boxy lamp with a screen to diffuse the light, but you can also get regular table lamps that can take the special bulbs. Some people even wear visors that aim the light into their eyes.

Full-spectrum light visors to treat SAD are easy to wear and really work. Light visor photo courtsey of Bio-Brite, Inc., (800) 621-LITE.

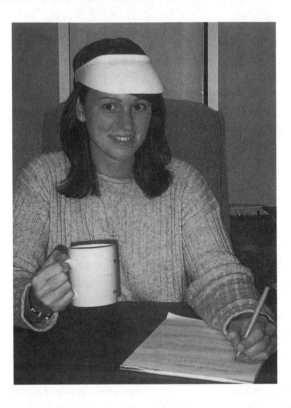

Getting more light by sitting or working in front of a full-spectrum light box is an effective way to treat SAD. Photo courtesy of Hughes Lighting Technologies, (800) 544-4825.

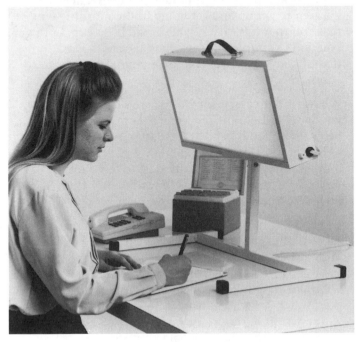

Wake Up and Smell the Melatonin

Light therapy alone works for about 80 percent of all SAD patients. The ones who don't respond to light therapy are often helped by prescription antidepressant drugs such as Prozac®. But recent research suggests that SAD people could skip the drugs and take supplements of the hormone *melatonin* instead. That's because your body produces melatonin only at night and uses the hormone to set your internal clock. By taking small amounts of melatonin supplements in the afternoon, instead of waiting until dark for your body to start producing it naturally, you can reset your internal clock and get back to a more normal schedule. The amount of melatonin you need to make this work is very small. In early studies, patients had good results from tiny doses.

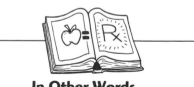

In Other Words...

You make the hormone **melatonin** only at night as part of your normal circadian rhythm. Melatonin controls a lot of your body's normal cycles, but it's especially important for your sleep/wake cycle. When the sun comes up in the morning, you stop making melatonin and wake up.

If you want to try melatonin for SAD, follow these steps:

1. First, be sure your problem really is SAD and not a physical illness or serious depression. Discuss taking melatonin with your doctor before you try it.

2. Take 0.1 mg of melatonin eight hours after your usual wakeup time. If you get up at 7 a.m., for example, take the melatonin at 3 p.m.

3. Take another 0.1 mg of melatonin two hours after that (at 5 p.m. if you got up at 7 a.m.).

4. Take another 0.1 mg of melatonin two hours after the second dose (at 7 p.m. if you got up at 7 a.m.).

5. Get up the next morning at your usual time and continue with the melatonin schedule. Stay on it for a week. By then you should find it much easier to get up in the morning.

The melatonin may make you very sleepy. If that happens, cut back on the number of doses. Skip the third and even the second dose if you need to.

You can buy melatonin supplements at any drugstore or health-food store. The smallest tablets are usually 0.3 mg, so you'll have to cut the tablet into thirds.

Don't Be SAD

If you're SAD in the winter, you're not alone. For information about where to buy lights and to find a support group near you, contact these organizations:

National Organization for Seasonal Affective Disorder (NOSAD)
P.O. Box 40133
Washington, DC 20016

Seasonal Studies Program
National Institute of Mental Health
Building 10, Room 4S-239
9000 Rockville Pike
Bethesda, MD 20892
Phone: (301) 496-2141 or (301) 496-0500

There Is a Time...

Jet lag from moving rapidly through several time zones is a guaranteed way to mess up your sleep for a couple of days. So is shift work, especially if you regularly rotate between day and night shifts. Researchers have found that light therapy can help you get over the jet lag or adjust to your new shift schedule faster and with less lost sleep. The timing is a little tricky, though, and so far this isn't a do-it-yourself technique. That's because how much time you spend under the light and when depends on your body temperature and the levels of some specific hormones in your blood. These normally move up and down over the course of your normal 24-hour cycle, so by measuring them, researchers know when to turn on the light and reset your body clock.

Right now, you'd probably have to go to a hospital-based sleep lab to have your internal clock tuned up. In the future, though, you might be able to do it at home while you sleep. As we've mentioned, researchers found that shining a light on the back of your knee works just as well on your internal clock as shining the light into your eyes and it looks like you have light receptors not just in your eyes but in your blood. It's possible that some day jet-lagged travelers will wrap a fiber-optic blanket around a leg, go to sleep, and wake up with their body clock reset to their new time zone.

Melatonin to the Rescue

Until light therapy for jet lag becomes something anyone can do, time-warped travelers can try melatonin to speed up the process of resetting their internal clocks. Melatonin is also helpful for shift workers adjusting to their new schedules. The usual dose is 3 mg the first night you're at your destination or trying to get to sleep after a shift change. Take it about two hours before you'd like to get to sleep—and don't plan to do anything else after you take it, because the melatonin will make you very sleepy. Keep using the melatonin for the next few days if you have trouble getting to sleep, but don't take it for more than five days. If you haven't adjusted by then, more melatonin won't help.

Shedding Light on Skin Problems

Back in the 1890s, a Danish doctor named Nils Finsen noticed that tuberculosis patients with skin sores got better when they were able to spend a lot of time in the sunshine. Dr. Finsen explored this further and found that it was the *ultraviolet* (*UV*) *light* in the sunlight that did the trick. He was rewarded with the Nobel Prize in Medicine in 1903.

Ever since then, light—particularly ultraviolet light—has been used to treat some skin problems. UV light is especially helpful for *psoriasis*, an annoying chronic skin condition. The drawback is that you'll need at least one or two treatments a week for a month or longer, so you'll be spending a lot of time at the doctor's office. There's also a good chance that in about a year you'll have to start the treatments all over again. Even so, it might be worth it—the results can sometimes be dramatic. If you have psoriasis, talk to your doctor about UV light therapy.

Light Up Your Health

Many studies have shown that healthy people exposed to bright light or *full-spectrum light* just feel better overall—they're less stressed and more relaxed. In fact, some school systems, factories, and offices have been experimenting with using full-spectrum lights instead of the usual fluorescent ones. The idea is to improve learning and productivity, but there's no firm evidence one way or the other to prove that it works. It doesn't hurt, however, and a lot of people say they prefer full-spectrum light. You can easily replace the regular bulbs in your light fixtures with full-spectrum bulbs from any well-stocked lighting center. The bulbs are on the expensive side, but they last a really long time.

There's less evidence that some alternative ideas for light therapy have any value. Some

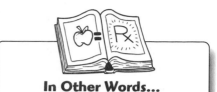

In Other Words...

Sunlight contains light at many different wavelengths. The light we see is called the **visible spectrum**, but sunlight also contains **ultraviolet (UV) light** at wavelengths too long for our eyes to pick up. UV radiation penetrates your skin, though—it's what makes your skin burn and tan.

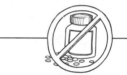

Hazardous to Your Health!

Ultraviolet light can give you a nice, healthy-looking tan—and too much can give you skin cancer and blinding cataracts. Protect yourself by wearing sun screen and dark glasses when you're outdoors in bright sunlight—even in the winter.

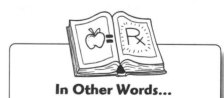

In Other Words...

Full-spectrum light is just that—artificial light that mimics the full color range of natural sunlight, including the ultraviolet end of the spectrum.

practitioners say a type of ultraviolet light called UVA-1 can help people with lupus, a chronic autoimmune disease. Others claim that irradiating your blood with ultraviolet light and then putting it back into your body can help treat cancer, infections, asthma, rheumatoid arthritis, and the symptoms of AIDS.

Some alternative practitioners believe that shining red light on parts of your body can help problems such as depression, chronic headaches, and sinus problems. If your shoulder hurts, for instance, shining red light on it is said to help, although nobody can quite explain why.

Rules, Rules, Rules

The American Medical Association recognized SAD as a medical disorder back in 1993, but the FDA hasn't quite caught up. According to the FDA, light boxes to treat SAD are experimental devices. Manufacturers aren't allowed to make any medical claims for their lights; on the other hand, you don't need a prescription to buy one. Even so, ask your doctor to write a letter to your health insurance company explaining why you need the special light. In most cases, your insurer will pay for the light.

Light therapy for psoriasis and some other skin problems is a standard medical approach—your insurance company will probably pay with no questions asked. They probably won't pay for other light therapy treatments, since some are considered experimental and others aren't part of mainstream medicine.

The Least You Need to Know

➤ Your daily cycle of body rhythms is affected by light.

➤ Some people get SAD—seasonal affective disorder—during the short, dark days of winter.

➤ SAD symptoms, such as depression, sleeping too much, overeating, and having trouble concentrating, are often helped by exposure to bright light.

➤ Light therapy can help relieve jet-lag symptoms and help shift workers adjust to schedule changes.

➤ Skin problems such as psoriasis are often helped by exposure to ultraviolet light.

Chapter 26

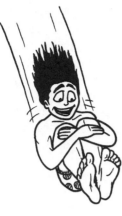

Hydrotherapy: Water, Water, Everywhere

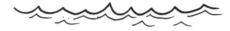

In This Chapter

➤ The importance of water for good health

➤ The many kinds of water therapy

➤ Water treatments for muscle and joint pain, circulatory problems, and other ailments

➤ Simple home hydrotherapy techniques

At the end of a long day, isn't it great to relax in a nice hot bath? As you play with your rubber ducky and soak away your tensions, you're doing something humans have always done—using water as a form of therapy. In fact, more than five thousand years ago, Hippocrates, the father of medicine, recommended bathing in natural hot springs as a treatment for a range of health problems. What Hippocrates advised then is still advised today by a lot of health professionals. So the next time someone tells you to go soak your head or take a long walk off a short pier, say yes! Some water therapy might be exactly what you need.

You're All Wet

You only have to see a baby splashing happily in the bath, or stand in line at a water park on a hot day, to realize how much humans naturally love water. There's more to water than just having fun in it. *Hydrotherapy*, or using water internally or externally as a treatment, can help a wide range of health problems.

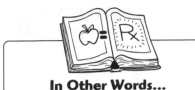

In Other Words...

Hydrotherapy is the use of water in some form as a treatment for a health problem, as a way to maintain general good health, or as a way to relax.

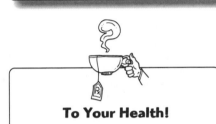

To Your Health!

Is your tap water safe to drink? As recent outbreaks of water-carried illness show, maybe not, even if it meets all federal and state standards. If you're worried about your drinking water or want more information on home water filters and other steps you can take, call the federal Environmental Protection Agency's safe drinking water hot line at (800) 426-4791.

Hydrotherapy comes in two basic forms: internal and external. *Internal* hydrotherapy usually means drinking water as a form of treatment. It can also mean internal cleansing using colon hydrotherapy (we discuss this more in Chapter 20, "Detoxification Treatments: What a Waste"). *External* hydrotherapy generally means applying water to your skin in some way—through a bath or compress, for instance.

Have Another Drink

Dr. Pressman always asks his patients to drink at least 64 ounces—eight 8-ounce glasses, or two quarts—of pure water every day. At first, a lot of patients find it hard to imagine drinking that much. After a week or so, though, they feel so much better that they can't imagine *not* drinking that much.

Why does drinking lots of water help your health? Because 60 percent of your body is made up of water. You need plenty of water to help regulate your body temperature, carry nutrients and oxygen to your cells, keep your skin and connective tissues supple, cushion your joints and organs, and carry wastes quickly out of your body.

Surveys show that only about 20 percent of all Americans really drink 64 ounces of water every day. Even worse, about 9 percent of Americans don't drink any water at all on an average day. The average American does get eight servings of fluids every day, but they mostly come in the form of milk, juice, and soda pop. Offsetting those fluids are the five servings of caffeine- or alcohol-containing drinks the average American drinks each day—beverages that rob your body of water. The result is that most people just aren't getting the benefits of enough water.

So swap the soda pop for spring water and trade your coffee for herbal tea. There's a good chance you'll see some quick improvements in your health: You'll feel more alert, you'll have fewer headaches, your skin will be smoother, and your elimination will improve. If you have arthritis, your joints may hurt less. And if you're troubled by frequent bladder infections or constipation, drinking more water may help quite a bit.

Bathing for Better Health

For centuries, the natural mineral springs in the little village of Spa in Belgium had a reputation for healing—the ancient Romans used to visit them. By the 19th century, the village had grown into a major health center. People came from all over Europe and the world to "take the waters" as a treatment for ailments of all sorts. The water treatments became so popular that the word *spa* came to mean any health resort.

A bath using *colloidal* oatmeal—oatmeal that has been finely ground into a powder—can be very soothing for skin irritations such as poison ivy or psoriasis. You can buy colloidal oatmeal at any drugstore or make your own by grinding ordinary oatmeal in a blender. Just add a handful to the bath water and soak away your itches.

Many of the water therapies developed at Spa and other places, including Dr. Kellogg's famed sanitarium at Battle Creek, Michigan, are still used today. Let's dive in and take a closer look.

Getting into Hot Water

Hot baths are relaxing in general. They're also very soothing for aching joints and sore muscles, and they're helpful for improving your circulation. The water should be no hotter than 110°F (40°C)—don't stay in for more than half an hour. Adding a few drops of a fragrant essential oil makes the bath more enjoyable (see Chapter 24, "Aromatherapy: The Nose Knows," for more information).

Sometimes *hyperthermia*—raising your body temperature—is used to treat infections and stimulate your immune system. The idea is to raise your body temperature from the normal 98.6°F to 102°F—just as your body does when you run an infection-fighting fever. Hyperthermia is done by immersing yourself in a very hot bath until your body temperature goes up. Hyperthermia is generally safe if you're a healthy adult, but it

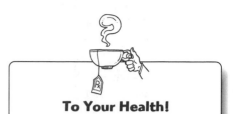

To Your Health!

By the time you feel thirsty, your body already needs water badly. The time to drink is before you get thirsty, especially when you're very active or if the weather is very hot or very cold. As you get older, you don't feel as thirsty, but you need water more than ever—80 ounces a day—because your kidneys don't work as efficiently.

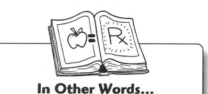

In Other Words...

Hyperthermia deliberately raises your body temperature from normal—98.6°F—to fever level—102°F—in order to fight infection and stimulate your immune system.

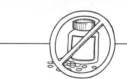

Hazardous to Your Health!

Use hyperthermia only if your doctor recommends it. Children, pregnant women, and older adults should not use hyperthermia. Do not use hyperthermia if you have diabetes, high blood pressure, or heart disease.

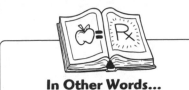

In Other Words...

A **sitz bath** is what it sounds like—
a bath you sit in, with the water
covering your pelvic region but not
your feet. In fact, the name comes
from the German word meaning
"seat" or "sit."

should really only be done if your doctor advises it.
Don't try it with kids or if you're pregnant. If you're an
older adult or have heart disease, high blood pressure, or
diabetes, skip it.

A *sitz bath* can be very helpful for relieving the discomfort of some problems in the pelvic area, including
bladder infections, vaginal irritations, hemorrhoids, and
anal fissures. Sit in a bathtub or large basin and add
enough hot water to cover the pelvic region up to your
belly button. (If you have to use the tub, hang your feet
over the side.) Sitz baths are short—don't stay in for
more than five minutes. Avoid sitz baths if you're in the
first three months of a pregnancy.

Stuck in Neutral

To take a neutral bath, you need a really big bathtub. That's because this bath involves
submerging yourself up to the neck in a tub full of water that's just below body temperature. (You can use a regular oral thermometer to check the water temperature.)
Stay in for 15 to 20 minutes; add more hot water as needed. Neutral baths are very
relaxing, so they're helpful for dealing with anxiety and insomnia; they're also helpful
for chronic pain and aching muscles and joints. A lot of women find that neutral baths
help them iron out the mood swings that come with PMS and the early stages of
menopause. Try it first thing in the morning to get your day started on an even keel.

Cooling Off

There's nothing quite like a cold shower to get you up and moving in the morning—
you'll feel invigorated all day. If you can't bring yourself to stand under a cold shower,
try a cold friction rub instead. Soak a washcloth or hand towel in cold water, wring it
out lightly, then rub yourself vigorously with it all over. Dip the washcloth in cold
water again as needed. Your skin will turn a rosy pink, and you'll feel a lot more awake
afterward.

Running Hot and Cold

Contrast therapies use alternating hot and cold water. The basic idea is that hot is
expanding and relaxing, while cold is contracting and stimulating. By alternating the
two, you alternate between the expansion and contraction. That gets your circulation
really moving, which in turn carries more nutrients to your cells and carries more
wastes away. If you apply heat to one part of your body while applying cold to another, you move blood from the cold region to the hot. This often helps relieve pain in
the cold region.

Contrast sitz baths are even more helpful for pelvic region problems than ordinary hot sitz baths. They're a little harder to organize, since you need two big basins. Fill one basin with hot water and the other with cold. Sit in the hot basin with your feet in the cold basin. After three minutes, switch—sit in the cold basin with your feet in the hot basin. Stay that way for just a minute or so. Repeat up to three times; end with your feet in the cold basin.

A similar approach often helps headaches, particularly sinus headaches. Sit with your feet and ankles in a basin of hot water and put a cold compress on your forehead. The hot water expands your feet and pulls blood downward; the cold compress helps push blood out of your head. The combination reduces the congestion in your head and relieves the headache. Just soaking your feet in alternating cold and hot water can help relieve swelling in the feet and legs.

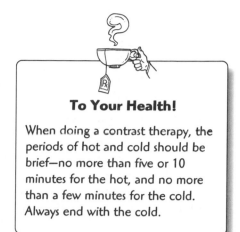

To Your Health!

When doing a contrast therapy, the periods of hot and cold should be brief—no more than five or 10 minutes for the hot, and no more than a few minutes for the cold. Always end with the cold.

Constitutional Hydrotherapy

Naturopathic physicians sometimes recommend a treatment known as *constitutional hydrotherapy* (also called a *wet sheet pack*). The treatment starts by wrapping you in a sheet soaked in cold water. You then lie on a table or bed and are covered with a heavy blanket. Over the next 30 to 60 minutes, you gradually warm up and then start to sweat. The contrasts in temperature improve your circulation and stimulate your immune system; the sweating removes toxins from your body. Constitutional hydrotherapy is sometimes suggested for viral illnesses such as chronic fatigue syndrome or as a detoxification treatment. Do this only if your doctor recommends it.

Getting All Steamed Up

Breathing in steam can help relieve a sore throat, laryngitis, chest congestion, and coughing. Fill a basin with very hot water, bend over it, and drape a towel over your head to trap the steam. Breathe deeply. Refill the basin as needed. For congestion and coughs, try adding a few drops of eucalyptus or tea-tree oil to the water (see Chapter 24 on aromatherapy for more information).

A sauna or Turkish bath is a steam bath without the steam. A small room is heated to above 100°F

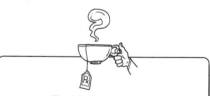

To Your Health!

Taking a steam bath—sitting in a very hot, steamy room—is amazingly relaxing. It's great for relieving cold symptoms, and because you sweat a lot, it can help detoxify your body. Stay in the steam bath for no longer than 20 minutes.

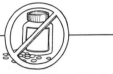

Hazardous to Your Health!

Do not take a sauna or steam bath if you are pregnant or have heart disease, high blood pressure, circulatory problems, diabetes, or asthma. Do not use a steam bath as a way to lose weight.

using dry heat. Just as a steam bath does, a sauna makes you sweat, which removes toxins from your system. In Scandinavia, where saunas are traditional, people alternate five or 10 minutes in the heat with a quick roll in the snow outside. Many health clubs offer sauna rooms; you'll have to substitute a quick dash under the cold shower for the snow. If you don't alternate, spend no more than 15 or 20 minutes in the sauna.

In Russia and Scandinavia, steam baths and saunas are also recommended for treating hangovers.

Hydrotherapy Help

Hydrotherapy has some serious medical applications. Water exercise in a pool is often prescribed for pregnant women, for people with arthritis, for disabled people, and as rehab for athletic injuries. The water supports most of your weight, and you can exercise without stressing your joints. Whirlpool treatments are helpful and very soothing for joint, muscle, and back injuries.

Water exercise classes for pregnant women and people with arthritis are often offered at health clubs and Ys. For other kinds of hydrotherapy, you'll need to work with a physical therapist.

Watered Down Health

Water treatments such as whirlpools, sitz baths, and water exercise programs are usual treatments in standard medicine—medical doctors often recommend them. The relaxing effects of saunas and steam baths are well understood, although pregnant women and anyone with a chronic health problem, such as heart disease, should stay away. Medical doctors are a lot more skeptical of naturopathic water treatments such as constitutional hydrotherapy. They feel these treatments don't really help and could be harmful for frail patients.

Rules, Rules, Rules

Many forms of hydrotherapy—whirlpool treatments, water exercises for arthritis, sitz baths, and the like—are widely accepted by doctors. Your insurance company will probably pay at least in part for hydrotherapy to treat problems like arthritis or a sports injury, if your doctor recommends it and the treatment comes from a licensed practitioner such as a physical therapist. Naturopathic doctors recommend hydrotherapy fairly often; if your insurance pays for naturopathic therapy, you might be covered for some of the hydrotherapy. Although hydrotherapy is an accepted part of European health treatment—many workers get paid visits to spas as a benefit—you're not likely to be reimbursed if you decide that what you really need is a week at a health resort.

The Least You Need to Know

➤ Hydrotherapy uses water in various ways to treat ailments, for relaxation, and as a way to maintain good health.

➤ Baths of various kinds and temperatures can help improve your circulation and stimulate your immune system.

➤ Sitz baths are very helpful for relieving painful symptoms of some problems in the pelvic region.

➤ Steam baths and saunas are very relaxing. They make you sweat, which helps detoxify your body.

➤ Hydrotherapy, such as water exercises for people with arthritis and whirlpool treatments for joint injuries, can be helpful for relieving pain and speeding healing.

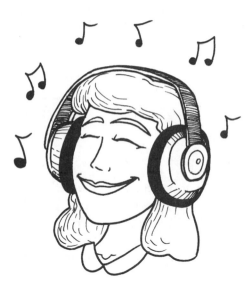

Chapter 27

Sound Therapy: Soothing the Savage Breast

In This Chapter

➤ Music's healing power

➤ How music therapy helps people with serious illnesses

➤ How music helps you relax—and makes you smarter

➤ Sound therapy and your health

Wherever you go today, you can't help but hear music. There's that awful syrupy stuff they play in elevators and hotel lobbies, the happy music they play in supermarkets and department stores, the loud music your teenager plays, and more. Then there's music you choose for yourself, in your office, your car, and at home.

Why all this musical bombardment? It's because music affects your mood. Those chirpy songs at the supermarket, for example, have been scientifically chosen to put you in the mood to buy. When you decide which radio station to listen to or which CD to play, you're affecting your own mood. And more and more evidence shows that you could be affecting your health as well.

Listening to Your Health

When you listen to music, it has a measurable effect on your body. If the music is slow, quiet, and instrumental, your heartbeat slows down and your blood pressure drops; if the music is faster, louder, and includes vocals, your heart beats faster and your blood pressure goes up.

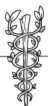

The Healing Arts

Music and medicine have gone together for thousands of years. In ancient Egypt, the melodies doctors used when they chanted incantations were part of the treatment. The ancient Greek philosopher Pythagoras believed that music helps restore the balance of the body and cure illness. In Tibet, the harmonic sounds of singing bowls are said to have a healing influence. And in many cultures, spiritual healers use drums, rattles, and other rhythm instruments as part of healing ceremonies.

Researchers have known about the relaxing and energizing effects of music for decades. More recently, they've come to realize that music can do more than just relax you—it can help you heal. Listening to music you enjoy could actually increase your levels of disease-fighting immune cells and help you recover from illness faster. Music also helps lower your blood pressure, breathing rate, and heart rate; this helps you relax and lets your body heal. And premature babies who hear quiet, rhythmic sounds and soothing music in their incubators gain more weight, have fewer complications, and go home days sooner.

Being in Tune with Your Body

Ever wonder why your dentist always has that relentlessly upbeat music playing in the waiting room? It's because numerous studies have shown that music helps people deal with pain better, and that it helps with dental pain best of all. Next on the music relief hit parade is pain from migraine headaches. Studies have shown that listening to music during a headache helps relieve the intense pain. Migraine sufferers who listen to music as a regular relaxation exercise have fewer headaches—and the ones they do get are shorter and less painful.

Music has also been shown to help reduce pain and anxiety for surgical patients, which in turn helps them recover faster. This is an old idea—as far back as 1914, surgeons were playing records in the operating room to calm patients who were about to have surgery. More recently, a 1997 study showed that surgery goes more smoothly for patients if they listen to music both before and during the operation. The study looked at people who were having cataracts in their eyes removed under local anesthesia. As they were waiting for the surgery to begin, their blood pressure soared. Just 10 minutes after they started listening to music of their choice, though, their blood pressure and heart rate went back down to normal levels. By the time the surgery started, they were feeling a lot less anxious.

And here's one other important use of music in the operating room: Studies show that when the surgical team listens to music, they work together better.

Getting on Your Nerves

The positive effects of *music therapy* on people with neurological disorders such as Parkinson's disease, Alzheimer's disease, and brain damage from strokes are amazing:

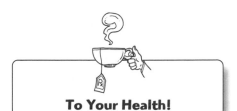

To Your Health!

If you really can't stand your dentist's choice of music, point out that pain studies show that patients who choose their own music get the most relief.

➤ **Parkinson's disease.** People with Parkinson's gradually lose their ability to start a movement—they become "frozen" and rigid and can't move. The sound of music helps many PD patients start moving. And if the music has a good rhythm, they walk to its beat in a more regular and steady way. Music therapists who work with PD patients make tapes of music with a steady beat. By listening to the tapes every day over several weeks, the patients are able to move and walk better. The effect lasts even after they stop listening.

➤ **Stroke and other brain damage.** Rhythmic music helps people with brain damage from a stroke or injury to walk faster and more easily—they tend to keep up with the beat of the music. The reason seems to be that the music helps their brains "organize" the complex actions needed for walking. Music therapy can also help a stroke victim's mental state, helping to lift the depression and anxiety that often go with brain damage.

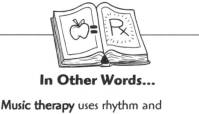

In Other Words...

Music therapy uses rhythm and melody to improve your psychological and emotional well-being—and sometimes also your physical well-being. Music therapy is becoming increasingly accepted by the medical community as a valuable complementary therapy.

➤ **Alzheimer's disease.** As this devastating disease of the elderly goes on, patients get less and less responsive—except when they hear music. Listening to music, especially music they loved in earlier days, can make people with a severe case of Alzheimer's sing along or even get up out of a wheelchair and dance. The music also seems to help these patients relax and interact more.

Music therapy is used to help treat people with severe depression, anxiety, and chronic pain. It's being used to help disabled, mentally handicapped, and autistic children communicate without words. Music also helps these kids improve their attention spans and their physical coordination. Some researchers believe that music therapy can also be very helpful for kids with learning disabilities and attention deficit disorder. That's why more and more music therapists today work in schools in the special education department.

The Mozart Effect

A study that made headlines in 1995 showed that listening to the delightful music of Wolfgang Amadeus Mozart for just 10 minutes helped college students score higher on intelligence tests. What got smaller headlines was that the effect only lasted for about 15 minutes—but hey, even 15 minutes of being smarter is good.

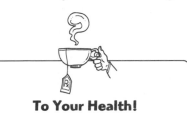

To Your Health!

A good book on the value of music for improving your mental and physical health is *The Mozart Effect*™, by Don Campbell (Avon Books, 1997). You can also get tapes and CDs with selections of Mozart's music chosen for their brain-improving effects.

Since then, the Mozart Effect has become a hot topic. Why does Mozart work better than, say, Nine Inch Nails? The reason seems to be the high frequencies in Mozart's music, which are in the bandwidth said to be the best for improving concentration.

Other composers and other types of music also have a positive effect. Gregorian chants have a frequency range similar to Mozart's music, for example, which could explain why they're so popular with college students today. A 1998 study showed that healthy people who listened to the music of Bach, Brahms, and Ravel scored higher on tests of overall mood. It's possible that the rhythm of the selections helps—the effect is greatest when the music is on the slow side, about 60 beats or less to a minute.

The Tomatis Method

The first researcher to point out the beneficial effects of Mozart's music was Alfred A. Tomatis, M.D. A French physician who has spent decades studying the relationship between sound and mental and physical health, Tomatis is the inventor of a device called the Electronic Ear, which is said to improve listening abilities. It's been used with good results in some programs for learning-disabled children.

Sound Ideas: Other Sound Therapy Techniques

Some researchers believe that specific sounds—whether you make them yourself or just listen to them—can help treat specific physical and emotional problems. Here's a rundown of the main ideas:

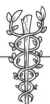

The Healing Arts

In 1997, Governor Zell Miller proposed that the state of Georgia provide a cassette or CD of classical music to the parents of every newborn—over 100,000 a year—in order to boost the baby's intelligence later in life. He played the final section of Beethoven's Ninth Symphony to the members of the legislature to make them smarter, but they still voted down his proposal.

➤ **Toning.** By making stretched-out vowel sounds that you let resonate through your whole body (toning), you release tension and energize yourself. Toning practitioners say it's like giving yourself an internal massage. The overall idea is that specific sound frequencies have a positive effect on your brain wave patterns. The same idea is behind chanting and other vocalization techniques.

➤ **Cymatics.** In cymatic therapy, you don't just hear the sound—you feel it through a special electronic device applied directly to your skin. Sir Peter Guy Manners, M.D., the inventor of cymatics, claims that disease causes disharmonies in the natural vibration pattern of the part of the body that is affected. By applying a range of audible sound frequencies to the area, cymatics restores harmony and balance. The cymatic instrument looks a little like a telephone handset. The treatment is painless and noninvasive, but there's no real evidence that it works.

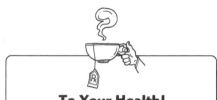

To Your Health!

Lots of New Age and ethnic musicians have recorded music that uses rhythms and frequencies designed for meditation and healing. Those same rhythms occur in the slower music of classical composers such as Mozart, Handel, Bach, Vivaldi, and Telemann. Music is very individual, though, so what works for one person may not work for you. Keep listening until you find what you like.

Some practitioners use other sound devices to treat health problems. We can't really say if their machines and methods work or not—you'll have to use your own judgment.

The Sound of Silence

Sometimes what you want isn't music, it's silence. In today's society, that's very hard to find, especially if you live in a city. Instead, you may have to mask the constant sounds of traffic and other noises with *white noise*. This is easy to do with anything that makes a soft, constant noise at the same low pitch, like an air conditioner or fan. You can also buy inexpensive white-noise generators—small machines about the size of a small clock radio that make a steady hum or whoosh. However you make it, the white noise masks the other noises around you and makes them far less distracting and annoying. White noise is very helpful for people who are light sleepers—it blocks noises that keep you up or wake you.

A delightful alternative to white noise is the sounds of nature, such as chirping crickets or waves breaking on a beach. Some of the more expensive white-noise generators also make several different natural sounds. You can buy recordings of natural sounds—there's a surprising number of these available at music stores and from catalogs. The recordings are very relaxing to listen to, and they're great for soothing you to sleep. They work well with babies and young children, too.

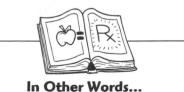

In Other Words...

White noise is any sort of steady, soft sound on a steady frequency and with no rhythm—the noise made by an air conditioner is a good example. White noise is useful for masking other sounds, such as traffic noises or conversation.

Finding Qualified Practitioners

Music therapists are a fun group—they can all sing and play the guitar or piano. Not only that, they carry around a lot of neat percussion instruments that they encourage you to play with.

About 70 American colleges and universities offer undergraduate or graduate degrees in music therapy. In addition to their degrees, music therapists do an internship and then take a national certifying exam sponsored by the Certification Board for Music Therapy. Those who pass become board-certified registered music therapists and can use the letters RMT-BC after their name. All told, there are about 5,000 registered music therapists in the United States.

To find a qualified music therapist near you, contact:

American Music Therapy Association (AMTA)
8455 Colesville Road, Suite 1000
Silver Spring, MD 20910
Phone: (301) 589-3300
Fax: (301) 589-5175
E-mail: info@musictherapy.org

AMTA was founded in 1998 with the merger of two national organizations—the National Association for Music Therapy and the American Association for Music Therapy.

Most music therapists work in hospitals, nursing homes, rehab centers, and schools, but some are in private practice. Their fees vary, but on average, an hour of music therapy costs about $50.

For more information on toning and other self-help sound therapy techniques, contact:

> **Sound Healers Association (SHA)**
> Box 2240
> Boulder, CO 80306
> Phone: (800) 246-9764
> Fax: (303) 443-6023
> E-mail: soundheals@aol.com

SHA offers courses, seminars, and an international directory of sound healers.

Rules, Rules, Rules

One reason AMTA was founded was to work for more recognition of music therapy as a valuable treatment for health problems. They've already made some headway—today their help is sometimes covered by medical insurance, especially if it's part of treatment in a clinical setting such as a rehab center. Medicare, for example, now pays for in-hospital music therapy in some cases. Coverage varies among different health insurance plans—check with your insurer.

The various types of sound therapy, like cymatics, aren't well understood by the medical community, and some of the theories are considered crackpot or worse. You'll have to pay for it yourself, and you're on your own when it comes to finding a qualified practitioner.

The Least You Need to Know

➤ Music has been used for thousands of years as part of medical treatment.

➤ Listening to music before, during, and after surgery or dental treatment helps patients relax and feel less pain.

➤ Listening to music relieves stress, lowers your blood pressure, slows your heartbeat, and promotes healing.

➤ Music can help patients with neurological problems such as Parkinson's disease, stroke damage, and Alzheimer's disease improve their mobility and feel less depressed and anxious.

➤ Some kinds of music, particularly Gregorian chants and the works of Mozart, have been shown to improve concentration and memory.

➤ Music therapists are professionals trained to use sound and rhythm as part of physical, emotional, and psychological healing.

Part 8

It's All in Your Mind

Modern medicine has created an artificial divide between your mind and your body. But how often have you caught a cold after a long period of stress? You know your mind and your body are intimately connected. The mind/body connection is the area where alternative medicine really differs from standard medicine—it's a big part of why people are turning to alternative treatments. Alternative medicine looks at the whole person—body, mind, and spirit.

In this section, we discuss ways to reduce the stress in your life through yoga, relaxation techniques, meditation, and more. And as you'll discover, less stress translates into better health.

Chapter 28

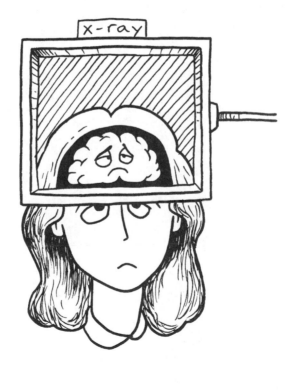

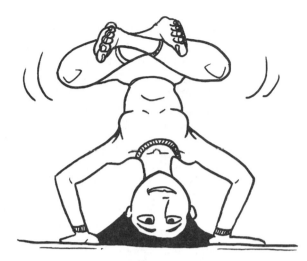

Yoga: Exercise Your Body—and Your Mind

We're going to talk about some pretty amazing things in this chapter, but here's the most amazing thing of all: The practice of yoga is more than five thousand years old, but it's still valuable today. In our stress-filled, hurried lives, yoga can provide an oasis of tranquillity that can translate into better physical and mental health. And for some people, yoga is more than just valuable—it's lifesaving. That's because yoga, combined with changes in your diet and your lifestyle, could actually reverse heart disease.

Body and Mind Together

In India, where it originated, *yoga* is seen as a complete system of physical and mental training done primarily for spiritual enlightenment. Here in the West, yoga has become very popular, but mostly as a form of gentle exercise that's great for stretching and toning your body—and that also just happens to do a lot for improving your emotional outlook and sharpening your mind.

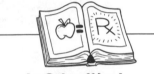

In Other Words...

The word **yoga** comes from the Sanskrit word meaning "union." That's because yoga unites your mind and your body. Sanskrit is the ancient language of India and Hinduism; now it's used only for sacred and scholarly writings. Yoga practices are an aspect of the Hindu religion, although yoga by itself is not a religion.

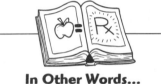

In Other Words...

Hatha yoga (pronounced *HAT-ha YOH-gah*) is the most popular form of yoga in Western culture, mostly because its emphasis is on strengthening the body. The name comes from the Sanskrit words *ha*, meaning "sun," and *tha*, meaning "moon." The combination word *hatha* is often translated as "balance."

Yoga combines physical exercise, breathing techniques, and meditation. The combination of mind and body can do great things for you. Many people start doing yoga as a way to help a particular physical problem, like back pain. They soon find that yoga makes them feel better overall. They're more relaxed yet also more energetic. They're less stressed and more focused and creative.

One of the most beautiful things about yoga is that anyone can do it. No matter how out of shape you are, no matter what your age, state of health, or physical limitations, you can benefit from yoga.

Hatha Yoga

Carved figures showing yoga poses have been found in ancient temples in India that are some 5,000 years old. Yoga as we know it, however, dates back to the second century B.C., when the great sage Patanjali laid out the path to enlightenment through yoga. Since then, different schools of yoga taking somewhat different approaches have developed. The one that's most commonly taught in the United States is called *hatha yoga*. It's an approach that focuses on the body, using physical postures, breathing techniques, and meditation.

The goal of hatha yoga is balance between the body and the mind. A tense mind leads to a tense body, and vice versa. The physical postures of hatha yoga, combined with breathing techniques, create relaxation and serenity.

Asanas: Posing the Question

Asanas are the postures, or yoga exercises, that are used to make your body stronger and more flexible. There are thousands of asanas, but you don't have to learn them all. There are about 20 basic postures that are commonly used; during a short yoga workout, you would use only about four or five of these. Serious yoga students go on to learn many more.

Although some of the asanas might look difficult, they're not, because your goal is only to do them as well as you can, not to do them perfectly, and especially not to do them better than anyone else in your class. Although you may want to push yourself a little bit, the asanas should never hurt—the old saying "no pain, no gain" has no place in yoga class. The asanas provide gentle stretching and improve flexibility. And though you're unlikely to break a sweat in yoga class, the asanas also improve strength and endurance.

We don't have the room to go into descriptions of the asanas here. They're easy to learn and easy to do—your yoga instructor will teach them to you and show you the correct way to do them. If you're learning yoga on your own, there are useful diagrams and pictures in all the books on the subject. Videos showing the asanas are extremely helpful. Yoga is so popular today that you can probably check out a video at your public library!

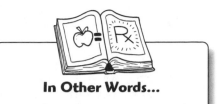

In Other Words...

Asanas (pronounced *AH-sah-nahs*) are the yoga physical postures, or exercises. Literally, *asana* means "posture." It comes from the Sanskrit root *as*, meaning "to stay."

Pranayama: Breathing Easier

A basic idea in hatha yoga (and in other forms of yoga) is *prana*, or life force. Yoga exercises are said to maximize the flow of prana in your body, which in turn gives you better health and more energy. Your breath is seen as one aspect of prana, so it stands to reason that learning to control your breathing would help regulate prana in your body.

Yoga uses *pranayama*, or breath-control exercises, as a way to channel your prana into and out of your body. If you're a Western-style skeptic about that idea, think of it this way: Deep, regular breathing sends a signal to your body, telling it to relax, and gets plenty of oxygen to your cells. Here's another way to look at it: Breath control equals mental control. Pranayama improves your mental clarity.

In yoga, pranayama is just as important as the asanas. Learning to control your breath takes some concentration, but once you focus, it's not hard. In fact, pranayama breathing exercises are where the famous "om" sound comes from—it's the sound you make as you breath out slowly after breathing in deeply.

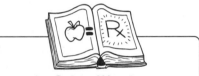

In Other Words...

Prana can be loosely translated as "life force." Prana flows in your body, but it's universal—it's found everywhere, in all things, living or inanimate. **Pranayama** (pronounced *PRAH-NAH-YAH-mah*), or breath-control exercises, are an important part of yoga, especially hatha yoga. By controlling your breath, you control the flow of prana into and out of your body.

Think About It

Meditation is an important part of yoga—some people would say it's really the main part. Every yoga session should begin with a brief period of emptying your mind of distracting thoughts, and should end with a good 10 minutes or more of additional meditation. We'll get into the details of meditation in the next chapter.

Yoga for Less Stress

In our high-achieving, competitive society, stress is inevitable. Here's where learning yoga can have amazing results. Yoga doesn't remove the stress from your life, but it teaches you to handle it better by letting you access your inner strength. Just doing your short, simple, daily routine of yoga postures, breathing exercises, and meditation can do wonders for reducing stress. The routine regulates your breathing, relaxes your muscles, floods your cells with fresh oxygen and nutrients, and increases your general feeling of well-being. And little by little, if you do the exercises regularly, you'll find yourself getting a different take on life. Situations that used to stress you out don't any more—or if they do, you cope better.

Yoga doesn't just teach you to do breathing exercises whenever you want to throttle your boss. The deep relaxation yoga helps you get over stress-related problems like anxiety, insomnia, panic attacks, and mild depression—inexpensively, without drugs, and while improving your health in general.

Weight Loss with Yoga

Forget yoga, we hear you saying—everyone knows that the best way to cope with stress is to eat a lot of chocolate chip cookies. We agree (we couldn't have gotten through writing this book without them), but getting fat is a big price to pay. Yoga is fabulous for losing weight and keeping it off. There isn't any particular yoga diet. You lose weight because yoga reduces stress, improves your body image and self-esteem, and strengthens your concentration and willpower. Try it—you have nothing to lose but some extra pounds.

The Yoga Way to Better Health

Yoga helps an amazing range of health problems. That's because anyone in any state of health can benefit from the gentle movement and relaxing breathing exercises of yoga. When we say anyone, we mean it—yoga can be done if you're in a wheelchair or can't even get out of bed.

Here's a rundown of how yoga helps:

➤ **Back and neck problems.** If your doctor has sent you to a physical therapist for back or neck problems, you've probably already done some yoga exercises. Yoga is great for stretching and strengthening the muscles in your back, shoulders, neck, abdomen, hips, and legs. When these muscles are in good shape, your back and neck troubles fade away.

➤ **Heart disease.** The amazing Dr. Dean Ornish uses yoga exercises and meditation as part of his program to reverse heart disease. It works. Why? Because yoga teaches you to relax your muscles, improves your breathing, and slows your heart rate. Yoga also improves your circulation overall and keeps your blood vessels flexible. If you've been diagnosed with heart disease, talk to your doctor before you try yoga.

➤ **High blood pressure.** When you're under stress, your blood pressure zooms. Yoga teaches you to relax, which can really lower your blood pressure. In fact, if you have mild high blood pressure, you may be able to get it under control just with yoga and some lifestyle and diet changes—no drugs. Discuss yoga for your high blood pressure with your doctor before you try it.

➤ **Arthritis.** Painful joints hurt even more when the muscles around them are all tensed up. Your yoga teacher will help you design an exercise routine that gently stretches your muscles without stressing your joints. The extra relaxation from breathing exercises and meditation helps reduce the pain even more.

➤ **Asthma.** Yoga in general, and the breath-control exercises in particular, are often very helpful for people with asthma. These people have fewer attacks, and the ones they do have are less severe.

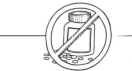

Hazardous to Your Health!

If you've had a spine-related injury, check with your doctor before you start a yoga program. And work with an experienced teacher so you do the postures correctly and don't hurt yourself further.

➤ **Chronic fatigue syndrome (CFS).** This baffling disease responds well to yoga. That's because yoga is very energizing. By doing their exercises in the morning, CFS patients can get through their day more easily and aren't as exhausted.

➤ **Pregnancy.** Yoga can help you get through a pregnancy with less stress and more energy. Talk to your doctor about yoga before you start, though, and don't go it alone. Find a teacher with experience in pregnancy yoga. Check with your birthing center—there may well be a yoga instructor on staff.

Other problems can be helped by yoga as well. Migraine headaches, allergies, breathing problems, diabetes, and digestive trouble all respond well.

Finding the Right Yoga Teacher for You

Yoga today is so popular that finding a teacher is easy—just check your Yellow Pages, the bulletin board at your health-food store or alternative health center, or with your health club or Y.

Finding the teacher who's right for you may be a little more difficult. Every teacher has a slightly different approach, and some are more experienced than others. Because there's no nationally recognized standard for yoga teachers, we suggest you follow these guidelines from the American Yoga Association:

➤ **Training.** Some yoga instructors get their training just by taking a few weekend seminars. They see yoga as just another approach to physical fitness. This amount of training usually isn't enough to make knowledgeable teachers. Ideally, your

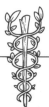

The Healing Arts

What's the difference between a yoga teacher and a guru? Literally, the Sanskrit word *guru* means "dispeller of darkness." A guru is a personal spiritual advisor who helps direct you toward spiritual growth and enlightenment. Not everybody needs a guru. If you connect well with your yoga teacher and respect his or her abilities, your teacher will provide you with the guidance you need to improve your yoga, especially when you're first starting out.

teacher has studied yoga for several years—and continues to study it under the guidance of a more experienced instructor.

➤ **Personal yoga practice.** Does your yoga teacher live the yoga lifestyle? Good teachers practice yoga themselves as a daily discipline.

➤ **Lifestyle factors.** Good yoga teachers apply yoga to their lifestyle and are vegetarians who don't smoke, drink, or use recreational drugs. They're also knowledgeable about nutrition and diet.

➤ **Flexibility.** A good yoga teacher takes an individual approach to each student—even in group classes—and works with you to vary the techniques according to your abilities. The class should be small enough so that the instructor has time for every student.

Yoga teachers are usually happy to answer your questions and will usually let you attend a sample class for free. If you're not comfortable in the class for any reason, find another teacher. You may need to check out two or three before you find one who's a good fit for you.

Yoga has a spiritual component, but it's not a religion. Avoid any teacher who pressures you to follow any sort of spiritual or religious practices or the teachings of any particular guru as part of your classes.

The American Yoga Association was established in 1968 as the first and only not-for-profit organization in the United States dedicated to education in yoga. For information about finding a qualified teacher, contact:

American Yoga Association
P.O. Box 19986
Sarasota, FL 34276
Phone: (941) 953-5859
Fax: (941) 364-9153

The association doesn't offer certification, but it does offer well-regarded training courses for yoga instructors.

Another good source of information about yoga and finding an instructor is:

> **International Association of Yoga Therapists**
> 20 Sunnyside Avenue
> Mill Valley, CA 94941
> Phone: (415) 868-1147
> E-mail: IAYT@yoganet.com

This organization emphasizes education and research in yoga.

Enjoying Your Yoga Class

One of the great things about yoga is that it's very inexpensive. You can generally attend an hour-long group yoga class for less than $25—and you don't need to buy any equipment or wear expensive outfits. A simple leotard is a good choice for class. It's comfortable and lets you and your teacher see the contours of your body well as you move through the poses. Yoga is done barefoot, so you don't need an incredibly expensive pair of elaborate exercise shoes.

Once you've found a compatible teacher, the most important part of the yoga class takes place in your head. Go in with an open mind and a positive, noncompetitive attitude. Don't overdo or push yourself beyond what's comfortable for you, no matter what anyone else in the class is doing.

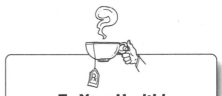

To Your Health!

Although yoga isn't strenuous and injuries are rare, be cautious, especially at first. If you have back, neck, or joint problems, be very careful, especially with asanas that twist your spine. It would be best in these cases to take yoga classes and work with your teacher to find the asanas that are best for you.

Designing Your Home Yoga Workout

Between classes, you can easily practice at home, because yoga doesn't need any fancy equipment. In fact, it doesn't need any equipment at all, although you might want to buy an inexpensive exercise mat or small area rug for your practice area.

You can do yoga anywhere—all you need is a patch of floor space free of clutter, preferably in a quiet place. Outside is nice if the weather permits, but stay indoors if it's cold. You want your muscles to be flexible, and cold tightens them up.

For the best results from yoga at home, try to do it regularly. You don't need to do all your asanas—it's best to rotate them around, doing three or four different ones each time. Twenty or 30 minutes, preferably every day or every other day, is a good home workout.

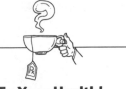

To Your Health!

A warm, draft-free area makes it much more comfortable to do yoga at home. You don't want to get chilled when you're meditating or working on a yoga pose. To stay warm, wear loose, comfortable clothes that don't bind at the waist, wrists, or ankles. If your feet are cold, wear ballet slippers or booties—anything that's comfortable and has a very thin sole.

Taking yoga classes is a great way to get started in yoga, but it's not the only way. There are tons of great yoga books and videotapes out there that will teach you the basics. One we recommend highly is *The Complete Idiot's Guide to Yoga*, by Joan Budilovsky and Eve Adamson. The American Yoga Association (see the previous section) has an excellent selection of books and videos.

Rules, Rules, Rules

As we explained earlier, you're on your own when it comes to finding a good yoga teacher. Ask around and attend classes until you find a teacher you like and who understands you.

Yoga as a treatment for stress-related problems, heart disease, back trouble, and other ailments is becoming more and more acceptable to many doctors. In fact, if you have high blood pressure or you've had a heart attack, your doctor may recommend yoga to you. You won't have far to go to find a class—today yoga is taught at many hospitals and health centers. In some cases, your health insurance may cover the costs if your doctor recommends yoga, but check before you sign up for a year's worth of lessons.

The Least You Need to Know

➤ Yoga is an ancient system combining physical postures, breath control, and meditation for better overall health.

➤ Hatha yoga, the form taught most often in the West, emphasizes the physical aspects of yoga.

➤ Yoga exercises are simple, gentle, and easy. They stretch and tone the muscles and build flexibility and strength.

➤ No matter what your age or state of health, you can do yoga. You don't need fancy equipment, classes are inexpensive, and you can easily do your workout at home.

➤ Doing yoga regularly is a great way to relax and deal with stress and stress-related problems like insomnia and high blood pressure.

➤ Yoga helps many physical problems, such as heart disease, arthritis, asthma, and chronic fatigue syndrome.

Chapter 29

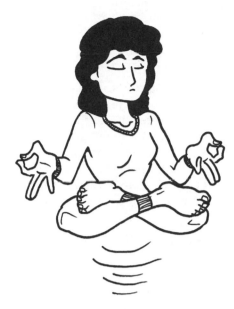

Relaxation and Meditation: Rising Above It All

In This Chapter

➤ Reducing stress with relaxation and meditation

➤ Helping heart disease and chronic illness with relaxation and meditation

➤ Easy relaxation and meditation exercises

➤ The different meditation styles

➤ Learning to meditate

Here's why healthcare costs so much: Studies show that at least 60 percent of all visits to doctors are for things like headaches, pain, digestive problems, and fatigue. The doctor examines you, runs some tests, prescribes some medication—the bills for all that add up. The problem is that most of the time you're not really sick—you're stressed out. What if you could find a way to manage your stress yourself? Then you wouldn't go to the doctor so often—and healthcare costs might go down. And what if the way you find is easy and doesn't cost anything? Then healthcare costs might go down a lot.

Are we dreaming? About healthcare costs going down, definitely. But there really is an easy and cost-free way to manage your stress and achieve better health: Learn some simple relaxation and meditation techniques.

Why You're Stressed Out

Why does *stress* have such a bad effect on your body? Because back in caveman days, if you ran across a threat—a saber-toothed tiger, say—you had two options: Run for it or stay put and fight it out. Either way, your body reacted to the threat by getting you ready. Your heart rate increased, your blood pressure jumped, you breathed faster, a flood of hormones sharpened your senses. Assuming that you outran the tiger or chased it off, you then felt totally exhausted. Within a few hours after that, your body returned to normal.

Today researchers call that reaction the *fight-or-flight response* to stress. It happens to all of us all the time, even though most of us aren't too likely to have to face large, hungry cats (well, okay, maybe your pet cat gets a little surly if you're slow filling the food bowl). Why? Because modern life is full of threats: family pressures, impossible bosses, traffic jams, money worries. And even though you're wearing a designer business suit and carrying a briefcase, your body still thinks it's wearing skins and fur and carrying a spear—and it still reacts as if you're facing a saber-toothed tiger. The problem is that the tiger doesn't go away. You leave the office only to get stuck in traffic on the way home and to have an argument with your teenager once you get there. Your body reacts each time and gets exhausted each time, but the stress is so constant you don't have a chance to return to normal in between.

The end result of long-term stress? It's a long, scary list: anxiety, depression, headaches, insomnia, high cholesterol, high blood pressure, heart palpitations, menstrual problems, muscle pain, back pain, digestive problems, skin rashes, and more. Stress also makes health problems such as asthma and diabetes worse. And stress can make you eat too much, drink too much, and abuse drugs.

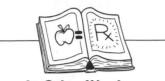

In Other Words...

Stress is a bit of a buzzword today, but let's use it in its specific sense here. Stress means any situation that forces you to make a rapid adjustment to changed circumstances. Bad things like fights with your spouse are stressful—and so are good things like going on a vacation.

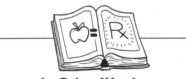

In Other Words...

When you're threatened or under stress, your body reacts with the **fight-or-flight response**. Your heart rate, blood pressure, and respiration rate go up; your muscles tense, you sweat, your digestion stops, your immune system is put on hold, and your emotional tension soars. You also produce large amounts of stress hormones, which damage your body in the long run.

Setting Your Mind at Ease

Let's get real here. The stress in your life isn't going to go away, so you're going to have find some way to manage it better. That's surprisingly simple to do once you've learned some very basic relaxation and meditation techniques. By using controlled breathing, conscious muscle relaxation, and mental focusing, you can achieve a state of deep relaxation that reverses the harmful effects of the fight-or-flight response.

Relaxation techniques and meditation are also very helpful for dealing with the stress of painful health conditions like arthritis or serious illnesses like cancer. Stress makes these conditions worse, which causes more stress, which makes the condition worse. You can break the downward spiral with relaxation and meditation techniques.

Does it work? It sure does.

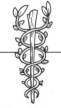

The Healing Arts

A 1998 study looked at 41 adults (with an average age of 67) from the same Midwestern town. Eighteen of the adults had been regular meditators for years; the other 23 didn't meditate. Whose cholesterol was 15 percent lower? You guessed it—the meditators. And although 15 percent might not sound like a lot, lowering your cholesterol level by just 10 percent makes a big dent in your chances of heart disease or a stroke.

Relaxation and meditation have been shown, in study after study, to help stress-related illness:

➤ Chronic-pain patients reduced their visits to the doctor by 36 percent.

➤ 80 percent of high blood pressure patients lowered their blood pressure and needed less medication.

➤ 100 percent of insomnia patients had improved sleep—and 90 percent no longer needed sleeping pills, or needed them less often.

➤ Women with severe PMS reduced their symptoms by more than 50 percent.

➤ Infertile women were less depressed, angry, and anxious—and had a 35 percent conception rate.

You may not make it into a dramatic statistic, but you too can improve your mental and physical health with relaxation and meditation. With training, you can learn to relax at will.

Progressive Muscle Relaxation

You've probably already noticed that having just 20 minutes or so of peace and quiet of any sort can do a lot to help you relax. By learning how to do progressive muscle relaxation, you can make the most of those 20 minutes. And if you do, you'll feel

363

emotionally calmed, mentally recharged, and physically energized. This basic technique was first developed in the 1930s and remains very popular today—it's the first
thing you learn in a relaxation class. You can do this anywhere, as long as there's room
to lie down. Take off your shoes and wear loose, comfortable clothing if possible.
Here's how:

1. Lie on your back on the floor or a bed, with your hands at your sides. Put a pillow
   under your head if you want.

2. Close your eyes and feel your body. Focus on your breathing for a few minutes—
   try to make it slow, deep, and even.

3. Tense the muscles in your right foot, hold for a few seconds, and release. Move
   up your leg and repeat: first your calf, then your thigh. Repeat the sequence with
   your left leg.

4. Tense and release your bottom on each side. Then tense and release your stomach
   muscles.

5. Make a fist with your right hand, then release. Move up your arm and repeat: first
   your forearm, then your upper arm. Repeat with your left arm.

6. Raise your shoulders up as far as you can, as if you were shrugging. Relax and
   repeat several times.

7. Gently roll your head from side to side several times.

8. Make faces: Yawn as widely as you can, stick out your lower jaw as far as you can,
   squeeze your eyes shut, raise your eyebrows.

9. Lie quietly and concentrate on your breathing again for a few minutes. When
   you're ready, get up.

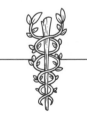

The Healing Arts

In 1991, a study in the *American Journal of Psychiatry* compared two groups of insomniacs.
The first group was treated with sleeping pills. The second group was taught muscle-
relaxing exercises. For the first week, the sleeping-pill group got more sleep. By the second
week, the relaxation group had caught up to the pill-takers. By the fifth week, the relaxers
were way ahead of the pill-takers, falling asleep faster and sleeping better. Added relaxation benefits? No cost, no "hangover," and no dependency.

When Dr. Pressman teaches progressive relaxation classes, invariably at least one person falls asleep. He's not a boring teacher—the students sack out because the technique really works. If you have insomnia, try it in bed when you're ready to sleep. This is also a great cure for a tension headache.

The Relaxation Response

In the 1960s, Dr. Herbert Benson of Harvard Medical School became very interested in the way just sitting quietly could help reduce the effects of stress. He called it the *relaxation response*—and learning how to do it has helped thousands and thousands of people lead healthier lives.

Dr. Benson's technique combines relaxation and meditation techniques with training in coping skills, exercise, and nutrition. The program is designed for people with chronic illness such as heart disease, high blood pressure, and diabetes. The goal is to reduce your symptoms, help you understand your disease better, regain a sense of control and well-being, and look at the factors— lifestyle, diet, stress, and so on—that make your symptoms worse.

Today Dr. Benson heads the world-famous Mind/ Body Medical Institute, which is part of Beth Israel Deaconess Medical Center in Boston. The Mind/Body Institute has branches at a number of major hospital centers across the country. For more information, contact:

> **Mind/Body Medical Institute**
> One Deaconess Road
> Boston, MA 02215
> Phone: (617) 632-9535
> Fax: (617) 632-7383
> E-mail: mbmi@bidmc.harvard.edu

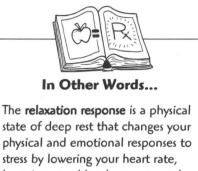

In Other Words...

The **relaxation response** is a physical state of deep rest that changes your physical and emotional responses to stress by lowering your heart rate, lowering your blood pressure, and relaxing your muscles.

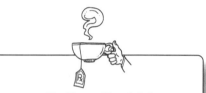

To Your Health!

Dr. Herbert Benson gave medical respectability to the mind/body connection. We recommend his books, especially the ground-breaking best-seller *The Relaxation Response* (Avon, 1976), *The Wellness Book* (Simon & Schuster, 1992), and *Timeless Healing: The Power and Biology of Belief* (Simon & Schuster, 1997).

You don't necessarily have to go to a Mind/Body center to learn the relaxation response. Many cardiac-care hospitals now teach the methods to heart patients. It's also used at many cancer hospitals to help patients better cope with their illness.

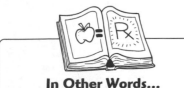

In Other Words...

Meditation uses various mental techniques to induce a state of deep relaxation, inner harmony, and focused awareness. It's often described as a state of "relaxed awareness," "altered consciousness," or "emptying the mind."

Meditation Approaches

Relaxation techniques concentrate on your physical body—the idea is that what relaxes the body also relaxes the mind. The opposite is also true—what relaxes the mind also relaxes the body. That's the idea behind the various types of *meditation*.

Meditation counteracts the fight-or-flight response. It slows your heart rate and lowers your blood pressure, slows your breathing, and relaxes your muscles. It also reduces the emotional overload of stress and restores clarity to your thinking.

In many religions, contemplation and prayer are forms of meditation. Here in the West, the spiritual element of meditation is less important than the practical desire to reduce stress and improve health. There are a lot of different meditation styles with roots in different parts of the world, but we only have room to discuss the three styles most popular in the West.

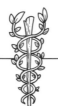

The Healing Arts

Can heart disease actually be reversed? The answer is yes—in some cases. In 1992, Dr. Dean Ornish showed that his program of diet, exercise, lifestyle changes, and meditation could indeed reverse heart disease for many patients. We can't say for certain that meditation does the trick—and all the meditation in the world won't help your heart if you don't also take the other steps—but it's the one thing that sets Dr. Ornish's program apart from similar ones that stress diet, exercise, and lifestyle.

Yoga for Your Brain

The physical exercises and breathing exercises of yoga go hand-in-hand with meditation (see Chapter 28, "Yoga: Exercise Your Body—and Your Mind," for more information). The purpose of yoga meditation is to attain total awareness through the cessation of thought. As you'll learn in yoga class, this is usually done through a combination of breath control and mental training. You can meditate anywhere, but some yoga poses are considered especially good for helping you sit in a relaxed way that lets your energy flow freely. The most famous is the lotus pose, where you sit cross-legged, with your ankles on your thighs. If that's too uncomfortable, just sitting cross-legged or even kneeling with your hands on your knees is fine.

Once you're comfortable, breath steadily and deeply and empty your mind of all thought. That's easy to say, but it's often hard to do. Yoga instructors usually tell you to just "push away" any thoughts and let your mind just rest. A few minutes of meditation is a good way to start and end your yoga workout.

Transcendental Meditation™

Remember when The Beatles went to India to study meditation with Maharishi Mahesh? Their visit brought Eastern meditation to Westerners in a big way. Riding on the crest of interest, Maharishi Mahesh brought his own brand of meditation to the West in the 1960s. Transcendental Meditation™—TM for short—is a form of meditation-based Hindu philosophy. As part of TM, you learn a *mantra* that you repeat silently while you meditate. The mantra helps you focus on your meditation and exclude outside thoughts.

TM is a simplified, seven-step approach to learning how to meditate. All it takes is 15 to 20 minutes, twice a day. Although TM has deep roots in Hinduism, it's not a religion, and you don't have to be interested in its spiritual aspects to benefit from doing it.

You can teach yourself TM from books and tapes, but you'll learn faster and better if you take a class. These are easy to find, because TM is probably the most popular form of meditation in the West. For more information on TM, and to find a qualified teacher near you, contact:

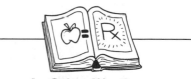

In Other Words...

A **mantra** is a sound or sounds used in meditation as the object or focus. The word comes from the Sanskrit words *man*, meaning "constant thinking," and *tra*, meaning "to be free." By repeating your mantra, you free yourself from thought but not from consciousness.

Maharishi International University
1000 North Fourth Street
Fairfield, IA 52556
Phone: (888) LEARN TM
E-mail: info@tm.org

TM is said to be particularly helpful for reducing stress and anxiety, lowering high blood pressure, and helping people get over drug and alcohol abuse.

Vipassana: Mindfulness

A traditional form of Buddhist meditation, *vipassana,* or mindful meditation, has recently arrived in the West—although it has been practiced in the East for over 2,500 years. Vipassana focuses on the present moment. During meditation, you learn to be mindful of the here and now. You're not dragged down by the past or afraid of the future. You face and accept all aspects of life and learn to keep your emotions on an even keel during life's normal—and even abnormal—ups and down. Because vipassana uses breath control and other meditation techniques to help you attain the right receptive frame of mind, you'll want to find a teacher to get you started. For more information, contact:

> **Vipassana Meditation Center**
> P.O. Box 24
> Shelbourne Falls, MA 01370
> Phone: (413) 625-2160
> Fax: (413) 625-2170

The First Step: A Basic Meditation Exercise

If you're wondering whether meditation will work for you, try this basic exercise. If you feel energized and relaxed when you're done (and we think you will), then you might want to start looking around for a meditation class.

Here's how to do a meditation exercise:

1. Start by finding a quiet place where you won't be interrupted for 20 minutes or so. Given our hectic lifestyles and busy families, this is probably the hardest thing about meditation!

2. Pick a focus word or a short phrase that has meaning to you. Words like peace, love, or God are common choices; short phrases like the first few words of a favorite prayer or poem work well. Go with whatever feels right to you.

3. Sit in a relaxed position in a comfortable chair with your hands resting lightly in your lap. Close your eyes and consciously relax your muscles.

4. Breathe naturally. Silently repeat your focus word as you exhale. Disconnected thoughts of work, family, life, and all sorts of other things will float into your mind. Gently push them away or let them pop like soap bubbles. Don't worry about whether you're meditating the right way or not—there is no right or wrong way, there's only your way.

5. After 10 or 20 minutes, stop. It's okay to open your eyes to check the time during your meditation, but don't use a timer. Sit quietly for a few minutes, then return to your usual activities.

That wasn't hard, was it? Did you notice how after just a few minutes your breathing got slower and deeper and you felt more relaxed and ready for the rest of the day? That's the beauty of meditation.

The Next Steps: Learning to Meditate

The basic meditation exercise we just gave you is a good start, but even that's hard for a lot of people. Most of us just aren't used to sitting still and being calm for even 20 minutes. Learning to meditate isn't easy, and trying to learn on your own can be so frustrating that you give up. The idea of meditation is *less* stress, not more, so we suggest finding a good teacher who will help you get started and guide you along the way.

Meditation is popular enough today that finding a teacher is fairly easy. Many yoga instructors, for instance, can help you learn to meditate (check back to Chapter 28 for more information). Transcendental Meditation™ courses are widely offered. Short meditation courses of various kinds are often taught at health clubs, Ys, alternative health centers, and even through community health centers and local hospitals. Also check your Yellow Pages and the bulletin board at your local health-food store.

A couple of national organizations promote meditation. For more information and help in finding classes and programs near you, contact:

Institute for Noetic Sciences
475 Gate Five Road, Suite 300
Sausalito, CA 94965
Phone: (415) 331-5650
Fax: (415) 331-5673

Insight Meditation Society
1230 Pleasant Street
Barre, MA 01005
Phone: (508) 355-4378
Fax: (508) 355-6398

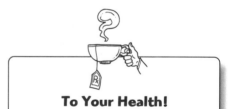

To Your Health!

Meditation classes are often taught in several short sessions, but you might want to look into a weekend retreat instead. You learn faster in a supportive environment, it's fun, and it's usually not too expensive.

Staying with It

How do you get to Carnegie Hall? Practice, practice, practice. It's the same with meditation. You'll really only get the benefits of it if you practice. Ideally, you should meditate twice a day, for about 15 or 20 minutes. To help meditation become a regular part of your daily routine, try to do it at the same time every day.

The benefits of meditation don't happen overnight, but they do start to show up with surprising speed. After just a few weeks of regular meditation, you may find yourself having a better overall outlook: calmer, more positive, and optimistic. That in turn helps you deal with everyday stress a lot better and helps you cope with unexpected stress better as well.

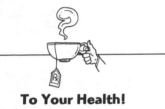

To Your Health!

Many people who meditate regularly say it also helps them deal with the people in their lives—family, friends, coworkers—with more understanding and less frustration.

The benefits of meditation for your health may take several weeks or even longer to kick in. Remember that everybody responds differently to meditation—and some people don't respond at all. Putting pressure on yourself is counterproductive, and you shouldn't feel you've failed if your health problems don't improve. Even if they don't, your emotional outlook on them might, and that alone makes meditation worthwhile.

If you're meditating to lower your high blood pressure, for example, you might be able to bring it down just a little, while other people could lower theirs a lot more. But when it comes to high blood pressure (and high cholesterol, being overweight, asthma, migraines, and a lot of other health problems), every little bit helps. Lowering your diastolic blood pressure reading (the second, lower number) by just two points lowers your chance of heart disease by 8 percent.

Rules, Rules, Rules

Short relaxation and meditation courses are usually very inexpensive and easy to find—your employer might even offer one for free. It's money well spent.

Meditation is widely accepted as a way to treat some health problems, particularly stress-related diseases. Your health insurance will probably cover at least some of the cost of taking meditation classes or going to a Mind/Body Institute program if your doctor recommends it.

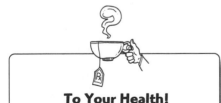

To Your Health!

You really need to be compatible with your meditation teacher and feel that he or she understands you. You might have to try a sample class with more than one teacher to find someone you can work well with.

There's no national standard or state licensing for meditation instructors. Since many yoga instructors also teach meditation, check back to Chapter 28 for more information on finding a qualified teacher. Instructors who use the trademarked Transcendental Meditation name have been trained in teaching the method, but always ask first—some people use the name loosely and aren't well-trained.

Meditation and Medicine

Most doctors would agree that relaxation and meditation techniques are very valuable for patients with stress-related or chronic illnesses. Meditation often helps patients need less pain medication and gives them a sense of control over their illness that reduces their feelings of anxiety and helplessness. Doctors are quick to point out that the techniques are not a substitute for medication and for diet and lifestyle changes. If you have high blood pressure, for instance, meditation may be helpful, but it's still important to take your medicine, stop smoking, and make any other needed lifestyle changes.

The Least You Need to Know

➤ Relaxation and meditation can help reverse the harmful effects of stress.

➤ Relaxation techniques focus on helping you consciously relax your body.

➤ Progressive muscle relaxation is a very effective, easy-to-learn technique for stress reduction.

➤ Meditation techniques, including yoga and Transcendental Meditation, focus on relaxing your mind through relaxed awareness.

➤ Relaxation and meditation techniques are very helpful for people with stress-related illnesses, chronic pain, and serious illnesses made worse by stress.

Chapter 30

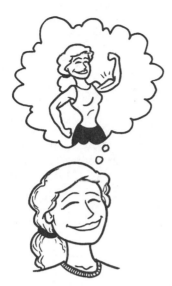

Use Your Head

A lot of the problems people go to the doctor about don't have just a physical cause. Insomnia, asthma, high blood pressure, digestive ailments, and many—maybe even most—other health problems are strongly affected by your emotions. In other words, "It's all in your head." Well, a lot of it, anyway. And if your head is where the problem is, that's where to solve it. Three approaches—hypnotherapy, guided imagery, and biofeedback—work so well that they're widely accepted by the medical profession.

Hypnosis: You're Getting Sleepy...

You've probably seen that scene in old movies when a patient is hypnotized by someone swinging an old-fashioned pocket watch back and forth and intoning, "You are getting sleepy...sleepy...sleepy." The patient promptly falls into a trance and reveals some crucial piece of information to the hypnotist. Or maybe you've seen the vaudeville bit, where the stage hypnotist gets a volunteer from the audience to run around acting like a chicken.

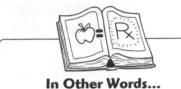

In Other Words...

Hypnosis is an artificially induced state of deep relaxation, altered perceptions, and greater openness to sensations and feelings. **Hypno-therapy** is the use of hypnosis to treat specific health or emotional problems. Both words come from the Greek word *hypnos*, meaning "sleep," but hypnosis isn't really sleep—it's usually described as a state of focused concentration.

There's a bit of truth to the *hypnosis* clichés, although not too many hypnotherapists these days have pocket watches, and stage hypnosis is pretty much a thing of the past.

Today *hypnotherapy*—guiding a patient into a relaxed trance state—is widely used as a way to help people deal with anxiety, chronic pain, cancer treatment, and much more. The beauty of hypnotherapy isn't just that it works amazingly well—it's that it works without drugs or fancy equipment, and only with the willing participation of the patient. That's because it's impossible to hypnotize someone against his or her will.

Hypnosis Today

There's nothing mysterious or sinister about hypnosis. A typical session takes place in a therapist's office. You sit in a very comfortable chair while the therapist helps you, through a variety of relaxation techniques and visualizations, to reach a state of deep relaxation. Even though you're so relaxed that your arms and legs feel very heavy and your eyes are closed, you're still aware of what's happening around you. Your breathing and heartbeat slow down, and you feel relaxed but focused. You're in a hypnotic state, sometimes called a *trance*.

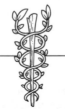

The Healing Arts

Back in the late 18th century, a Viennese physician named Franz Mesmer believed that magnetic forces flow through your body. Following that logic, he had patients sit in a comfortable chair and spoke soothingly to them while passing an iron rod along their bodies. The theory was that the iron would somehow realign their magnetic fluids, just as a magnet can be used to move iron filings. His patients had some miraculous cures, but magnetism had nothing to do with it. Dr. Mesmer had inadvertently stumbled on the basic principles of hypnotherapy—and to this day, hypnotism is sometimes called **mesmerism**, and when we're fascinated by something, we say we're *mesmerized*.

When you're hypnotized, your rational mind is on hold. Your subconscious—the part of your mind that has a big effect on how you feel things like anxiety or pain—takes over. And because your subconscious is very receptive, your hypnotherapist can make positive suggestions to you about your physical or emotional problem. After anywhere from 30 to 60 minutes of this, the hypnotherapist gradually brings you back to full awareness. The subconscious suggestions you received stay with you, though, and have a positive effect in the days that follow.

Hypnotherapy for Health

The medical uses of hypnotherapy have been recognized for decades. There's probably more evidence showing its value than for any other alternative technique. The very conservative *American Medical Association* (AMA) first approved the use of hypnosis back in 1957. Today many hospitals and cancer centers have hypnotists on staff. Hypnosis helps seriously ill patients deal better with the stress of hospitalization and treatment. Studies show, for instance, that when patients are hypnotized several times before an operation and told they won't have much pain afterward, they really don't. They need far less pain medication, and they heal faster. There are even documented cases of people having major surgery using only hypnosis as anesthesia.

We wouldn't go *that* far, but let's look at some of the other uses of hypnosis:

➤ **Relieving pain.** Chronic pain from severe burns and other injuries, especially ones that affect the nerves, can often be helped by hypnosis. Less severe pain, like from dental work, is also helped by hypnosis.

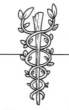

The Healing Arts

Hypnotherapists claim that 90 percent of the population can be hypnotized. For reasons we still don't really understand, some people can be hypnotized more deeply—sometimes much more deeply—than others, but just about anybody who's willing can be at least lightly hypnotized. Can you? You'll need someone's help to try this rule of thumb: Roll your eyes back as far as you can while slowly lowering your eyelids. When your eyes are half closed, the more white that shows, the easier you will be to hypnotize.

➤ **Conquering fears.** It's one thing to dislike spiders, and another to be so afraid of them that you never leave your house. Hypnosis can help you get over phobias (extreme fears). It can even help you relax about going to the dentist.

➤ **Breaking bad habits.** Hypnosis gets high marks from people who want to quit smoking, lose weight, or give up alcohol or drugs.

➤ **Helping stress-related problems.** Some health problems, such as asthma, migraines, irritable bowel syndrome, and eczema, get worse when you're under stress. Hypnosis helps you cope better and keeps your symptoms from acting up.

➤ **Childbirth.** By relieving fear and anxiety, hypnosis can help pregnant women get through childbirth quicker and with less pain.

Hypnosis works on anyone, no matter what their age—it's often used to help kids who have a problem with bed-wetting.

Self-Hypnosis Techniques

Self-hypnosis is a good way to help chronic pain or a chronic health problem such as asthma. It's also good for boosting your confidence, keeping yourself away from a bad habit, or just for overall relaxation.

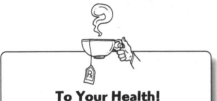

To Your Health!

During self-hypnosis, it's important to give yourself a focused, positive message, like "I don't need cigarettes any more."

We don't have room here to discuss the best ways to hypnotize yourself. It's fairly easy to learn, though, especially if a trained hypnotherapist teaches you how. In fact, teaching you self-hypnosis is often part of hypnotherapy. You can also get books and tapes that teach the basic methods.

Paging Dr. Mesmer

Hypnotherapists aren't licensed or certified by any state. Most hypnotherapists are licensed in some other healthcare area, though, like medicine, psychotherapy, or counseling, and use hypnosis as part of their treatment. Most medically trained hypnotherapists are certified by the American Society of Clinical Hypnosis or The Milton H. Erickson Foundation. For more information, and to find a trained hypnotherapist near you, contact:

American Society of Clinical Hypnosis (ASCH)
2200 East Devon Avenue, Suite 291
Des Plaines, IL 60018
Phone: (847) 297-3317
Fax: (847) 297-7309
E-mail: 70632.1663@compuserve.com

The Milton H. Erickson Foundation
3606 North 24th Street
Phoenix, AZ 85016
Phone: (602) 956-6196
Fax: (602) 956-0519
E-mail: office@erickson-foundation.org

About 4,000 hypnotherapists belong to ASCII. To be certified by either organization, practitioners need at a minimum a master's degree in a health or mental health field.

Can Hypnosis Be Misused?

It can be and it has. Some sensational court cases recently relied on "recovered memories" of murder, sexual abuse, and other crimes as evidence—memories that were "recovered" through hypnosis and later turned out to be false. The AMA and other groups have come down hard on using hypnosis in this way, calling it a misuse of hypnosis. In 1994, the AMA warned that "The use of recovered memories is fraught with problems of potential misapplication." Hypnosis can sometimes release intense emotions. Untrained hypnotherapists may not know how to respond well to this and could unintentionally do more harm. If you're interested in hypnotherapy, we urge you to work with an experienced, trained therapist. And we agree with the AMA: "The use of hypnosis for entertainment purposes is vigorously condemned."

Guided Imagery: Healing from Within

Imagine yourself on a beautiful beach somewhere, soaking up the warm sunshine and watching the palm trees wave against a clear blue sky. It's relaxing just to think about it, isn't it? Take this sort of thinking to the next level, and you have *guided imagery* or *visualization*—the technique of imagining sensations that affect your body or your emotional outlook.

A Guided Tour

The success of guided imagery, like hypnosis, depends a lot on how willing you are. The more open you are to the process, the more likely it is to help you. A typical guided imagery session takes place in a therapist's office. You sit in a very comfortable chair while the therapist helps you, through a variety of relaxation techniques and visualizations, to reach a state of deep relaxation that lets images form freely in your mind. It's not

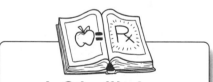

In Other Words...

Guided imagery is the technique of imagining sights, sounds, emotions, and other sensations in order to affect your body, help you relax, and promote healing. It's sometimes known as **visualization**, because you usually visualize images as part of the techniques.

unlike the sensation you feel just before you fall asleep, but you're fully awake even though you're deeply relaxed. At that point, the therapist will ask you to visualize what's bothering you or what you want to achieve. You'll be encouraged to imagine the problem or goal symbolically or as a sensation. You might imagine a burning pain, for instance, as a flaming torch or hot coal. Then you'll be asked to imagine the solution—putting ice on the hot coal, say. The session might last anywhere from half an hour to an hour. Afterward, whatever issue you worked on may well be resolved. Your burning pain, for example, might be much better or even gone. And the good thing is that it will probably stay gone.

Imagining Success

Guided imagery is often used as a way to improve your performance, whether it's in sports, on stage, or at the office. The basic idea is to imagine yourself performing that action, whatever it is—used this way, guided imagery is sometimes called *mental rehearsal*. Many serious athletes use it to visualize themselves in detail—going through every motion of a complex gymnastics routine perfectly, for example. Musicians, dancers, singers, actors, and other performers also use guided imagery to imagine themselves performing. For both athletes and performers, guided imagery builds confidence, improves concentration, and reduces or even eliminates stage fright.

Guided Imagery and Your Health

Have you ever said about a bad headache, "It's like a steel band around my head?" If you imagined slicing through the steel band with a magic sword, would that make your headache go away? It very well might. This sort of visualization for better health is one of the most interesting uses of guided imagery. Let's take a closer look at some of the ways it's being used:

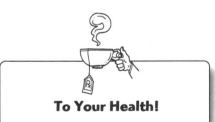

To Your Health!

Guided imagery works for just about any stressful situation. The technique is a good way to prepare for important job interviews, presentations to the board of directors, speeches, and so on.

➤ **Childbirth.** As part of natural childbirth classes, pregnant women use guided imagery to imagine themselves going through delivery.

➤ **Asthma.** Visualization techniques can help people with asthma relax during an attack and get over it faster. It can also help them learn to recognize and deal with the emotional factors that can trigger an attack.

➤ **Irritable bowel syndrome (IBS).** Stress makes IBS worse. By using guided imagery to reduce stress levels, people with this difficult disease can handle their symptoms better and even avoid flare-ups caused by emotional factors.

➤ **Cancer treatment.** Chemotherapy and radiation for cancer are difficult experiences; guided imagery can help patients deal with the stress and side effects better. By visualizing their cancer cells and imagining ways to attack them, cancer patients feel they help their treatment work better and keep the cancer from coming back. So many patients claim it works that guided imagery for cancer treatment is now being actively studied. So far, though, there's nothing solid to report.

➤ **Immune enhancement.** Just as cancer patients visualize destroying their cancer cells, sick people can use guided imagery to visualize their immune system attacking the germs. You might picture your white blood cells as giant blobs smothering evil-looking germs, for example. Another approach is to visualize yourself perfectly well again.

➤ **Chronic pain.** Guided imagery works so well for treating pain, especially chronic pain, that we feel it should be a central part of any treatment. That's because it works quickly, inexpensively, and without drugs.

During a guided imagery session, you might imagine an active situation—smothering germs—or allow a passive image to form. Someone with asthma, for example, might find that when he lets his mind float freely, he sees barbells sitting on his lungs. By imagining himself tossing the weights away, he may help his condition.

Finding a Guide

The best way to get started in guided imagery is by working with a trained therapist. There's no state licensing or certification for guided imagery therapy. A lot of licensed healthcare providers, like psychotherapists and counselors, do guided imagery with patients as part of their treatment. Some guided imagery therapists have been trained in an approach called *Interactive Guided Imagery* and belong to the Academy for Guided Imagery, the organization that promotes it. For more information, and to find a Certified Interactive Imagery Guide, contact:

> **Academy for Guided Imagery**
> P.O. Box 2070
> Mill Valley, CA 94942
> Phone: (800) 726-2070
> Fax: (415) 389-9342

Your therapist will probably teach you ways to do guided imagery on your own. There are a lot of do-it-yourself books and tapes on the subject. The Academy for Guided Imagery offers a good selection.

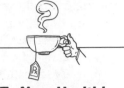

Biofeedback: Listening to Yourself

Every time you step on the scale and say to yourself, "I've got to cut back on the fudge ripple ice cream," you're doing a simple form of *biofeedback*. That's because biofeedback trains you to use signals from your own body as a way to improve your health.

Biofeedback Basics

The basic idea behind biofeedback is that it's possible to consciously alter unconscious body processes, like your blood pressure, heart rate, and even brain activity. To do that, though, you need some way of knowing if what you're doing is having any effect. That's where the various types of biofeedback machines come in. These devices use sensors that painlessly monitor your muscle tension, skin temperature, heartbeat, breathing, blood pressure, and sometimes your brain and convert the information into sounds, lights, meters, or images on a computer screen. By relaxing, focusing on the feedback, and consciously attempting to change it in the desired way—make it brighter or louder, for example—you learn to control whatever your health problem is. People with high blood pressure, for example, can learn to consciously bring it down.

Beating Stress with Biofeedback

Biofeedback is often recommended as a way to change your habitual reactions to stress. If your way of handling stress is to tighten the muscles of your lower back, you might have gotten so used to it that it seems normal. When you see your muscle tension displayed on a computer screen, though, you realize just how tense you really are. And when you learn relaxation techniques to loosen the muscles, you can see exactly how well they work.

Many stress-related health problems are helped quite a bit by biofeedback. High blood pressure, tension headaches, migraines, asthma, anxiety, insomnia, and irritable bowel syndrome, among other problems, respond well.

More Help from Biofeedback

Some very specific health problems can also be helped by biofeedback. The most important is urinary incontinence, or inability to control your bladder. This difficult condition affects as many as one-third of all people over age 65. It makes normal living difficult, and it also causes a lot of embarrassment, shame, and frustration. Biofeedback can be very effective for helping people regain control over the muscles and nerves of the bladder.

People with Raynaud's disease, a circulatory condition that causes painful spasms in the small arteries of the hands when they get cold, also benefit from biofeedback. They learn to consciously improve the circulation to their hands, which stops the spasms.

Biofeedback also helps people with paralysis and movement disorders regain function in the affected parts. It's often used for stroke patients.

Biofeedback ADDs Up

One of the hottest areas in biofeedback today is helping kids with *attention deficit disorder* (ADD) and *attention deficit hyperactivity disorder* (ADHD). These kids have trouble sitting still and focusing on their schoolwork and other activities; they can become very disruptive in and out of school.

The medical approach to ADD/ADHD is to medicate the children with Ritalin®—an approach that many concerned parents rightly don't want to take. An alternative is biofeedback training using the child's own brain waves. Kids with these disorders typically show more of the brain waves associated with "daydreaming" and lack of attention than normal. A standard device is used to painlessly project the child's brain waves onto a computer screen. By using their brain waves to play computer games, the kids actually learn to control their brain-wave state and create more of the waves associated with focused attention. The kids learn the difference between attention and distraction, which helps them calm down and learn to concentrate. There aren't that many good studies to show that it works, but there are a lot of grateful parents. If your kid has been diagnosed with ADD or ADHD, it might be worth looking into biofeedback.

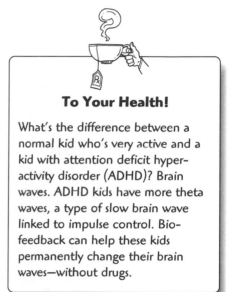

To Your Health!

What's the difference between a normal kid who's very active and a kid with attention deficit hyperactivity disorder (ADHD)? Brain waves. ADHD kids have more theta waves, a type of slow brain wave linked to impulse control. Biofeedback can help these kids permanently change their brain waves—without drugs.

Finding Feedback

As with hypnosis and guided imagery, there's no state licensing or certification for biofeedback therapists. It's usually done by people licensed in other health-related fields, like psychotherapists, counselors, and physical therapists. Most practitioners have been certified by the Biofeedback Certification Institute of America. For more information, and to find a trained biofeedback therapist near you, contact:

> **Biofeedback Certification Institute of America (BCIA)**
> 10200 West 44th Avenue, Suite 304
> Wheat Ridge, CO 80033-2840
> Phone: (303) 420-2902
> Fax: (303) 422-3394

Biofeedback practitioners really need to know what they're doing. Work only with one who's certified by BCIA.

Rules, Rules, Rules

Hypnosis, guided imagery, and biofeedback are all pretty well recognized by the medical and mental-health professions as being valuable treatments for some problems. If your health insurance covers psychotherapy or counseling, it may cover some of the costs for hypnosis and biofeedback if they're administered by a licensed health-care professional. If your doctor has recommended biofeedback to treat a specific health problem, such as urinary incontinence, your insurance will probably cover it. You're less likely to be covered for guided imagery—check with your health plan first. On the other hand, in 1997 Blue Shield of California, a major health insurer in that state, formed an alliance with the Academy for Guided Imagery to offer stress-management training to members.

The Least You Need to Know

➤ Hypnotherapy is a safe, drug-free treatment for chronic pain and physical problems related to stress, such as headaches and insomnia.

➤ Hypnotherapy is also useful for changing bad habits and helping you to diet and quit smoking.

➤ Guided imagery teaches you to visualize your health problems and imagine ways to banish them.

➤ Guided imagery is helpful for problems such as chronic pain and irritable bowel syndrome, and for improving your immune system. Many cancer patients use guided imagery as a way to visualize killing cancer cells.

➤ You can learn to control your body's internal activities by using biofeedback devices. Biofeedback can help you learn to control high blood pressure, muscle tension, and other stress-related health problems.

➤ Biofeedback is used to treat specific health disorders, such as urinary incontinence. Today it's being used to help kids with attention deficit disorder learn to calm down and concentrate.

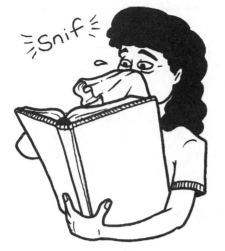

Quick Reference Chart for Health Problems

If You Have This Health Problem...	See These Chapters
Acne	20, 24
Allergies	4, 6, 9, 11, 13, 16–18, 20–22, 28
Anxiety	5, 7, 11, 13–17, 20, 22–24, 26–30
Arthritis	4–10, 13, 15–20, 22–23, 25–26, 28–29
Asthma	4, 6, 9–10, 15–18, 20–22, 25–26, 28–30
Attention deficit disorder	3, 27, 30
Back pain	3, 5–8, 10, 12, 15–17, 19–22, 27–30
Bruises	13, 15–16
Burns	9, 24
Cancer	4–7, 9, 15–22, 29–30
Carpal tunnel syndrome	21
Chronic fatigue syndrome	4–6, 13, 16–17, 19–22, 26, 28
Chronic pain	3, 5–7, 10, 12–13, 15–17, 19–23, 26–30
Colds	5, 13, 15–16, 20, 24
Constipation	11–12, 15–16, 20, 26
Dental problems	7
Depression	3, 6–7, 11, 13–17, 20, 22, 24–25, 27, 29
Diabetes	5, 7–9, 13, 15–19, 24, 26, 28–29
Diarrhea	5–6, 13, 15–16, 18–20
Environmental illness	20
Headaches	10–12, 15, 24, 27, 29–30

continues

If You Have This Health Problem...	See These Chapters
Heart disease	3–9, 13, 15–18, 20, 22–23, 26–30
Heart failure	8, 13, 15–17
Hemorrhoids	15, 20, 26
Herpes	9, 15, 17, 24
High blood pressure	4–6, 8–10, 15–19, 22, 26–30
High cholesterol	5, 15–20, 29
Immune system	3–7, 9–10, 13, 15–18, 20, 24, 26, 29–30
Insomnia	5, 10–13, 15–16, 20, 22–26, 28–30
Intermittent claudication	8
Irritable bowel syndrome	6, 17, 20–22, 30
Jet lag	25
Leaky gut syndrome	20
Macular degeneration	17
Menopause	4, 13–14, 16–17, 19, 26
Menstrual problems	3, 5–6, 10–12, 15–16, 20, 24, 29
Migraines	10, 15, 21, 27–28
Osteoporosis	7, 17
Pregnancy	15, 22, 26, 28
Premenstrual syndrome (PMS)	5–6, 12–13, 15–17, 20, 26, 29
Prostate problems	4, 12–13, 15, 17
Psoriasis	5, 13, 22, 24–26
Seasonal affective disorder	25
Skin rashes	5, 15
Toxic bowel	20
Varicose veins	11, 15, 17
Wound healing	5, 11, 13, 16–17

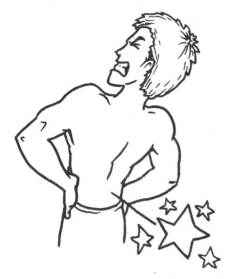

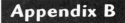

Common Health Problems

Some common health problems come up again and again in this book. Rather than explain them each time, we decided to list them separately for easy reference.

If you are currently taking any drug—prescription or over-the-counter—that your doctor has recommended, don't stop! Alternative treatments might help you need less of the drug or even stop it eventually, but never change the dose or stop taking a drug on your own! Always talk to your doctor before starting an alternative treatment, and always talk to your doctor about changing your medication.

Anxiety

Tension or apprehensiveness in the face of major stress is a perfectly normal form of anxiety. Sometimes anxiety can get out of control, however, leaving you feeling vaguely worried or fearful for no obvious reason; sometimes the anxiety escalates into an overwhelming sense of dread and fear. Real physical symptoms accompany anxiety: Tense muscles, shortness of breath, rapid heartbeat, dry mouth, inability to concentrate, and insomnia are the usual signs.

Arthritis

There are over 100 different kinds of arthritis, but we'll stick to the two most common kinds: osteoarthritis and rheumatoid arthritis.

Osteoarthritis, also sometimes called *degenerative arthritis*, is the most common form of arthritis—nearly 16 million Americans suffer from it. It happens when the smooth layers of cartilage that act as a pad between the bones in a joint become thin, frayed, worn, or pitted. The result is pain, swelling, stiffness, and limited movement in the affected joints. Most people get osteoarthritis just from living long enough—it comes from years of wear and tear on the joints, especially weight-bearing joints such as the hips and knees. *Rheumatoid arthritis* is a chronic inflammatory disease that causes pain, stiffness, swelling, deformity, and permanent loss of function in the affected joints. In addition, you might have general symptoms such as fatigue, weakness, and loss of appetite. Rheumatoid arthritis is one of the most severe forms of arthritis. It affects over two million Americans, two-thirds of whom are women.

Asthma

Periodic attacks of wheezing and difficulty breathing are the classic symptoms of asthma, a chronic inflammatory condition of the lungs. If you have asthma, the airways of your lungs are unusually sensitive to things in the air, like pollen, smoke, air pollution, and chalk dust. Some asthma sufferers are also sensitive to certain foods.

When you have an asthma attack, the linings of your airways swell up, narrowing the airways and making it hard for you to breathe. The muscles that surround the airways then can go into spasms, which makes breathing even harder. The inflamed linings of your airways also produce mucus, which clogs them up. These reactions combine to make breathing very difficult. In addition, you might feel a painless tightening in your chest and wheeze, sometimes very noticeably, when you breathe.

Even mild asthma is cause for concern, because it can suddenly get much worse. If your doctor has prescribed an asthma medicine—even an over-the-counter one—don't stop taking it. Talk to your doctor about alternative treatments for asthma before you try them.

Atherosclerosis

Atherosclerosis happens when fatty deposits called *plaque* build up inside your arteries—often an artery that nourishes your heart or leads to your brain. Clogged arteries set you up for a heart attack, angina, or a stroke.

Chronic Fatigue Syndrome

Chronic fatigue syndrome (CFS) is a mysterious and difficult-to-diagnose illness. CFS has a wide range of symptoms that vary considerably from patient to patient. Fatigue (extreme tiredness) is the clearest symptom of CFS. You may have CFS if you've had severe unexplained fatigue for over six months, especially if rest doesn't help and the fatigue interferes with your normal life. In addition, CFS symptoms may include severe fatigue, headaches, muscle and joint pain, tender lymph nodes, low-grade fever, sore throat, unrefreshing sleep, difficulty in concentrating, forgetfulness, and depression. Researchers still don't know what causes CFS, and right now there's no diagnostic test for it.

Congestive Heart Failure

When your heart is weakened by disease or by a faulty valve and can no longer pump blood efficiently through your body, you have congestive heart failure. Symptoms include breathlessness; tiredness; and swelling in the feet, ankles, and legs.

Crohn's Disease

Crohn's disease (also sometimes called ileitis) is a chronic disorder that causes inflammation or ulceration in the small intestine and sometimes also in the large intestine. The most common symptoms of Crohn's disease are abdominal pain, often in the lower right part of the abdomen, and diarrhea. Some patients also have bleeding, weight loss, and fever. Although most people with Crohn's disease develop it as children or young adults, the cause is unknown. The disease tends to come and go, with flare-ups and symptom-free periods (often for years), but most people who have Crohn's disease have it all their lives.

Depression

Mild depression—feeling a little down once in a while for a few hours, or even a few days—is very common. It's often a perfectly normal response to stress, poor health, or unhappy news like a divorce or losing your job. Symptoms of mild depression include insomnia, irritability, fatigue, stomach upsets, and trouble concentrating. You might not realize at first that depression is causing your physical symptoms.

Severe depression is another story. When you're severely depressed, you feel down all day, every day; lose interest in pleasurable activities; lose or gain a lot of weight; feel really tired all the time; have feelings of hopelessness, worthlessness, and guilt; and even think of suicide. Unlike mild depression or a passing feeling of sadness, severe depression is a serious medical condition. Without treatment, the condition can last for weeks, months, or years. According to the National Institutes for Mental Health, in any six-month period, nine million American adults suffer from a depressive illness.

If you feel deeply depressed for more than a week, talk about it with your doctor or someone else you can trust. Depression can sometimes follow a distressing emotional event, such as divorce or a death in the family, but often it just happens, as any other illness does.

Diabetes

Some 13 to 14 million Americans have *noninsulin-dependent* diabetes. This happens when your cells, for unknown reasons, become resistant to *insulin*, a hormone made in your pancreas. Insulin carries glucose (sugar) into your cells, where it then can be burned for fuel. When your cells are resistant to insulin, the glucose can't get in. It builds up in your blood instead, while your cells literally starve. This form of diabetes

387

usually begins in adults over the age of 40 and is most common after age 55. Diabetes can lead to serious complications. It's the single biggest cause of kidney disease, for example; it's also a leading cause of blindness. Diabetics have double the risk of the general population for heart attack and stroke. Diabetics also sometimes get a painful nerve condition, usually in the legs, called diabetic neuropathy.

Fibromyalgia

Fibromyalgia symptoms include painful, achy muscles and joint pain that go on for several months, along with fatigue, headaches, sleep problems, and a range of other problems that vary quite a bit from patient to patient. Fibromyalgia is another of those mysterious illnesses that has no known cause and is hard to diagnose.

Heart Disease

In this book, we've used heart disease in a general sort of way, but what we usually mean is *coronary artery disease*—blockages caused by plaque in the arteries that nourish your heart muscle. For more information, see "Atherosclerosis."

High Blood Pressure

Every time your heart beats (about 60 to 70 times a minute when you're resting), it pumps blood out through large blood vessels called arteries. Blood pressure is the force of that blood as it pushes against the walls of your arteries. Your blood pressure is at its highest when your heart beats and pushes the blood out—doctors call this the *systolic pressure.* When the heart is at rest between beats, your blood pressure falls. This is called *diastolic pressure.* Blood pressure is always given as two numbers: first the systolic and then the diastolic pressure.

Normal blood pressure ranges from below 130 to 140 systolic and below 85 to 90 diastolic. If your blood pressure is less than 140/90, it's normal. High blood pressure, or *hypertension,* is anything above 140/90. High blood pressure gets more serious as the numbers get higher. Your risk of heart attack, stroke, and kidney disease goes up along with your blood pressure.

High Cholesterol

Cholesterol is a waxy fat your body needs to make your cell membranes and many hormones, among other important roles. Most of your cholesterol is made in your liver, but you get some from eating animal foods. Just like oil and water, cholesterol and blood don't mix. To get the cholesterol to where it has to go, your liver coats it with a layer of protein. The protein keeps the cholesterol together so that it doesn't just float around in your blood. The technical name for the cholesterol-protein package is *lipoprotein.* There are several different kinds of lipoproteins, but the two most important are *low-density lipoprotein* (LDL) and *high-density lipoprotein* (HDL). Most of the cholesterol in your blood is carried as LDL cholesterol; only about one-third to one-fourth is carried as HDL cholesterol. But too much LDL cholesterol in the blood can lead to *atherosclerosis* ("clogging" of the arteries), which can lead to heart disease, stroke, and other problems. That's why LDL cholesterol is often called "bad" cholesterol. HDL cholesterol actually helps remove cholesterol from the blood—that's why it's often called "good" cholesterol. Ideally, you want to have a relatively low LDL level and a relatively high HDL level.

To measure your blood cholesterol levels, your doctor sends a sample of your blood to a laboratory, where the amounts of LDL and HDL in it are measured. The results come back as milligrams per deciliter, abbreviated as mg/dl (a deciliter is one-tenth of a liter). Usually there are two numbers: your total cholesterol (LDL plus HDL) and also your LDL separately. In general, if your total cholesterol is below 200 mg/dl, you don't have to worry. If it's above 200 mg/dl but below 240 mg/dl, you have borderline high cholesterol. If it's above 240 mg/dl, you have high cholesterol.

Insomnia

Insomnia—the inability to fall asleep or stay asleep—is the most common sleep complaint. About 50 million adult Americans have trouble getting a good night's sleep. If you take longer than 30 to 45 minutes to fall asleep, wake often during the night, or wake up early and can't get back to sleep, you have insomnia. Illness, anxiety, stress, indigestion, a headache, some medications (prescription and over-the-counter), jet lag from travel, shift work, and so on can all trigger occasional insomnia. Long-term insomnia (lasting more than three weeks) can be a symptom of serious illness, chronic drug or alcohol abuse, too much caffeine, or depression.

Irritable Bowel Syndrome

Crampy pain, gassiness, bloating, diarrhea, and changes in bowel habits are often signs of irritable bowel syndrome (IBS), an ailment that affects at least 10 to 15 percent of all American adults. In fact, IBS is second only to the common cold as a cause of missed work days. In the past, IBS was often called *colitis* or *spastic colon*, but these terms are no longer used. IBS should not be confused with ulcerative colitis, which is a more serious disease, or with Crohn's disease.

Migraine

The severe pain of a migraine headache is usually felt on just one side of your head. You also usually have some other unpleasant symptoms, such as nausea, vomiting, aversion to light, and cold hands and feet. A typical migraine lasts for about six hours and can really incapacitate you. Warning signs, called the *prodrome*, or *aura*, often start an hour or two before the headache strikes. The warning signs are usually visual—

many people see flashing lights or zigzag patterns. Only about 20 to 30 percent of all migraine headaches begin with an aura, however. Migraines are a fairly common type of headache—some 16 to 18 million Americans, 70 percent of them women, get them.

Premenstrual Syndrome (PMS)

Premenstrual syndrome, better known as PMS, is a general term for a variety of symptoms that some women get one to two weeks before the start of their menstrual periods. Somewhat less than half of all women have PMS to some degree. For most, the symptoms are minor inconveniences and can be dealt with easily. For about 10 percent of PMS sufferers, however, the symptoms can be a real problem, interfering with family relationships and work.

Over 150 PMS symptoms have been identified, but most fall into four groups:

> ➤ Nervous tension, irritability, anxiety, mood swings
> ➤ Weight gain, swelling of hands or feet, breast tenderness, abdominal bloating
> ➤ Headache, craving for sweets, increased appetite, pounding heart, fatigue, dizziness, fainting
> ➤ Depression, forgetfulness, crying, confusion, insomnia

Stress

Stress means any situation that forces you to make a rapid adjustment to changed circumstances. Bad things like losing your job are stressful—and so are good things like starting a great new job. When you're stressed out, your body responds with physical changes. Your blood pressure and heart rate go up; you may have headaches, back pain, digestive problems, or feel tired all the time. On the emotional level, you could have insomnia, feel anxious, and be unable to relax. In general, being under stress for long periods of time can weaken your immune system and make you more vulnerable to illness. Stress can also worsen some chronic problems, such as asthma, eczema, and psoriasis.

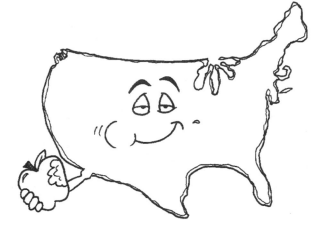

National Organizations

These organizations are national umbrella groups involved with alternative medicine. They're good sources of general information. Many organizations can also refer you to alternative medicine practitioners near you.

American Academy of Pain Management
13947 Mono Way, Suite A
Sonora, CA 95370
Phone: (209) 533-9744

American Association of Naturopathic Physicians (AANP)
601 Valley Street, Suite 105
Seattle, WA 98109
Phone: (206) 298-0215
Fax: (206) 298-0129
E-mail: webmaster@naturopathic.org

American Botanical Council (ABC)
P.O. Box 201660
Austin, TX 78720
Phone: (800) 373-7105
Fax: (512) 331-1924

American College for Advancement in Medicine (ACAM)
23121 Verdugo Drive, Suite 204
Laguna Hills, CA 92653
Phone: (800) 532-3688
Fax: (949) 455-9679

American Dietetic Association (ADA)
216 West Jackson Boulevard
Chicago, IL 60606
Phone: (312) 899-0040
Nutrition hot line: (800) 366-1655
Fax: (312) 899-1772

American Holistic Medical Association (AHMA)
6728 Old McLean Village Drive
McLean, VA 22101-3906
Phone: (703) 556-9728
Fax: (703) 556-8729
E-mail: HolistMed@aol.com

American Holistic Nurses' Association (AHNA)
P.O. Box 2130
Flagstaff, AZ 86003-2130
Phone: (800) 278-AHNA
Fax: (520) 526-2752

Foundation for the Advancement of Innovative Medicine (FAIM)
Two Executive Boulevard, Suite 204
Suffern, NY 10901
Phone: (914) 368-9797
Fax: (914) 368-0942
E-mail: faim@rockland.net

Herb Research Foundation
1007 Pearl Street, Suite 200
Boulder, CO 80302
Phone: (303) 449-2265
Fax: (303) 449-7849

National Acupuncture and Oriental Medicine Alliance
14637 Starr Road SE
Olalla, WA 98359
Phone: (253) 851-6896
Fax: (253) 851-6883

National Certification Commission for Acupuncture and Oriental Medicine (NCCAOM)
11 Canal Center Plaza, Suite 300
Alexandria, VA 22314
Phone: (703) 548-9004
Fax: (703) 548-9079

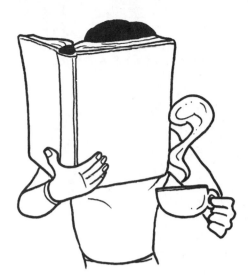

Read All About It

The health headlines aren't always what they seem. Often a new "discovery" gets front-page coverage, but later developments that cancel it out get stuck on the back pages. The best way to stay current with new developments is with magazines and newsletters that focus on alternative health and holistic living. Your local library will probably carry some of these titles.

Newsletters

Bottomline/Health
55 Railroad Avenue
Greenwich, CT 06830
(203) 625-5900

Consumer Reports on Health
101 Truman Avenue
Yonkers, NY 10703
(800) 234-2188

Dr. Atkins' Health Revelations
1101 King Street, Suite 400
Alexandria, VA 22314
(800) 336-4893

Health & Healing
4321 Birch Street, Suite 100
Newport Beach, CA 92660
(800) 826-1550

Let's Live Nutrition Insights
320 North Larchmont Boulevard
Los Angeles, CA 90004
(800) 225-6473

Longevity Research Update
Longevity Research Center
P.O. Box 12619
Marina del Rey, CA 90295
(310) 821-2409

Men's Health Confidential
33 East Minor Street
Emmaus, PA 18098
(800) 666-2303

Townsend Letter for Doctors and Patients
911 Tyler Street
Port Townsend, WA 98368
(360) 385-6021

Tufts University Diet & Nutrition Newsletter
53 Park Place
New York, NY 10007
(212) 608-6515

Magazines and Journals

Alternative and Complementary Therapies
Two Madison Avenue
Larchmont, NY 10538
(914) 834-3100

Alternative Medicine Digest
1640 Tiburon Boulevard, Suite 2
Tiburon, CA 94920
(800) 333-4325

American Health
28 West 23rd Street
New York, NY 10010
(212) 366-8900

Aromatherapy Quarterly
P.O. Box 421
Inverness, CA 94937
(415) 663-9519

Fitness
110 Fifth Avenue
New York, NY 10011
(212) 499-2000

Health
Two Embarcadero Center, Suite 600
San Francisco, CA 94111
(415) 248-2700

Healthy & Natural Journal
100 Wallace Avenue, Suite 100
Sarasota, FL 34237
(941) 366-1153

Herbalgram
American Botanical Council
P.O. Box 201660
Austin, TX 78720
(800) 373-7105

Integrative Medicine
655 Avenue of the Americas
New York, NY 10010
(888) 437-4636

Let's Live
320 North Larchmont Boulevard
Los Angeles, CA 90004
(800) 225-6473

Life Extension
Life Extension Foundation
P.O. Box 229120
Hollywood, FL 33022
(888) 715-5433

Macrobiotics Today
George Ohsawa Macrobiotic Foundation
P.O. Box 426
Oroville, CA 95965
(800) 232-2372

Massage
1315 West Mallon Avenue
Spokane, WA 99201
(509) 324-8117

Men's Health
33 East Minor Street
Emmaus, PA 18098
(800) 666-2303

Natural Health
17 Station Street
Brookline, MA 02147
(617) 323-1000

Natural Medicine Journal
828 High Ridge Road
Stanford, CT 06905
(203) 595-0006

New Age Journal
42 Pleasant Street
Watertown, MA 02172
(617) 926-0200

Prevention
33 East Minor Street
Emmaus, PA 18098
(800) 441-7761

Qi: The Journal of Traditional Eastern Health and Fitness
P.O. Box 18476
Anaheim Hills, CA 92817
(800) 787-2600

The Scientific Review of Alternative Medicine
59 John Glenn Drive
Amherst, NY 14228
(800) 421-0351

Vegetarian Times
Four High Ridge Park
Stamford, CT 06905
(203) 321-1755

Yoga Journal
2054 University Avenue, Suite 601
Berkeley, CA 94704
(800) 334-8152

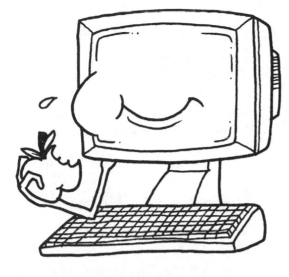

Alternative Health Online

A vast amount of health information is now available online through the World Wide Web. The information highway is littered with misinformation and commercialism, though, so use your common sense. Trust the information you find on a Web site only if the sponsor or owner of the site is clearly identified, the contributors are named with their credentials, the information is backed up by citations to legitimate studies, and the links go to other credible sites. Also check that the site is updated regularly. If a site pushes a particular treatment, supplement, or other product, be very wary.

The sites we've listed here provide solid information from reputable sources. The addresses are as up-to-date as we can make them, but things change quickly on the Web. Some of these sites may vanish, but you can be sure many more will arrive.

General Sites about Alternative Medicine

The Alternative Medicine Home Page
www.pitt.edu/~cbw/altm.html

American Holistic Health Association (AHHA)
www.ahha.org

Ask Dr. Weil
www.drweil.com

Dr. Bower's Complementary and Alternative Medicine Home Page
www.galen.med.virginia.edu/~pjb3s/Complementary_Practices.html

Foundation for the Advancement of Innovative Medicine (FAIM)
www.healthy.net/pan/chg/faim

HealthAtoZ
www.healthatoz.com

Healthfinder™
www.healthfinder.gov

Office of Alternative Medicine,
National Institutes of Health
www.altmed.od.nih.gov/oam

Prevention's Healthy Ideas™
www.healthyideas.com

Quackwatch
www.quackwatch.com

Wellness Web
www.wellweb.com

Acupressure

American Oriental Bodywork
Therapy Association
www.healthy.net/pan/pa/bodywork

Acupuncture

Acupuncture.com: The Online
Resource for Traditional Chinese
Medicine
www.acupuncture.com

American Academy of Medical
Acupuncture
www.medicalacupuncture.org

National Certification Commission
for Acupuncture and Oriental
Medicine/National Acupuncture
and Oriental Medicine Alliance
www.nccaom.org

Applied Kinesiology
www.icakusa.com

Alexander Technique

Complete Guide to the Alexander
Technique
www.alexandertechnique.com

North American Society of Teachers
of the Alexander Technique
(NASTAT)
www.prairienet.org/alexandertech/

Ayurvedic Medicine

About Ayurveda
www.ayur.com

Ayurvedic Health Center Online
www.ayurvedic.org

The Ayurvedic Institute
www.ayurveda.com

Living Wholeness
www.wholeness.com

Chinese Herbs

Acupuncture.com: The Online
Resource for Traditional Chinese
Medicine
www.acupuncture.com

Chiropractic

Chiropractic OnLine (American
Chiropractic Association)
www.amerchiro.org

International Chiropractors
Association
www.chiropractic.org

Colon Hydrotherapy

International Association for Colon
Hydrotherapy (I-ACT)
www.healthy.net/iact

Feldenkrais Method

Feldenkrais Guild® of North America
(FGNA)
www.feldenkrais.com

Flower Remedies

Flower Essence Society
www.flowersociety.org

Hellerwork

Hellerwork International, LLC
www.hellerwork.com

Herbs

American Botanical Council
www.herbalgram.org

Herb Research Foundation
www.herbs.org

Holistic Medicine

American Holistic Medical
Association
www.ahmaholistic.com

Homeopathy

Homeopathic Academy
of Naturopathic Physicians
www.healthy.net/HANP

Homeopathic Educational Services
www.homeopathic.com

National Center for Homeopathy
www.homeopathic.org

Hypnotherapy

The Milton H. Erickson Foundation
www.erickson-foundation.org

Light Therapy

Mental Health Net
www.depression.cmhc.com

Resources for Seasonal Affective
Disorder (SAD)
www.sunflower.org/~cfsdays/sat.ht

Massage Therapy

American Massage Therapy
Association
www.inet.amtamassage.org

Associated Bodywork and Massage
Professionals
www.abmp.com

Touch Research Institute
www.miami.edu/touch-research

Myotherapy

Bonnie Prudden Myotherapy
www.bpmyo.com

Naturopathy

American Association
of Naturopathic Physicians
www.naturopathic.org

Council on Naturopathic Medical
Education
www.cnme.org

Nutrition

American Dietetic Association
www.eatright.org

Price-Pottenger Nutrition
Foundation
www.healthy.net/ppnf

Osteopathy

access AOA (American Osteopathic
Association)
www.am-osteo-assn.org

American Academy of Osteopathy
www.aao.medguide.net

Oxygen Therapies

American College of Hyperbaric
Medicine
www.hyperbaricmedicine.org

Oxygen and Ozone Therapies
www.oxytherapy.com

Pain Management

American Academy of Pain
Management
www.aapainmanage.org

Polarity Therapy

American Polarity Therapy
Association (APTA)
www.polaritytherapy.org

Reflexology

Home of Reflexology
www.reflexology.org

Reflexology Research
www.reflexology-research.com

Relaxation Response

The Mind/Body Medical Institute
www.med.harvard.edu/programs/
mindbody

Rolfing

Rolf Institute of Structural
Integration
www.rolf.org

Shiatsu

American Oriental Bodywork
Therapy Association
www.healthy.net/pan/pa/bodywork

Sound/Music Therapy

American Music Therapy Association
www.musictherapy.org

Sound Healers Association
www.healingsounds.com

Therapeutic Touch

American Holistic Nurses'
Association
www.ahna.org

Healing Touch International
www.healingtouch.net

Traditional Chinese Medicine

Acupuncture.com: The Online
Resource for Traditional Chinese
Medicine
www.acupuncture.com

Transcendental Meditation™

The Transcendental Meditation Program
www.tm.org

Yoga

Yoga Internet Resources
www.tiac.net/users/mgold/www/
yoga.html

Yoga Journal
www.yogajournal.com

Yoga Research Center
www.members.aol.com/yogaresrch

YOYOGA! with Joan
www.yoyoga.com

Glossary

Acupoint   In traditional Chinese medicine (TCM), a shorthand way of saying *acupuncture point*—a specific point along an acupuncture meridian.

Acupressure   In TCM, gentle but firm hand or finger pressure on points along the meridians.

Acupuncture   In TCM, the insertion of very fine needles into selected parts of the skin to relieve pain and other symptoms of illness or injury.

Adverse drug reaction (ADR)   Any unpleasant, unintended, and undesired effect of a drug used as a medical treatment.

Aggravation   A temporary worsening of your symptoms from taking a homeopathic remedy. Aggravations happen when your body's healing powers start working. They make you feel worse for a few hours, but after that, you'll probably start to feel a lot better.

Agni   In Ayurvedic medicine, your digestive ability, but also the way you absorb other things, like air or experiences.

Alexander Technique   A movement system that restores your range of motion through awareness of your body and correct movement.

Allopathic medicine   See *standard medicine*.

Alternative medicine   A broad term covering a range of healing therapies. It's usually defined as those treatments and healthcare approaches not generally used by doctors and hospitals and not generally reimbursed by medical insurance companies.

Ama   In Ayurvedic medicine, waste or impurity.

Amino acid   A small molecule that has an amino group—a chemical fragment containing nitrogen—and an acid group—a chemical fragment containing carbon, oxygen, and hydrogen. Proteins are made from strings of amino acids.

Anma   An ancient form of traditional Oriental massage still practiced in Japan today.

Antioxidants   Enzymes that protect your body by capturing free radicals and escorting them out of your body before they do any more damage.

Applied kinesiology (AK)   A branch of chiropractic that uses muscle testing, along with other standard methods of diagnosis, to find imbalances that harm your health. Pronounced *kin-EASY-ology*.

Aromatherapy   The use of pleasant-smelling essential oils to treat physical and emotional problems.

Asanas   In yoga, physical postures, or exercises. Pronounced *AH-sah-nahs*.

Ashi points   In traditional Chinese medicine, tender spots on your body.

Atherosclerosis   Fatty deposits called *plaque* build up inside your arteries—often an artery that nourishes your heart or leads to your brain.

Attention deficit disorder (ADD)   Inability to sit still and concentrate.

Ayurveda   The traditional medical system of India based on disease prevention through balance and harmony.

Bach Flower Remedies™   Brand name for flower essences discovered by Dr. Edward Bach.

Bacterial overgrowth   See *dysbiosis*.

Benign prostate hypertrophy (BPH)   A condition caused by an enlarged prostate gland, which presses on the urethra and causes a need to urinate frequently.

Biofeedback   Learning to use signals from your body as a way to improve your health. Biofeedback uses information about your internal functions, such as your blood pressure or heart rate, as a way to train you to control them.

Bodywork   General term for any system of movement, touch, and sometimes deep massage designed to help you improve your body's structure and function.

Bruxism   The grinding of your teeth in your sleep.

Caffeine   An alkaloid chemical found in many plants and first isolated from coffee in 1820. A mild stimulant that improves alertness and concentration.

Carotenes   Orange- or red-colored substances that give vegetables like carrots and squash their color.

Carrier oils   Light, bland vegetable oils such as sweet almond oil, apricot kernel oil, fractionated coconut oil, jojoba oil, or grapeseed oil. They're used as a base for the volatile and aromatic essential oils, especially for massage oils and skin preparations.

Catalase   An enzyme your body makes to break down hydrogen peroxide into water and an atom of oxygen.

Cerebral insufficiency   Poor blood circulation to the brain, causing senility, memory loss, and depression.

Chelation   Using special chemicals administered intravenously to remove calcium and heavy metals from your body. Often used as a treatment for clogged arteries, poor circulation, and high blood pressure. Pronounced *key-LAY-shun.*

Chiropractic   Healing art that gives special attention to the role of the skeleton and muscles in health. Chiropractic care works with your body's natural strengths to restore and maintain your health—without drugs or surgery.

Chlorophyll   Complex pigment that makes green plants green.

Cholesterol   A waxy fat your body uses to make cell membranes and hormones, among other things. Too much cholesterol in your blood can cause atherosclerosis.

Circadian rhythm   Your body's 24-hour internal clock.

Colon hydrotherapy   Use of small amounts of water to remove wastes from the lower portion of your colon. Also sometimes called a *high colonic* or *colonic irrigation.*

Colonic irrigation   See *colon hydrotherapy.*

Complementary medicine   The use of alternative treatments in addition to—not instead of—standard medical treatment. Usually applied to alternative practices, such as acupuncture and chiropractic, widely accepted by medical doctors and health insurers. Sometimes called *integrative medicine.*

Compress   Cloth soaked in an herbal infusion or decoction and placed directly on the skin. Sometimes called a *fomentation.*

Constipation   Having fewer bowel movements than normal or having stools that are hard, dry, and difficult to pass. Also called *irregularity.*

Constitutional type   In homeopathic theory, your body type, your personality, and your basic temperament. Your constitutional type corresponds to a specific homeopathic remedy.

Cranial osteopathy   Gentle osteopathic manipulation of the skull bones to diagnose illness, relieve pain, and help problems such as chronic fatigue and hyperactivity. Also sometimes called *craniosacral therapy* or *cranial therapy.*

Decoction   Strong tea made by combining an herb with cold water in a small pot, bringing the mixture to a boil, and simmering for 10 to 20 minutes.

Deqi   The Chinese term for stimulating the acupuncture needles once they are in place. Deqi breaks up the obstructions in the meridians and lets the Qi flow smoothly again. Pronounced *deh-chee.*

Detoxification pathways   General term for all the various ways your body removes wastes and toxins from your system.

Diabetes   Inability to use glucose for fuel in your cells, sometimes because you no longer make the hormone insulin, but more often because your cells have become resistant to insulin.

Diabetic neuropathy   A complication of diabetes that causes numbness, tingling, and pain in the nerves of the feet and legs; it sometimes spreads to the nerves of the arms and trunk.

Diarrhea   Frequent passing of loose, watery stools.

Diastolic pressure   Your blood pressure when your heart is at rest between beats—the lower number in your blood pressure reading.

Dietary fiber   The indigestible parts—mostly cell walls—of plant foods.

Diuretic   A drug or herb that makes your kidneys produce more urine. Diuretics remove water from your body.

D.O.   Doctor of Osteopathy. A D.O., also called an *osteopath*, can do everything an M.D. can, including prescribe drugs, perform surgery, and admit you to the hospital.

Dosha   In Ayurvedic medicine, your "vital energy," "governing principle," or "metabolic body type." Your dosha is the combination of physical, mental, and emotional characteristics that makes up your individual Ayurvedic constitution. See also *kapha*, *pitta*, and *vata*.

Dysbiosis   Illness occurring when the friendly bacteria naturally found in your intestines are overwhelmed by the unfriendly bacteria that also live in your intestines. Also sometimes called *bacterial overgrowth*. If the problem is primarily in the large intestine, it's sometimes called *toxic bowel*.

EDTA   Ethylene diamine tetra acetic acid, an organic molecule that chelates with some kinds of metallic ions, like calcium, lead, iron, mercury, copper, and zinc.

Environmental illness (EI)   Illness caused by an overload of toxins in the body. The symptoms include depression, forgetfulness, headaches, fatigue, rashes, and loss of appetite.

Environmental toxins   Harmful poisons found all around us, including dioxin, carbon monoxide, formaldehyde, lead, pesticides, and other dangerous substances.

Enzymes   Complex chemical substances your body makes to help speed up chemical reactions in your body.

Essential fatty acids   Fatty acids your body must have to function normally and make cell walls, hormones, neurotransmitters, and other substances.

Essential oils   Natural chemicals extracted from plants by distillation. Essential oils aren't greasy or oily; they feel very much like water and evaporate very quickly.

Feldenkrais Method™   A bodywork system that combines gentle touch and movement training to help you increase your range and ease of motion and improve your flexibility and coordination.

Fight-or-flight response   Your body's response to stress. Your heart rate, blood pressure, and respiration rate go up; your muscles tense; you sweat; your digestion stops; your immune system is put on hold; and your emotional tension soars. You also produce large amounts of stress hormones.

Flavonoids   The substances found in fruits and vegetables that give them their colors and flavors. Many flavonoids are also powerful antioxidants.

Flower essences   Homeopathic remedies made from wild flowers. Each flower essence helps a specific emotional problem.

Fluoridation   The practice of adding tiny amounts of the mineral fluoride to municipal water supplies. In small amounts, fluoride strengthens your teeth and protects them against decay.

Free radicals   Unstable, destructive oxygen atoms created by your body's natural processes and also by the effects of toxins such as cigarette smoke and air pollution.

Freeform amino acid supplements   Dietary supplements that contain only those particular amino acids in their pure form. Because the aminos are already in their simplest form, you absorb them into your body right away.

Fructooliosaccharides (FOS)   Natural sugars found in honey, garlic, and artichoke flour that help nourish desirable bacteria in your intestines.

Full-spectrum light   Artificial light that mimics the full color range of natural sunlight, including the ultraviolet end of the spectrum.

Functional medicine   Another name for *orthomolecular medicine*.

Gingivitis   A gum disease causing red, swollen gums that bleed easily.

Ginseng   Generic name for several different types of roots used in traditional Chinese medicine.

Glutathione   Your body's most abundant natural antioxidant enzyme.

Guided imagery   Technique of imagining sights, sounds, emotions, and other sensations in order to affect your body, help you relax, and promote healing. Sometimes known as *visualization*.

Halitosis   Bad breath.

Hatha yoga   The most popular form of yoga in Western culture, mostly because its emphasis is on strengthening the body. Pronounced *HAT-ha YOH-gah*.

Healing crisis   Feeling worse, not better, after a few days of an alternative treatment. A healing crisis is normal and usually lasts for only a day or two—after that, you'll probably start to feel much better.

Heart failure   A condition occurring when your heart is damaged or weak and can't pump blood efficiently.

Heavy metals   Metals, including aluminum, arsenic, cadmium, lead, mercury, and nickel, that are harmful to your health in all but tiny amounts.

Hellerwork™ Bodywork therapy using deep massage, along with retraining in basic movements.

Hemorrhoids Itchy, enlarged, or swollen veins in the rectum. Also called *piles*.

Herb Plant parts used for cooking or medicine—roots, stems, leaves, seeds, fruits, and even bark.

Herpes A group of viruses. Herpes simplex, type one, causes cold sores. Herpes simplex, type two, causes genital herpes. Herpes zoster causes chicken pox and shingles.

High blood pressure Blood pressure—the pressure of your blood against your arteries as your heart beats and contracts—that is too high. Also called *hypertension*.

High colonic See *colon hydrotherapy*.

High-density lipoprotein (HDL) "Good" cholesterol, because it can help remove LDL ("bad") cholesterol from your blood.

Homeopathy A holistic medical system that uses very, very tiny doses of a drug to produce symptoms similar to the illness. The remedies stimulate your natural healing powers.

Hormones Chemical messengers your body makes to tell your organs what to do. Hormones regulate many activities, including your growth, blood pressure, heart rate, glucose levels, and sexual characteristics.

Hydrogen peroxide A chemical substance made up of two hydrogen atoms and two oxygen atoms. Your body naturally makes some hydrogen peroxide—you need it for a lot of normal body functions, including making hormones and neurotransmitters.

Hydrotherapy Use of water—internally or externally—as a health treatment. Internal hydrotherapy usually means drinking water as a form of treatment. External hydrotherapy generally means applying water to your skin in some way—through a bath or compress, for instance.

Hyperbaric oxygen therapy (HBOT) Medical treatment giving a patient oxygen at higher pressure (hyperbaric) than normal. Used for serious problems, such as carbon monoxide poisoning, and to help wounds from surgery heal faster.

Hypertension See *high blood pressure*.

Hyperthermia Deliberately raising your body temperature from normal—98.6°F—to fever level—102°F—in order to fight infection and stimulate your immune system.

Hypnosis An artificially induced state of deep relaxation, altered perceptions, focused concentration, and greater openness to sensations and feelings.

Hypnotherapy Use of hypnosis to treat specific health or emotional problems.

Infusion A strong drink made by steeping a larger amount of an herb in boiling water for between 10 and 20 minutes.

Insomnia   Inability to fall asleep or stay asleep.

Insulin   A hormone made by your pancreas and needed to carry glucose into your cells for fuel.

Integrative medicine   See *complementary medicine*.

Intravenous infusion   Dripping a liquid into a vein using a thin needle.

Jet lag   Fatigue and insomnia caused by traveling rapidly through time zones.

Jing   In traditional Chinese medicine, your "vital essence," or your ability to change, grow, and adapt on a long-term basis.

Juice fast   See *therapeutic fast*.

Kapha   In Ayurvedic medicine, the dosha that controls your structure. Kapha dosha types are cool, damp, and slow. Kapha people have heavy, solid bodies and a tendency to put on weight.

Ki   The Japanese word for "Qi," or "life energy." Pronounced *key*.

Leaky gut syndrome   Damage to the villi of the small intestine that allows large molecules of undigested food to enter your bloodstream. Your body reacts as if the molecules are invaders, causing symptoms such as skin rashes, digestive upsets, joint pain, and fatigue.

Light therapy   Any treatment that uses natural or artificial light.

Linoleic acid   Essential fatty acid found in fish and many plants.

Linolenic acid   Essential fatty acid found in seeds, including corn kernels, and also egg yolks and some fish.

Low-density lipoprotein (LDL)   "Bad" cholesterol, because excess amounts in your blood can lead to clogged arteries, heart disease, and stroke.

Macrobiotics   A dietary and philosophical approach to life that emphasizes balance and simplicity. The macrobiotic diet emphasizes whole grains and vegetables.

Mantra   A sound or sounds used in meditation as the object or focus. The mantra helps you focus on your meditation and exclude outside thoughts.

Massage   Manipulation of your soft tissues (skin and muscles) in order to improve your circulation, help you relax, and relieve pain and soreness.

Masseuse   Professional massage therapist.

Meditation   Any of a variety of mental techniques that induces a state of deep relaxation, inner harmony, and focused awareness.

Megavitamin therapy   See *orthomolecular medicine*.

Melatonin   A hormone made by your pineal gland and used to regulate your sleep/wake cycle.

Mercury amalgam fillings   The "silver" fillings most people have for dental cavities. The mixture, or amalgam, is made of mercury, tin, copper, silver, and sometimes zinc.

Meridians   In traditional Chinese medicine, the invisible pathways or channels in your body through which your Qi flows. Blockages in the meridians interrupt the smooth flow of Qi and cause illness.

Migraine   A very severe headache usually felt on just one side of your head. Other symptoms include nausea, vomiting, sensitivity to light, and cold hands and feet.

Mineral   An inorganic chemical element, such as calcium or potassium, that your body must have in very small amounts for normal health. You must get your minerals from the foods you eat and any supplements you take.

Mother tincture   The mixture of water, herbs, and sometimes alcohol that is the basis for any homeopathic remedy.

Moxa   Also known as mugwort (*Artemisia vulgaris*), moxa is a traditional Chinese herb said to help promote healing.

Moxibustion   In acupuncture, stimulating the needles with heat by burning a small cone of dried moxa leaves on the end of the needle.

Musculoskeletal system   The framework that supports your entire body—your bones, muscles, joints, ligaments, and other connective tissues.

Music therapy   The use of rhythm and melody to improve your psychological, emotional, and sometimes physical well-being.

Myotherapy   Any treatment that affects your muscles. There are many types of myotherapy, including physical therapy, massage, and many kinds of bodywork.

Naturopath   See *naturopathic physicians*.

Naturopathic medicine   See *naturopathy*.

Naturopathic physicians   General practitioners trained as specialists in natural medicine. Also called *naturopaths*.

Naturopathy   A medical system that treats health problems by using the body's natural ability to heal. Modern naturopathy includes a wide range of therapies, such as herbs, homeopathy, acupuncture, and nutrition. Also called *naturopathic medicine*.

N.D.   Doctor of Naturopathic Medicine.

Neat   Undiluted.

Needling   See *deqi*.

Neurotransmitter   A chemical you make to transmit messages along your nerves and among your brain cells.

Neutral bath   A full-body bath in water just below body temperature.

Nutritional supplement   Any product you take, like a vitamin or mineral, in addition to your normal diet. Nutritional supplements are used to improve overall health and sometimes to help specific health problems.

OMP   See *Oriental medicine practitioner.*

Oriental medicine   See *traditional Chinese medicine.*

Oriental medicine practitioner (OMP)   A healthcare professional trained in traditional Chinese medicine. In the United States, most OMPs are licensed acupuncturists.

Orthomolecular medicine   Treating the underlying causes of illness with large doses of vitamins, minerals, and other supplements. Also called *megavitamin therapy* or *functional medicine.*

Osteopath   A Doctor of Osteopathy (D.O.).

Osteopathic manipulative therapy (OMT)   Overall term for a variety of hands-on physical techniques used to diagnose and treat musculoskeletal problems.

Osteopathy   A branch of medicine that believes that your body structure—your bones and muscles—and the rest of your body functions operate together. Osteopathy believes that imbalances in your body structure cause disease, and that restoring the balance will restore health.

Oxidative therapy   Hydrogen peroxide treatments.

Periodontist   Dentist who specializes in treating gum diseases.

Periodontitis   Infection of the bone supporting your teeth.

Pineal gland   A small gland found inside your brain. It produces melatonin and regulates your internal clock.

Pitta   In Ayurvedic medicine, the dosha that controls your metabolism. Pitta dosha types are warm, oily, and intense. They have medium bodies and are alert and intelligent.

Placebo effect   Positive results from a harmless treatment or dummy drug that has no real action. The word comes from the Latin word meaning "I will please."

Plaque   Fatty deposits of cholesterol, calcium, and other substances that build up inside your arteries and block them.

Polarity Therapy™   Stimulating and balancing your body's energy fields through gentle touch to the sacrocranial system.

Potency   In homeopathic theory, the dilution of the remedy. The more dilute a remedy is, the more potent it is.

Poultice   Small amount of an herb soaked in water and placed directly on the skin.

Prakruti   In Ayurvedic medicine, your natural dosha or combination of doshas—your inborn, natural constitution. Put more philosophically, your prakruti is your essential nature.

Prana   In Ayurvedic medicine and yoga, your "life energy" or "life force." Prana enters your body through your food and through your breathing.

Pranayama   In yoga, breath control exercises. Pronounced *PRAH-NAH-YAH-mah*.

Prostate gland   A small male organ wrapped around the urethra.

Protein   An organic substance made up of hydrogen, oxygen, carbon, and nitrogen. Proteins are made from strings of amino acids.

Provings   Tests done by Dr. Hahnemann, the founder of homeopathy, to discover the effects of various drugs.

Qi   In traditional Chinese medicine, the invisible but fundamental energy that flows through everything and everyone in the universe—the life force of all living and nonliving things. Sometimes written *chi* or *ch'i* and pronounced *chee*.

Qigong   In traditional Chinese, the concept of "energy cultivation" or "energy development." More loosely, it can be translated as "energy flow." Qigong exercises keep your Qi flowing.

Quack   Someone who pushes false or useless health treatments or remedies.

Quackery   False or useless health treatments.

Rectum   The last portion of your digestive tract.

Reflex points   In reflexology, the points on your feet and hands that correspond to other parts of your body. Massaging the points releases energy blocks and stimulates your natural healing powers.

Reflexology   A form of Touch Therapy that uses pressure on specific points of the feet (and also hands) to affect other parts of the body.

Reiki   Japanese word (pronounced *ray-key*) meaning the energy found in all living and nonliving things. Reiki practitioners channel that energy to themselves or others as a healing technique.

Relaxation response   Physical state of deep rest that changes your physical and emotional responses to stress by lowering your heart rate, lowering your blood pressure, and relaxing your muscles.

Retina   The thin, light-sensitive layer of cells at the back of your eye.

Rolfing   A form of deep-tissue massage that realigns and balances your body.

SAD   See *seasonal affective disorder*.

Seasonal affective disorder (SAD)   Type of depression that affects people in the winter when the days are short and dark. The symptoms of SAD generally go away when the longer, sunnier days of spring begin.

Serotonin   Neurotransmitter that carries impulses in the parts of your brain that control your mood and emotions. If you have plenty of serotonin, you feel calm and confident. If you don't have enough, you might feel depressed and anxious, and you might also crave carbohydrates and overeat.

Shen In traditional Chinese medicine, your "spirit" or "mind."

Shiatsu Also sometimes written *shiatzu*, the Japanese version of acupressure.

Sitz bath Bath taken in water that covers your pelvic region but not your feet.

Spinal manipulation Basic principle of chiropractic. By gently moving misaligned vertebrae back into place, spinal manipulation relieves pain and other symptoms.

Standard medicine The medicine medical doctors learn in medical school and practice in hospitals. It's oriented toward treating illness, usually through drugs or surgery. Also called *allopathic medicine.*

Standardized herbs Herbs that have been lightly processed to make sure that each dose has the same basic amount of the major active ingredients.

Stool Human solid waste; feces.

Stress Any situation that forces you to make a rapid adjustment to changed circumstances.

Subluxation Misaligned vertebrae (the bones that make up your spine) that cause back and neck pain.

Succussation Preparing a homeopathic remedy by repeatedly shaking it very vigorously and banging it against a hard surface. The process releases the energy of the drug.

T'ai chi In traditional Chinese medicine, a system of gentle, flowing Qigong exercises designed to keep your Qi moving.

TCM See *traditional Chinese medicine.*

Tea Mild drink made by steeping a small amount of an herb in boiling water for a few minutes.

Temporomandibular joint syndrome (TMJ) Pain, headaches, clicking or popping noises when you chew, and other symptoms caused when the hinge-like joint that connects your lower jaw to your skull gets out of line.

Therapeutic fast Consuming only juice and no solid food for a short period—one to three days—as a way to rejuvenate and cleanse your system. Also called *juice fast.*

Therapeutic Touch A healing approach that "sweeps away" energy blockages and transfers the healer's energy to the patient.

Thumb walking A basic reflexology technique that uses the thumb to apply steady, gentle pressure to the reflex point.

Tincture Concentrated herbal remedy made by soaking an herb in pure grain alcohol or vinegar instead of water.

TMJ See *temporomandibular joint syndrome.*

413

Topical   Applied directly to the skin.

Toxic bowel   Excess of unfriendly bacteria in the large intestine. See also *dysbiosis*.

Trace minerals   Minerals you need in very, very, very tiny amounts.

Traditional Chinese medicine (TCM)   The system of medicine that has been used in China and other parts of Asia, including Japan and Korea, for thousands of years. It's also sometimes called *Oriental medicine*.

Trager Approach™   Mind/body therapy that uses gentle touch and movement to release deep-seated physical and mental patterns.

Transcendental Meditation™ (TM)   Simplified form of meditation based on Hindu philosophy. TM uses a mantra that you repeat silently while you meditate.

Trigger point massage   Use of strong finger pressure and deep massage to work on trigger points—muscle knots caused by stress, tension, or injury.

Triphala   A popular Ayurvedic herbal remedy made from the dried, powdered fruits of three different Indian herbs.

Tuina   A form of traditional Chinese massage. Pronounced *twee-nah*.

Ultraviolet (UV) light   Light wavelengths too long for your eyes to pick up. UV radiation penetrates your skin—it's what makes your skin burn and tan.

Urethra   The tube that carries urine from your bladder out of your body.

Vata   In Ayurvedic medicine, the dosha that controls your movement. Vata dosha types are cold, dry, light, and mobile. Vata people tend to be slim, with prominent features and dry skin.

Vikruti   In Ayurvedic medicine, your daily constitution.

Villi   Tiny, fingerlike projections lining your small intestine and designed to increase the total area available to absorb nutrients.

Visualization   See *guided imagery*.

Vitamin   An organic chemical compound essential for normal health in very small amounts. You must get all your vitamins from outside your body—from the foods you eat and any supplements you take.

White noise   Any sort of steady, soft sound on a steady frequency and with no rhythm. White noise is useful for masking other sounds, such as traffic noise or conversation.

Yin and Yang   The basic idea of balance behind all traditional Chinese medicine. Yin and Yang are the opposing, balancing forces of the universe.

Yoga   An ancient Indian technique combining physical exercise, breathing techniques, and meditation.

Index